Current Trends in
Histocompatibility

VOLUME 2
BIOLOGICAL AND CLINICAL
CONCEPTS

CURRENT TRENDS IN HISTOCOMPATIBILITY

Volume 1   Immunogenetic and Molecular Profiles

Volume 2   Biological and Clinical Concepts

Current Trends in
Histocompatibility

VOLUME 2
BIOLOGICAL AND CLINICAL CONCEPTS

Edited by

Ralph A. Reisfeld
and
Soldano Ferrone

Scripps Clinic and Research Foundation
La Jolla, California

PLENUM PRESS • NEW YORK AND LONDON

Library of Congress Cataloging in Publication Data

Main entry under title:

Current trends in histocompatibility.

   Includes index.
   CONTENTS: v. 1. Immunogenetic and molecular profiles. – v. 2. Biological and
clinical concepts.
   1. Histocompatibility. 2. HLA histocompatibility antigens. I. Reisfeld, Ralph A.
II. Ferrone, Soldano, 1940-
QR184.3.C87   616.07′9   80-18211
ISBN 0-306-40481-8 (v. 2)

© 1981 Plenum Press, New York
A Division of Plenum Publishing Corporation
233 Spring Street, New York, N. Y. 10013

Printed in the United States of America

Contributors

Zuhair K. Ballas, Basic Immunology Program, Fred Hutchinson Cancer Research Center, Seattle, Washington 98104

Jack R. Bennink, The Wistar Institute of Anatomy and Biology, Philadelphia, Pennsylvania 19104

B. Bergholtz, Tissue Typing Laboratory, Rikshospitalet (The National Hospital), Oslo, Norway

B.A. Bradley, Department of Immunohaematology, University Medical Center, Leiden, The Netherlands

Kent C. Cochrum, Department of Surgery, University of California, San Francisco, California 94143

Gunther Dennert, Department of Cancer Biology, The Salk Institute, San Diego, California 92112

Peter C. Doherty, The Wistar Institute of Anatomy and Biology, Philadelphia, Pennsylvania 19104

Rita B. Effros, The Wistar Institute of Anatomy and Biology, Philadelphia, Pennsylvania 19104

Mark Frankel, The Wistar Institute of Anatomy and Biology, Philadelphia, Pennsylvania 19104

E. Goulmy, Department of Immunohaematology, University Medical Center, Leiden, The Netherlands

Leonard J. Greenberg, Department of Laboratory Medicine and Pathology, University of Minnesota Medical School, Minneapolis, Minnesota 55455

Deanne M. Hanes, Department of Surgery, University of California, San Francisco, California 94143

Christopher S. Henney, Basic Immunology Program, Fred Hutchinson Cancer Research Center, Seattle, Washington 98104

Barry D. Kahan, Division of Organ Transplantation, Department of Surgery, The University of Texas Medical School at Houston, Houston, Texas 77030

David H. Katz, Department of Cellular and Developmental Immunology, Scripps Clinic and Research Foundation, La Jolla, California 92037

Ronald H. Kerman, Division of Organ Transplantation, Department of

Surgery, The University of Texas Medical School at Houston, Houston, Texas 77030

Lionel A. Manson, The Wistar Institute of Anatomy and Biology, Philadelphia, Pennsylvania 19104

Faramarz Naeim, Department of Pathology, University of California, Los Angeles, California 90024

H. Nousiainen, Tissue Typing Laboratory, Rikshospitalet (The National Hospital), Oslo, Norway

Keiko Ozato, Basic Immunology Program, Fred Hutchinson Cancer Research Center, Seattle, Washington 98104; present address: Immunology Branch, National Cancer Institute, Bethesda, Maryland 20014

G.G. Persijn, Eurotransplant Foundation, University Medical Center, Leiden, The Netherlands

Per Platz, Tissue-Typing Laboratory of the Blood-Grouping Department, State University Hospital (Rigshospitalet), DK-2100 Copenhagen Ø, Denmark

Lars P. Ryder, Tissue-Typing Laboratory of the Blood-Grouping Department, State University Hospital (Rigshospitalet), DK-2100 Copenhagen Ø, Denmark

Arne Svejgaard, Tissue-Typing Laboratory of the Blood-Grouping Department, State University Hospital (Rigshospitalet), DK-2100 Copenhagen Ø, Denmark

E. Thorsby, Tissue Typing Laboratory, Rikshospitalet (The National Hospital), Oslo, Norway

J.J. van Rood, Department of Immunohaematology, University Medical Center, Leiden, The Netherlands

Harald von Boehmer, Basel Institute for Immunology, 4005 Basel 5, Switzerland

Roy L. Walford, Department of Pathology, University of California, Los Angeles, California 90024

Rolf M. Zinkernagel, Department of Immunopathology, Scripps Clinic and Research Foundation, La Jolla, California 92037; present address: Department of Pathology, Universitatsspital, 8091 Zürich, Switzerland

Preface

Information about histocompatibility antigens is expanding so rapidly that it is difficult to remain abreast of all advances. In these volumes, we have made an effort to bring together the most current work on topics that have generated most of the recent advances and discussions. We have asked each author to present and interpret his most current work, and we have judiciously refrained from imposing our own prejudices and viewpoints. Although there is obvious overlap in some individual topics, we have encouraged this to provide the reader with as many different and sometimes opposing viewpoints as possible. This approach will, we hope, give a broad overview of current ideas in the field.

We wish to thank all contributors for their timely and exciting manuscripts, and we sincerely hope that the reader will benefit from these volumes.

R.A. Reisfeld
S. Ferrone

La Jolla

Contents

I. Role of Histocompatibility Antigens in Cell–Cell Interaction

Chapter 4

Hapten Recognition by Cytotoxic T Cells: The Modifying
Influence of the Major Histocompatibility Complex 59

Christopher S. Henney, Zuhair K. Ballas, and Keiko Ozato

Chapter 5

New Thoughts on the Control of Self-Recognition, Cell Interactions,
and Immune Responsiveness by Major Histocompatibility
Complex Genes 81

David H. Katz

Chapter 6
The Role of Cell-Surface Antigens in Progressive Tumor Growth
(Immunological Surveillance Re-revisited)
Lionel A. Manson

Chapter 7
Self-*HLA-D*-Region Products Restrict Human T-Lymphocyte
Activation by Antigen
E. Thorsby, B. Bergholtz, and H. Nousiainen

Chapter 8

Rolf M. Zinkernagel

II. Clinical Aspects of Transplantation: Association with Disease

Chapter 9

Kent C. Cochrum and Deanne M. Hanes

Chapter 10

HLA-Linked Regulation of Immune Responsiveness in Man:
Role of *I*-Region-Gene Products 177
Leonard J. Greenberg

Chapter 11

Clinical Histocompatibility Testing in Renal Transplantation:
Potential Keys to Alloimmune Specificity and Reactivity 201
Ronald H. Kerman and Barry D. Kahan

Chapter 12

Chapter 13

Chapter 14

I

Role of Histocompatibility Antigens in Cell–Cell Interaction

1

Histocompatibility Antigens and the T-Cell Repertoire

Harald von Boehmer

1. Introduction

Considering the numerous reviews dealing with the major histocompatibility complex (MHC) and its influence on T cells, it is not tempting to write yet another article on the subject. The experimental data that I am going to summarize are in principle compatible with several theoretical models. I therefore shall not attempt to discriminate among them. Our own view has been stated before (von Boehmer *et al.*, 1978b).

2. *H-2* Restriction

2.1. *H-2* Restriction of T Cells

Cell-surface structures encoded by genes in the MHC influence the T-cell receptor repertoire: the interaction of T cells with other cells is restricted by H-2 antigens (Katz *et al.*, 1973a; Rosenthal and Shevach, 1973; Zinkernagel and Doherty, 1974). The cell interactions require an apparent dual specificity of T cells: one for antigens (x) and one for H-2 antigens (s).

In a normal, nonchimeric animal, the repertoire of H-2 restriction is mainly directed against self H-2: T-cells from strain a depleted by various methods of alloreactivity to strain b can respond to antigen x on cells a

Harald von Boehmer • Basel Institute for Immunology, 4005 Basel 5, Switzerland.

3

but not on cells b (Schmitt-Verhulst and Shearer, 1977; von Boehmer *et al.*, 1978a; Bennink and Doherty, 1978; Sprent, 1978). Exceptions to these findings have also been reported (Wilson *et al.*, 1977; Doherty and Bennink, 1979).

Specificity for allogeneic restriction elements can, however, be acquired when T-cell differentiation occurs in an X-irradiated semiallogeneic host (von Boehmer *et al.*, 1975; Waldmann and Munro, 1975; von Boehmer and Haas, 1976; Zinkernagel, 1976a; Pfitzenmaier *et al.*, 1976; Miller *et al.*, 1976). The genotype of the radioresistant portion of the thymus determines the repertoire of *H-2* restriction (phenotype of *H-2* restriction) (Zinkernagel, 1978; Bevan and Fink, 1978; Waldmann *et al.*, 1979) (Table 1). Exceptions to this rule have also been reported (Kindred and Loor, 1974; Matzinger and Mirkwood, 1978).

The restricting elements recognized by T helper cells are encoded in the *I* region (Katz and Benacerraf, 1975) and those recognized by cytotoxic T lymphocytes (CTL) in the *K* or *D* region of *H-2* (Doherty *et al.*, 1976).

2.1.1. The Apparent Dual Specificity of T Cells Is the Result of Endogenously Produced Receptors

The apparent dual specificity of T cells does not require passive arming with receptors from other cells (Burnet, 1978): *H-2*-restricted CTL specific for male antigen or hapten can be cloned and recloned under conditions of limiting dilution and grown for several months without losing their specificity and cytotoxic potential (von Boehmer *et al.*, 1979). The dual specificity of T cells, therefore, is the result of endogenous receptor production.

2.1.2. T Cells Unrestricted by Either K, D, or I-region Products

CTL that operate unrestricted by *K*- or *D*-region products exist (Wagner *et al.*, 1975, 1978; Teh *et al.*, 1978; Forman and Flaherty, 1978;

TABLE 1. *H-2* Restriction

H-2 genotype of T cells*		*H-2* genotype of thymus*		*H-2* phenotype of restriction*·†	
a	a	a	a	a+	b−
a	b	a	b	a+	b+
a	a	a	b	a+	b+
a	b	a	a	a+	b−

* (a, b) *H-2* alleles.
† (+) Can or (−) cannot be used as restricting element.

Klein and Chiang, 1978; Fischer Lindahl, 1979; Kastner and Rich, 1979). Such unrestricted CTL recognize determinants *not* encoded in *K* or *D*. It seems, however, that in the majority of cases unrestricted CTL recognize determinants encoded within or near the MHC. It has been suggested that such cell-surface structures function as "transmembrane signal transmitters" (Langman, 1978; Snell, 1978).

No evidence has been reported that T helper cells can function unrestricted by *I*-region products. The question whether T-cell interactions with cells expressing allogeneic K, D antigens or T help for B cells expressing allogeneic *I*-region antigens is unrestricted cannot be answered because we do not know what *H-2* restriction means in molecular terms. There are, however, several reports that *H-2*-restricted killer cells specific for x lyse allogeneic target cells expressing neither x nor the appropriate restriction element(s) (Bevan, 1977; Finberg *et al.*, 1978). We found that an H-Y-specific killer-cell clone restricted to D^b lysed efficiently male as well as female target cells expressing allogeneic $H-2D^d$ antigens.

2.2. B Cells Are Not *H-2*-Restricted

Antibodies raised against antigens present on the surface of other cells are not H-2 restricted. It is clear that the majority of antibodies specific for cell-surface antigens x (Ly, Thy 1, H-Y, haptens) combine with such antigens regardless of what H-2 antigens are expressed on the cells. Thus, putative neoantigens formed by noncovalent association of *H-2* and x have not been defined yet by serology.

3. *H-2* Linked *Ir* Genes

3.1. Influence on the T-Cell Repertoire

H-2 genes control the T-cell repertoire not only for restricting elements (s), but also for non-H-2 antigens (x). This is referred to as "*H-2*-linked responsiveness." The observation of this phenomenon antedates that of *H-2* restriction. It now seems likely that immune-response (*Ir*)-gene products and the restricting elements (s) are identical: T cells restricted to certain *H-2* gene products are able to recognize some but not other antigens (x). Thus, the repertoire of restriction dictates in some way the repertoire of x recognition. This is nicely documented in experiments in which T cells from a responder-strain × nonresponder-strain F_1 hybrid collaborate with B cells from the high-responder parental strain only. If, however, both parental strains are responders, F_1 T cells collaborate with both types of B cells (Katz et al., 1973b). Similar observations have been made with F_1 T cells induced to proliferate by antigen-pulsed parental macrophages (Shevach and Rosenthal, 1973). Yet another example is the cytotoxic T-cell response to H-Y antigen, in which the ability of mice to respond is coupled to the repertoire of restriction (Simpson and Gordon, 1977; von Boehmer et al., 1977). These experiments, however, could not determine whether the H-2 genotype of T cells was decisive in determining responsiveness. In fact, in early experiments when H-2 restriction was not current, it was concluded that the genotype of T cells and not that of the thymus epithelium determined responsiveness (Tyan and McDevitt, 1970). In these experiments, low-responder cells were allowed to differentiate in an animal grafted with a low- and high-responder thymus graft. Such animals were still low responders, presumably because T cells restricted to high-responder I-region determinants could not find appropriate B cells or macrophages to interact with.

More recent experiments have shown that "H-2-linked responsiveness" is independent of the H-2 genotype of the T cells but is dependent on the phenotype of their restriction: T cells of low-responder genotype, when differentiated in X-irradiated recipients expressing H-2-gene products of high-responder genotype, acquire concomitantly with a new repertoire of restriction responsiveness to the antigen x in question (Table 2) (von Boehmer et al., 1978b; Miller, 1978; Kappler and Marrack, 1978). Ir genes as well as genes encoding restricting elements map in the I region for T helper cells and in the K or D region for T killer cells (Katz and Benacerraf, 1975; von Boehmer et al., 1978b).

TABLE 2. H-2-Linked Ir Genes

H-2 genotype of T cells*		H-2 genotype of thymus*		H-2 phenotype of restriction*,†	Responsiveness to antigens x under Ir-gene control?
a	a	a	a	a+	Yes
				b−	—
a	b	a	b	a+	Yes
				b+	No
b	b	a	b	a+	Yes
				b+	No
a	b	b	b	a−	—
				b+	No

* (a) Responder and (b) nonresponder alleles.
†(+) Can or (−) cannot be used as restricted element.

3.2. H-2-Gene Complementation

3.2.1. T Cells Restricted to Ia Antigens

Two low-responder strains can complement each other to produce a high-responder F_1 hybrid. One extensively studied case is the proliferative T-cell response to GLφ (Schwartz et al., 1976) or the T-dependent antibody response to the same antigen (Dorf and Benacerraf, 1975). The B10 as well as the B10.A strain are both low responders, while the F_1 hybrid is a high responder. One of the complementing genes maps in the IA region, the other in the IE region. All F_1 hybrids or recombinants expressing IA^B as well as IE^k are high responders (Table 3). F_1 high-responder T cells can be induced to proliferate only by F_1 high-responder macrophages, not by macrophages of either parent pulsed with GLφ (Schwartz et al., 1979). Chimeric mice constructed by injecting equal proportions of stem cells from both low-responder parental strains into X-irradiated F_1 hybrids failed to respond to GLφ, presumably because F_1 macrophages were not present (Schwartz et al., 1979). T cells from such chimeras could be primed by and respond to antigen-pulsed F_1 macrophages (Schwartz et al., personal communication). Essentially identical results were obtained when the T-dependent antibody response to GLφ was studied in allophenic mice constructed of two low-responder strains (Warner et al., 1977). The clue as to what might be so "special" on F_1 macrophages came from recent experiments by Jones et al. (1978): Unique IA^b-encoded specificities were found on cells of (B10 × B10.A)F_1 hybrids as well as on cells of the B10.A(5R) recombinant. They were absent on the surface of cells in either B10 or B10.A mice and required for their expression on the cell surface an IE^k-encoded protein. This observation fits nicely with experiments demonstrating unique mixed-lymphocyte reaction (MLR) determinants on (B10 × B10.A)F_1 hybrid cells (Fathman and Nabholz, 1977). In the case of the response to GLφ, it is likely that a unique restricting element on F_1 hybrid cells is the Ir-gene product.

3.2.2. Cytotoxic T Cells

A different type of Ir-gene complementation has been found in the responses of CTL to H-Y antigen. In this type, strains B10.A(5R) and B10.A both do not generate CTL specific for H-Y, whereas the F_1 hybrid does. The genes required map to the left of IB^B (presumably IA^b) and to K^k. The complementation in this case is not due to the presence of unique restricting elements on F_1 hybrid cells, because the K^k allele is

TABLE 3. *Ir*-Gene Complementation in Responses to GLϕ[a]

H-2 genotype of responding T cells and thymus		*H-2* genotype of macrophages or B cells		Responses to GLϕ (proliferation or antibody production)
IA^b	IE^b	IA^b	IE^b	−
IA^k	IE^k	IA^k	IE^k	−
IA^b	IE^k	IA^b	IE^k	+
IA^b	IE^k	IA^b	IE^b	−
IA^b	IE^k	IA^k	IE^k	−

[a] According to Schwartz *et al.* (1979).

sufficient for expression of the restriction element recognized by CTL (von Boehmer *et al.*, 1977; Simpson and Gordon, 1977). It appears that the generation of H-Y-specific CTL requires H-Y-specific T helper cells. For H-Y-specific T helper cells, a permissive restricting element is encoded in IA^b (von Boehmer *et al.*, 1977), but not in IA^k, whereas for H-Y-specific CTL, a permissive restricting element is encoded by K^k, but not by K^b or D^d (von Boehmer *et al.*, 1977; Simpson and Gordon, 1977). It appears that in all homozygous mice tested so far, with one exception (Simpson and Gordon, 1977), IA^b is the only permissive allele for H-Y-specific help, whereas there are several permissive alleles for H-Y-specific CTL. It has been postulated that there are several other permissive alleles for help in (k × d) (k × s) (k × a)F_1 hybrids as well as in homozygous H-2 mice (Hurme *et al.*, 1978). We have been unable to confirm these results: the effect of such alleles on the H-Y response is, according to our results, at least 30- to 100-fold weaker than that of IA^b on the basis of cell input at day 0 of culture. The postulates of distinct permissive alleles for H-Y-specific T helper cells and H-Y-specific CTL is consistent with the following experimental evidence: F_1 T cells of responder genotype (CBA × B6) that have differentiated from stem cells in X-irradiated recipients B10.A(5R) (permissive for help but nonpermissive for CTL) or CBA (nonpermissive for help but permissive for CTL) do not respond to H-Y antigen (von Boehmer *et al.*, 1978b; von Boehmer and Haas, 1979) (Table 4). If, however, cells from both types of chimeras are injected together into X-irradiated (CBA × B6)F_1 hybrids and primed by (CBA × B6) male cells, they can complement each other and generate in culture H-Y-specific CTL restricted to K^k (von Boehmer and Haas, 1979). Thus, the complementing *Ir* genes control two different classes of T cells required for the CTL response to H-Y.

On the other hand, B10.A(5R) T cells of nonresponder genotype that had differentiated in X-irradiated (CBA × B6) recipients of responder genotype acquired with their "new" repertoire of restriction the ability to respond to H-Y antigen. CBA T cells of low-responder genotype differentiated in (CBA × B6) hosts (von Boehmer *et al.*, 1978b) did not, however, respond to H-Y. This suggested that H-Y-specific CTL must express IA^b antigens for interaction with IA^b-restricted T helper cells (von Boehmer *et al.*, 1978b). This concept was originally proposed by Zinkernagel *et al.* (1978). Further supportive evidence came from experiments in which the responsiveness to H-Y was tested in chimeras constructed by injecting B6 as well as CBA stem cells in X-irradiated (CBA × B6)F_1 hybrid hosts: all H-Y-specific CTL were of B6 origin, whereas CTL specific for allogeneic H-2 antigens were derived from both B6 and CBA (Table 5).

TABLE 4. *Ir*-Gene Complementation in CTL Responses to H-Y

H-2 genotype of responding T-cells*	*H-2* genotype of thymus	H-2 phenotype of restriction for help*		H-2 phenotype of restriction for CTL*	CTL response to H-Y
b b d	b b d	*IA*^b		K^b , D^d	−
k k k	k k k	*IA*^k		K^k , D^k	−
b b b × k k k	b b b × k k k	*IA*^b	*IA*^k	K^b, K^k , D^b, D^k	+
① b b b × k k k	b b d	*IA*^b		K^b , D^d	−
② b b b × k k k	k k k	*IA*^k		K^k , D^k	−
① + ②	b b b + k k k	*IA*^b	*IA*^k	K^b, K^k , D^d, D^k	+

* The three letters (k, b, d) correspond to the haplotype designation in the *K*, *IA*, and *D* region. Permissive alleles for H-Y-specific help and H-Y-specific CTL are italicized.

TABLE 5. Acquisition of H-Y Specificity by T Cells of Low-Responder Genotype

$H\text{-}2$ genotype of responding T cells	$H\text{-}2$ genotype of thymus	$H\text{-}2$ phenotype of restriction for help	$H\text{-}2$ phenotype of restriction for CTL	CTL response for H-Y	$H\text{-}2$ genotype of CTL
b b d	b b b × k k k	IA^b, IA^k	K^b, K^k, D^b, D^k	+	b b d
k k k	b b b × k k k	IA^b, IA^k	K^b, K^k, D^b, D^k	−	—
b b b + k k k	b b b × k k k	IA^b, IA^k	K^b, K^k, D^b, D^k	+	b b b

3.3. The B-Cell Repertoire Is Not Directly Influenced by *H-2*-Linked *Ir* Genes

T-dependent antibody production is indirectly controlled by *Ir* genes influencing the repertoire of T helper cells. It appears, however, that in mice unresponsive to antigen x, antibodies specific for x can be elicited when x is conjugated to a carrier to which the T cells can respond (Green *et al.*, 1969; Dunham *et al.*, 1972; Kapp *et al.*, 1973). There is no evidence for a direct influence of *H-2*-linked *Ir* genes on the B-cell repertoire.

4. Frequency of Cells Specific for Allogeneic H-2 Antigens

4.1. Allospecific T Cells

The frequency of T cells responding to stimulation by allogeneic H-2 antigens is high: one in 30 lymphocytes from chicken can form pocks on the chorioallantoic membrane of an allogeneic embryo (Simons and Fowler, 1966). Similarly, the frequency of T cells able to respond to allogeneic stimulation by generation of CTL is high: at least one in 1000 lymphocytes from a mouse is able to generate CTL specific for a set of allogeneic H-2 antigens (Skinner and Marbrook, 1976; Fischer Lindahl and Wilson, 1977; Teh *et al.*, 1977).

4.2. Allospecific B Cells

The frequency of B cells specific for a set of alloantigens has not been determined directly. It is, however, more difficult to obtain alloantibodies than allospecific T cells. The reason for this is not clear, but the difficulty may reflect a lower frequency of allospecific B cells than of allospecific T cells.

5. T-Cell Repertoire for Restricting Elements vs. the Repertoire for Allogeneic H-2 Antigens

Several experiments have suggested that the repertoire of T cells for allogeneic H-2 antigens differs from the repertoire specific for restricting elements: Cross-reactive lysis was found to differ between allogeneic and *H-2*-restricted CTL (Blanden *et al.*, 1976; Zinkernagel, 1976b; Simpson *et al.*, 1978); for instance, third-party T cells stimulated with cells from wild-type (*H-2^b*) produced cross-reactive lysis on target cells from a mutant (H-$2K^{ba}$), while H-2-restricted CTL from wild-type mice stimulated with syngeneic virus-infected cells lysed only wild-type but not mutant target cells (Blanden et al., 1976; Zinkernagel, 1976b). H-2-restricted wild-type CTL induced by syngeneic trinitrophenyl (TNP)-coupled cells, however, cross-reacted on TNP-coupled mutant targets (Forman and Klein, 1977). More recent experiments indicate that the epitope density of x antigens on target cells is an important parameter for detection of cross-reactive lysis of H-2-restricted CTL: hapten-specific CTL restricted to K^K showed high cross-reactive lysis on densely, but not sparsely, coupled target cells expressing D^s or D^k antigens or antigens encoded in the H-2^r haplotype and weak cross-reactive lysis on densely coupled targets expressing K^s antigens or antigens encoded in the H-2^b or H-2^d haplotypes (Haas et al., 1979). It was found by other authors that CTL specific for K^k alloantigens also produced relatively strong cross-reactive lysis on targets expressing D^s alloantigens (Nabholz et al., 1974) and D^k antigens (Fischer Lindahl, personal communication) or antigens encoded in the H-2^r haplotype (Fischer Lindahl et al., 1975). Thus, more detailed studies are required to decide whether the T-cell repertoire for restricting elements differs from that for H-2-encoded alloantigens.

6. T-Cell vs. B-Cell Repertoire

6.1. Probing of the Repertoire by Responsiveness

When the repertoire of T cells and B cells is probed by testing responses to various antigens in different animals, it is clear that it differs in T and B cells: (1) Effector T but not B cells are restricted by H-2 antigens. (2) The repertoire of T but not of B cells is influenced by H-2-linked Ir genes. (3) The frequency of allospecific T cells appears to be higher than that of B cells.

6.2. Probing of Repertoire by v-Gene Markers on Responding Cells

A series of experiments has indicated that T and B cells use at least partly similar v-gene products when responding to antigen (x): Antiidiotypic antibody could be used to prime T and B cells for a response to streptococcal carbohydrate (Eichmann and Rajewsky, 1975). T cells from the primed mice would be entirely inhibited in vitro by the same antiidiotypic antibodies (Black et al., 1976). Similar observations have been made when in studies of T- and B-cell responses to phosphorylcholine (Cosenza *et al.,* 1976). The expression of idiotype markers was linked to expression of allotypic markers. Interestingly, idiotypic markers present on light chains of carbohydrate-specific antibodies could not be demonstrated on T helper cells (Krawinkel *et al.,* 1976). In fact, it has been suggested that different subsets of T cells use either V_H- or V_L-encoded structures for antigen recognition, while B cells use both (Lonai *et al.,* 1978). If this were true, it would lead to a vastly different but partly overlapping repertoire in T and B cells. Binz *et al.* (1978) have found allotype-linked idiotypic markers on allospecific T cells. In contrast, Bellgrau and Wilson (1979) were unable to demonstrate polymorphism of T-cell receptors specific for a set of alloantigens; i.e., they could not find evidence for allotype- or *H-2*-linked idiotypic markers in their system. The analysis of T-cell idiotypes by serology does not at present explain the influence of *H-2*-gene products on the T-cell repertoire, but it suggests that *v*-genes contributing to receptors on antigen-specific T and B cells are encoded on the same chromosome.

7. Conclusions

The apparent dual specificity of T cells is the result of endogenous receptor production. The repertoire of *H-2* restriction of T cells is largely determined by the *H-2* genotype of the radioresistant portion of the thymus. T cells acquire their repertoire of restriction specificities during differentiation from stem cells irrespective of their own *H-2* genotype. The repertoire of restriction of T helper cells is specific for IA antigens and of T killer cells for K and D antigens. *H-2*-linked *Ir* genes specify the restriction elements (s). At present, there is no need to postulate that *H-2*-linked *Ir* genes encode the *v*-region of T-cell receptors specific for antigens (x).

References

Bellgrau, D., and Wilson, D., 1979, Immunological studies on T cell receptors. II. Limited polymorphism of idiotypic determinants on T cell receptors specific for major histocompatibility complex alloantigens, *J. Exp. Med.* **149:**234.

Bennink, J.R., and Doherty, P.C., 1978, T cell population specifically depleted of alloactivity potential cannot be induced to lyse H-2 different virus-infected target cells, *J. Exp. Med.* **148:**128.

Bevan, M., 1977, Killer cells reactive to altered-self can also be alloreactive, *Proc. Natl. Acad. Sci. U.S.A.* **74:**2094.

Bevan, M.J., and Fink, P.J., 1978, The influence of thymus H-2 antigens on the specificity of maturing killer and helper cells, *Immunol. Rev.* **42:**3.

Binz, H., Wigzell, H., and Bazin, H., 1978, T cell idiotypes are linked to immunoglobulin heavy chain genes, *Nature (London)* **264**:639.

Black, S.J., Hämmerling, G., Berek, C., Rajewsky, K., and Eichmann, K., 1976, Idiotypic analysis of lymphocytes *in vitro*. I. Specificity and heterogeneity of T and B lymphocytes reactive with anti-idiotypic antibody, *J. Exp. Med.* **143**:846.

Blanden, R.V., Dunlop, M.B.C., Doherty, P.C., Kahn, H.I., and McKenzie, I.F.C., 1976, Effects of four H-2K mutations on virus induced antigens recognized by cytotoxic T cells, *Immunogenetics* **3**:541.

Burnet, F.M., 1978, Clonal selection and after, in: *Theoretical Immunology* (G.I. Bell, A.S. Perelson, and G.H. Pimbley, eds.), p. 63, Marcel Dekker, New York.

Cosenza, H., Augustin, A.A., and Julius, M.H., 1976, Idiotypes and anti-idiotypes as probes in analysis of immunoregulation, *Cold Spring Harbor Symp. Quant. Biol.* **41**:709.

Doherty, P.C., and Bennick, J.R., 1979, Vaccinia specific cytotoxic T cell responses in the context of H-2 antigens not encountered in the thymus may reflect aberrant recognition of a virus-H-2-complex, *J. Exp. Med.* **149**:150.

Doherty, P.C., Blanden, R.V., and Zinkernagel, R.M., 1976, Specificity of virus-immune effector T cells for H-2K or H-2D compatible interactions. Implications for H-antigen diversity, *Transpl. Rev.* **29**:89.

Dorf, M.E., and Benacerraf, B., 1975, Complementation of H-2 linked Ir genes in the mouse, *Proc. Natl. Acad. Sci. U.S.A.* **72**:3671.

Dunham, E.K., Unanue, E.R., and Benacerraf, B., 1972, Antigen binding and capping by lymphocytes of genetic nonresponder mice, *J. Exp. Med.* **136**:403.

Eichmann, K., and Rajewsky, K., 1975, Induction of T and B cell immunity by anti-idiotypic antibody, *Eur. J. Immunol.* **5**:661.

Fathman, C.G., and Nabholz, M., 1977, *In vitro* secondary MLR II: Interaction of MLR determinants expressed by F_1 cells, *Eur. J. Immunol.* **7**:370.

Finberg, R., Buralkoff, S.J., Contor, H., and Benacerraf, B., 1978, The biological significance of alloreactivity: T cells stimulated by Sendai virus coated syngeneic cells specifically lyse allogeneic target cells, *Proc. Natl. Acad. Sci. U.S.A.* **75**:51.

Fischer Lindahl, K., 1979, Unrestricted killer cells recognize on antigen controlled by a gene linked to Tla, *Immunogenetics* **8**:71.

Fischer Lindahl, K., and Wilson, D.B., 1977, Histocompatibility antigen activated cytotoxic T lymphocytes. II. Estimates of the frequency and specificity of precursors, *J. Exp. Med.* **145**:508.

Fischer Lindahl, K., Peck, A.B., and Bach, F.H., 1975, Specificity of cell-mediated lympholysis for public and private H-2 determinants, *Scand. J. Immunol.* **4**:541.

Forman, J., and Klein, J., 1977, Immunogenetic analysis of H-2 mutations. VI. Cross-reactivity in cell-mediated lympholysis between TNP-modified cells from H-2 mutant strains, *Immunogenetics* **4**:183.

Forman, J., and Flaherty, L., 1978, Identification of a new CML target antigen controlled by a gene associated with the Qa-2 locus, *Immunogenetics* **6**:227.

Green, I., Paul, W.E., and Benacerraf, B., 1969, Genetic control of immunological responsiveness in guinea pigs to 2;4 dinitrophenyl conjugate of poly-L-arginine protamine and poly-L-ornithine, *Proc. Natl. Acad. Sci. U.S.A.* **64**:1095

Haas, W., Pohlit, H., and von Boehmer, H., 1979, Cytotoxic T cell responses to haptenated cells. II. On the role of H-2 genes, *Eur. J. Immunol.* **9**:868.

Hurme, M., Chandler, P.R., Hetherington, C.M., and Simpson, E., 1978, Cytotoxic T cell responses to H-Y: Mapping of Ir genes, *J. Exp. Med.* **147**:758.

Jones, P.P., Murphy, D.B., and McDevitt, H.O., 1978, Two-gene control of the expression of a murine Ia antigen, *J. Exp. Med.* **148**:925.

Kapp, J.A., Pierce, C.W., and Benacerraf, B., 1973, Genetic control of immune responses *in vitro*. I. Development of primary and secondary PFC responses to the random terpolymer L-glutamic acid ^{60}-L-alanine^{30}-L-tyrosine^{10} (GAT) by mouse spleen cells, *J. Exp. Med.* **138**:1107.

Kappler, J.W., and Marrack, P., 1978, The role of H-2 linked genes in helper T cell function. IV. Importance of T-cell genotype and host environment in I-region and Ir gene expression, *J. Exp. Med.* **148**:1510.

Kastner, D., and Rich, R., 1979, H-2 nonrestricted cytotoxic responses to an antigen encoded telomeric to H-2, *J. Immunol.* **122**:196.

Katz, D.H., and Benacerraf, B., 1975, The function and interrelationships of the T cell receptors, Ir genes and other histocompatibility gene products, *Transplant. Rev.* **22**:175.

Katz, D.H., Hamaoka, T., and Benacerraf, B., 1973a, Cell interactions between histocompatible T and B lymphocytes. II. Failure of physiologic cooperative interactions between T and B lymphocytes from allogeneic strains in humoral response to hapten–protein conjugates, *J. Exp. Med.* **137**:1405.

Katz, D.H., Hamaoka, T., Dorf, M.E., Maurer, P.H., and Benacerraf, B., 1973b, IV. Involvement of the immune response (Ir) gene in the control of lymphocyte interactions in responses controlled by the gene, *J. Exp. Med.* **138**:1213.

Kindred, B., and Loor, F., 1974, Activity of host-derived T cells which differentiate in nude mice grafted with co-isogeneic or allogeneic thymuses, *J. Exp. Med.* **139**:1215.

Klein, I., and Chiang, C.L., 1978, A new locus (H-2T) at the D end of the H-2 complex, *Immunogenetics* **6**:235.

Krawinkel, V., Crammer, M., Berek, C., Hämmerling G., Black, S.J., Rajewsky, K., and Eichmann, K., 1976, On the structure of the T cell receptor for antigen, *Cold Spring Harbor Symp. Quant. Biol.* **41**:285.

Langman, R.E., 1978, The role of the major histocompatibility complex in immunity: A new concept in the functioning of a cell-mediated immune system, *Rev. Physiol. Biochem. Pharmacol.* **81**:1.

Lonai, P., Ben-Neriah, Y., Steinman, L., and Givol, D., 1978, Selective participation of immunoglobulin V region and major histocompatibility complex products in antigen binding by T cells, *Eur. J. Immunol.* **8**:827.

Matzinger, P., and Mirkwood, G., 1978, In a fully H-2 incompatible chimera, T cells of donor origin can respond to minor histocompatibility antigens in association with either donor or host H-2 type, *J. Exp. Med.* **148**:84.

Miller, J.F.A.P., 1978, Restrictions imposed on T lymphocyte reactivities by the major histocompatibility complex: Implications for T cell repertoire selection, *Immunol. Rev.* **42**:76.

Miller, J.F.A.P., Vadas, M., Whitelaw, A., and Gamble, J., 1976, Role of major histocompatibility complex gene products in delayed type hypersensitivity, *Proc. Natl. Acad. Sci. U.S.A.* **73**:2486.

Nabholz, M., Vives, J., Young, H.M., Meo, T., Miggiano, V., Rijnbeck, A., and Shreffler, D., 1974, Cell mediated lysis *in vitro*: Genetic control of killer cell production and target cell specificities in the mouse, *Eur. J. Immunol.* **4**:378.

Pfitzenmaier, K., Starzinski-Powitz, A., Rodt, H., Röllinghoff, M., and Wagner, H., 1976, Virus and TNP-hapten specific T cell mediated cytotoxicity against H-2 incompatible target cells, *J. Exp. Med.* **143**:999.

Rosenthal, A.S., and Shevach, E.M., 1973, Function of macrophages in antigen recognition by guinea pig T lymphocytes. I. Requirement for histocompatible macrophages and lymphocytes, *J. Exp. Med.* **138**:1194.

Schmitt-Verhulst, A.M., and Shearer, G.M., 1977, Specificity of CML and MLR clones responding to chemically modified syngeneic and allogeneic cells, *J. Supramol. Struct. Suppl.* **1**:206.

Schwartz, R.H., Dorf, M.E., Benacerraf, B., and Paul, W.E., 1976, The requirement for two complementing Ir-GLφ immune response genes in the T-lymphocyte proliferative response to poly (Glu^{53}-Lys^{36}-Phe^{11}), *J. Exp. Med.* **143**:897.

Schwartz, R.H., Yono, A., Stimpfling, J.H., and Paul, W.E., 1979, Gene complementation in the T lymphocyte proliferative response to poly (Glu^{55}, Lys^{36}, Phe^9)$_n$: A demonstration that both immune response gene products must be expressed in the same antigen presenting cell, *J. Exp. Med.* **149**:40.

Shevach, E.M., and Rosenthal, A.S., 1973, The function of macrophages in antigen recognition of guinea pig T lymphocytes. II. Role of the macrophage in the regulation of genetic control of the immune response, *J. Exp. Med.* **138**:1213.

Simons, M.J., and Fowler, R., 1966, Chorioallantoic membrane lesions produced by incubation of adult fowl small lymphocytes, *Nature (London)* **209**:588.

Simpson, E., and Gordon, R.D., 1977, Responsiveness to H-Y antigen: Ir gene complementation and target cell specificity, *Immunol. Rev.* **35**:59.

Simpson, E., Mabraaten, L., Chandler, P., Hetherington, G., Hurme, M., Brunner, C., and Bailey, D., 1978, Cross-reactive cytotoxic responses: H-2 restricted are more specific than anti-H-2 responses, *J. Exp. Med.* **148**:1478.

Skinner, M.A., and Marbrook, J., 1976, An estimation of the frequency of precursor cells which generate cytotoxic lymphocytes, *J. Exp. Med.* **143**:1562.

Snell, G.D., 1978, The major histocompatibility complex: Its evolution and involvement in cellular immunity, *Harvey Lectures 1977–1978*, Academic Press, New York.

Sprent, J., 1978, Role of H-2 gene products in the function of T helper cells from normal and chimeric mice measured in vivo, *Immunol. Rev.* **42**:108.

Teh, H.S., Harley, E., Philipps, R.A., and Miller, R.G., 1977, Quantitative studies on the precursors of cytotoxic lymphocytes, *J. Immunol.* **118**:1049.

Teh, H.S., Latarte, M., Philipps, R.A., and Miller, R.G., 1978, Characterization of the target cells antigen in I region-mediated lympholysis, *Cell. Immunol.* **37**:397.

Tyan, M.L., and McDevitt, H.O., 1970, Antibody responses to two synthetic polypeptides: The role of the thymic epithelial reticulum, *J. Immunol.* **105**:1190.

von Boehmer, H., and Haas, W., 1976, Cytotoxic T lymphocytes recognize allogeneic tolerated TNP-conjugated cells, *Nature (London)* **261**:139.

von Boehmer, H., and Haas, W., 1979, Distinct *Ir* genes for helper and killer cells in the cytotoxic response to H-Y antigen, *J. Exp. Med.* **150**:1134.

von Boehmer, H., Hudson, L., and Sprent, J., 1975, Collaboration of histoincompatible T and B lymphocytes using cells from tetraparental bone marrow chimeras, *J. Exp. Med.* **142**:989

von Boehmer, H., Fathman, C.G., and Haas, W., 1977, H-2 gene complementation in cytotoxic T cell responses of female against male cells, *Eur. J. Immunol.* **7**:443.

von Boehmer, H., Haas, W., and Pohlit, H., 1978a, Cytotoxic T cells recognize male antigen and H-2 as distinct entities, *J. Exp. Med.* **147**:1291.

von Boehmer, H., Haas, W., and Jerne, N.K., 1978b, MHC linked immune responsiveness is required by lymphocytes of low responder mice differentiating in the thymus of high responder mice, *Proc. Natl. Acad. Sci. U.S.A.* **75**:2439.

von Boehmer, H., Hengertuer, H., Nebholz, M., Levuhardt, W., Schreier, M.H., and Hees, W., 1979, Time specificity of a continuously growing killer cell clone specific for H-Y antigen, *Eur. J. Immunol.* **9**:592.

Wagner, H., Götze, D., Ptschelinzew, L., and Röllinghoff, M., 1975, Induction of cytotoxic T lymphocytes against I-region coded determinants: *In vitro* evidence for a third histocompatibility locus in the mouse, *J. Exp. Med.* **142**:1477.

Wagner, H., Starzinski-Powitz, A., Röllinghoff, M., Goldstein, P., and Jakob, H., 1978, T-cell mediated cytotoxic immune responses to F 9 teratocarcinoma cells: Cytolytic effector T cells lyse H-2 negative F 9 cells and syngeneic spermatogonia, *J. Exp. Med.* **147**:251.

Waldmann, H., and Munro, A.J., 1975, Cooperation across the histocompatibility barrier, *Nature (London)* **258**:728.

Waldmann, H., Pope, H., Bettles, C., and Davies, A.J.S., 1979, The influence of thymus on the development of MHC restrictions established by T helper cells, *Nature (London)* **277**:137.

Warner, C.M., McIvor, J.L., Maurer, P.H., and Merryman, C.F., 1977, The immune response in allophenic mice to the synthetic polymer L-glutamic acid, L-lysine, L-phenylalanine. II. Lack of gene complementation in two nonresponder strains, *J. Exp. Med.* **145**:766.

Wilson, D.B., Lindahl, K.I., Wilson, D.H., and Sprent, J., 1977, The generation of killer cells to trinitrophenyl-modified allogeneic targets by lymphocyte populations negatively selected to alloantigens, *J. Exp. Med.* **145**:361.

Zinkernagel, R.N., 1976a, H-2 restriction of virus specific cytotoxicity across the H-2 barrier: Separate effector T cell specificities are associated with self H-2 and with the tolerated allogeneic H-2 in chimeras, *J. Exp. Med.* **144**:933.

Zinkernagel, R.M., 1976b, H-2 compatibility requirement for virus-specific T cell-mediated cytolysis: The H-2K structure involved is coded by a single cistron defined by H-2K^b mutant mice, *J. Exp. Med.* **142**:437.

Zinkernagel, R.M., 1978, Thymus and lymphophemopoietic cells: Their role in T cell maturation, in selection of T cells' H-2 restrictions-specificity and in H-2 linked Ir gene control, *Immunol. Rev.* **42**:224.

Zinkernagel, R.M., and Doherty, P.C., 1974, Activity of sensitized thymus-derived lymphocytes in lymphocytic choriomeningitis reflects immunological surveillance against altered self components, *Nature (London)* **251**:547.

Zinkernagel, R.M., Callahan, G.M., Althage, A., Cooper, J., Streilein, P.W., and Klein, J., 1978, The lymphoreticular system in triggering virus-plus-self specific cytotoxic T cells: Evidence for T help, *J. Exp. Med.* **147**:897.

2

Continuously Proliferating Allospecific T-Cell Lines

A Model to Study T-Cell Functions and Receptors

Gunther Dennert

1. Introduction

Studies of the function and specificity of thymus-derived lymphocytes (T cells) have met with increasing difficulties in recent years. The main reason is that T cells perform many different regulatory and effector functions in both cell-mediated and humoral immunity, each of which functions is apparently executed by a distinct subset of T cells. This was, for instance, shown by functional assays in which T cells primed for one function were assayed for other functions (Dennert, 1976). By combining functional assays with serological procedures, it was established that T cells with specific functions may display specific Ly antigens (Cantor and Boyse, 1975). This very promising approach to the separation of T-cell subsets has yet to be fully exploited, since it is difficult to prepare sufficient amounts of Ly-specific antibody for experimentation. But the recent success in preparing hybridomas producing specific antibody has opened new avenues for the preparation of unlimited amounts of specific antibodies (Köhler and Milstein, 1976). Other procedures aimed at enriching or even purifying T-cell populations have had little success. For instance, fractionation of T cells by adsorption to and

Gunther Dennert • Department of Cancer Biology, The Salk Institute, San Diego, California 92112.

elution from matrices to which antigen was attached have yielded disappointing results (Rubin and Wigzell, 1973), with the exception of alloantigen-specific cytotoxic T cells (Golstein *et al.*, 1971).

It appears, therefore, that new procedures are needed to study T-cell functions on both the cellular and the molecular level. Recently, two different approaches have been pursued with differing success. In one, an attempt was made to make use of the finding that plasma cells secreting specific antibody and hybridized with myeloma cell lines give raise to continuous cell lines that may continue to produce antibody (Köhler and Milstein, 1976). Hybrids derived from somatic crosses between specific T-cell populations and T-lymphoma lines were therefore constructed and assayed for specific activity (Hämmerling, 1977). Unfortunately, this approach has so far met with only some success. While hybrids with suppressor activity in the *in vitro* humoral immune response were derived, continuous hybrid lines with cytotoxic activity have not been obtained so far. The reasons for these failures could be severalfold and are obviously difficult to analyze.

The second approach is based on the initial observation that T cells sensitized to alloantigens may under certain culture conditions continue to proliferate in secondary or tertiary culture (Cerottini *et al.*, 1974). Making use of this finding, we have established and characterized a number of different allospecific T-cell lines, which appear to proliferate permanently *in vitro* provided antigenic stimulation is present (Dennert and De Rose, 1976; Dennert and Raschke, 1977; Dennert, 1979). An interesting and potentially important variation of this procedure has recently been introduced by a number of laboratories (Gillis and Smith, 1977; Nabholz *et al.*, 1978). In this procedure, allospecific T cells were sensitized in a mixed-lymphocyte culture and stimulated for several weeks with alloantigens. Subsequently, these T cells could be induced to proliferate in the absence of alloantigen provided they were cultured in conditioned medium prepared from lymphocytes stimulated with the T-cell mitogen concanavalin A (Con A). In this review, I would like to discuss the generation, maintenance, and characterization of T-cell lines initiated by alloantigenic stimulation and evaluate the possible usefulness of allospecific T-cell lines for the study of T-cell functions and receptors.

2. Properties of Allospecific T-Cell Lines

2.1. Initiation of Allospecific T-Cell Lines

The initiation of long-term cultures of allospecific T cells follows standard tissue-culture procedures. Mixed-lymphocyte cultures containing 10^6/ml responder mouse spleen cells and equal numbers of irradiated allogeneic stimulator spleen cells are set up in Click's minimal essential medium or RPMI 1640, supplemented with 5% fetal calf serum and 5 × 10^{-5} M β-mercaptoethanol (Dennert and De Rose, 1976), in 20-ml Falcon tissue-culture bottles. Culture flasks are incubated in the upright position in 5% CO_2 in air at 37°C. The success of long-term culture of T cells appears to depend, at least in part, on the type of fetal calf serum used. Care is therefore advised in the selection of sera allowing optimal T-cell proliferation. The cultures must be fed at least every 2 weeks (Dennert and Raschke, 1977) by replacing the tissue-culture supernatant with fresh medium containing 10^6/ml irradiated spleen stimulator cells. For optimal cell proliferation and maintenance of high cytolytic activity, weekly feeding and stimulation with allogeneic cells are required (Dennert and Raschke, 1977). To avoid crowding, the cultures are split 1:2 once a cell density of 5 × 10^5/ml is reached. Long-term cultures have been derived from a number of different mouse strains (BALB/c, DBA/2, C57Bl/6, and C_3H), and differences in longevity of these cultures have not been seen.

2.2. Requirements for Cell Proliferation in Long-Term T-Cell Cultures

Long-term T-cell cultures proliferate when challenged with spleen stimulator cells for about 3–5 days, after which time the cells start dying. Some "quiescent" cells, however, have been shown to survive in these cultures for about 5–6 weeks and will proliferate on restimulation (MacDonald et al., 1974). Specific conditions appear necessary to stimulate "quiescent" cells. For instance, T-cell mitogens such as phytohemagglutinin (PHA) and Con A are not able to stimulate cell proliferation in long-term cultures (Table 1) (Dennert and De Rose, 1976). Very similar results were also reported by Andersson and Häyry (1973). The reason for this is not known, but it is possible that either allospecific T cells in long-term cultures are not responsive to these two mitogens or that they induce autokilling. This latter possibility is supported by the observation that allospecific T killer cells lyse each other in the presence of lectins (Dennert and De Rose, 1976). Various cell types carrying serologically detectable H-2 antigens on their cell surface were tested for their ability to induce cell proliferation. Interestingly, cells such as C57Bl/6 erythrocytes or EL4 tumor cells that carry H-2 antigens do not stimulate cell proliferation, while spleen cells do (Table 1). It emerged that the failure of these two cell types to stimulate cell proliferation was due to a lack of lymphocyte-activating determinants on these cells. In agreement with this, tumor cells such as the BALB/c myeloma cell line S194, which stimulates syngeneic or allogeneic spleen cells (Table 2) in a primary mixed-lymphocyte tumor-cell culture, also stimulate the proliferation of

TABLE 1. Failure of Tumor Cells, Erythrocytes, and T-Cell Mitogens to Induce Proliferation of Allospecific T Cells

Responder cells[a]	Stimulator cells[b]	[^{3}H]-TdR incorporation[c]
C·B6·9·75	—	52 ± 4
—	5 × 10^6 C57Bl/6 spleen cells (H-2^b)	183 ± 27
—	10^6 EL4 (H-2^b)	38 ± 1
—	5 × 10^6 C57Bl/6 red cells (H-2^b)	68 ± 4
C·B6·9·75	5 × 10^6 C57Bl/6 spleen cells	9,420 ± 166
C·B6·9·75	10^6 EL4	80 ± 2
C·B6·9·75	5 × 10^6 C57Bl/6 red cells	63 ± 9
C·B6·9·75	2 × 10^7 C57Bl/6 red cells	56 ± 6
C·B6·9·75	8 × 10^7 C57Bl/6 red cells	61 ± 1
BALB/c spleen	—	230 ± 50
BALB/c spleen	2 µg/ml Con A	7,238 ± 30
BALB/c spleen	1 µg/ml PHA	5,923 ± 334
C·B6·9·75	—	52 ± 3
C·B6·9·75	5 × 10^6 C57Bl/6 spleen cells	32,747 + 285
C·B6·9·75	0.5 µg/ml PHA	173 ± 31
C·B6·9·75	1 µg/ml PHA	141 ± 2
C·B6·9·75	2 µg/ml PHA	132 ± 2
C·B6·9·75	4 µg/ml PHA	152 ± 10
C·B6·9·75	8 µg/ml PHA	183 ± 4
C·B6·9·75	0.5 µg/ml Con A	163 ± 12
C·B6·9·75	1 µg/ml Con A	163 ± 3
C·B6·9·75	2 µg/ml Con A	161 ± 0
C·B6·9·75	4 µg/ml Con A	63 ± 1
C·B6·9·75	8 µg/ml Con A	65 ± 6

[a] 10^5 responder cells/ml; (C·B6·9·75) BALB/c anti-C57Bl/6 initiated September 1975.
[b] Stimulator cells were irradiated with 1000 rads.   [c]20-hr labeling on day 2.

long-term cultures. However, C57Bl/6 long-term cultures stimulated repeatedly with BALB/c spleen cells are not as efficiently stimulated with S194 as compared to cultures repeatedly stimulated with S194 (Table 2). Similarly, cultures stimulated with S194 respond much better to S194 than to BALB/c spleen cells (Table 2). This shows that a large population of the C57Bl/6 responder cells are sensitized to distinct antigens on S194 and BALB/c spleen stimulator cells, which are not shared by both. The lymphocyte-activating determinants on BALB/c spleen cells and BALB/c S194 therefore appear to be different (Dennert et al., 1977).

The finding that lymphocyte-activating determinants are important for the proliferation of allospecific T-cell lines led to the mapping of antigenic determinants responsible for the proliferative response. Results showed that apparently the serologically detectable H-2 specificities coded in the D end of the H-2 complex (Dennert and Raschke, 1977) are not involved. A BALB/c line sensitized to C67Bl/6 does not respond if

TABLE 2. Stimulation of Cell Proliferation by S194 Tumor Cells

Responder cells[a]	Stimulator cells	[³H]-TdR incorporation on day 3
C57Bl/6 spleen	—	375 ± 3
—	S194	185 ± 8
C57Bl/6 spleen	S194	3,320 ± 289
B6·C·7·76	—	70 ± 7
—	BALB/c spleen	79 ± 6
—	C57Bl/6 spleen	87 ± 1
B6·C·7·76	BALB/c spleen	13,675 ± 1176
B6·C·7·76	C57Bl/6 spleen	154 ± 16
B6·C·7·76	S194	1,584 ± 208
B6·S194·9·76	—	62 ± 5
B6·S194·9·76	S194	2,278 ± 614
B6·S194·9·76	BALB/c spleen	1,350 ± 40
B6·S194·9·76	C57Bl/6 spleen	86 ± 8

[a] B6·C·7·76 (C57Bl/6 anti-BALB/c) was 4 months in culture and B6·S194·9·76 (C57Bl/6 anti-S194) was 1 month in culture at the time of this experiment.

challenged with HTG spleen cells (Table 3). It appears, rather, that gene products coded for in the K and I regions are able to stimulate cell proliferation, since a C_3H line sensitized to SJL is stimulated to proliferate not only by ATH and B10 HTT but also by ATL stimulator cells (Table 3).

The stimulation of cell proliferation could be the result of interaction of either all cells in the culture or only a fraction of cells with the stimulator cells. In the latter case, one could imagine that a subpopulation of cells in the cultures responds to the lymphocyte-activating determinants followed by secretion of a lymphokine able to stimulate division in a second subset of T cells. It was therefore interesting to explore whether culture supernatants of lymphocytes stimulated in various ways are able to induce cell proliferation. Results presented in Table 4 show that cell supernatants of spleen cells stimulated with Con A cause some stimulation of allospecific T-cell lines, while supernatants from spleen cells stimulated in a mixed-lymphocyte culture by the T-cell mitogen PHA, or by the bone-marrow-derived lymphocyte (B-cell) mitogen bacterial lipopolysaccharide (LPS), show no stimulating effects. Comparison of proliferation caused by spleen stimulator cells with that caused by supernatants of Con-A stimulated cells reveals almost a 20-fold difference (Table 4). Cell supernatants therefore stimulate poorly in comparison to spleen cells. In fact, allospecific T-cell lines that were in culture for 2–3

TABLE 3. Contribution of *H-2*-Region Genes in the Stimulation of T-Killer-Cell Lines

Allospecific T-cell line[a]	Stimulator cells[b]	H-2 haplotype	[³H]-TdR incorporation on day 3	
C·B6·2·76	—		38 ±	2
—	BALB/c	(ddddddd)	47 ±	3
—	C57Bl/6	(bbbbbbb)	41 ±	5
—	HTG	(ddddddb)	47 ±	3
C·B6·2·76	BALB/c	(ddddddd)	175 ±	16
C·B6·2·76	C57Bl/6	(bbbbbbb)	9248 ±	419
C·B6·2·76	HTG	(ddddddb)	435 ±	57
C₃·S·2·77	—		64 ±	3
—	C₃H	(kkkkkkk)	69 ±	10
—	SJL	(sssssss)	67 ±	2
—	ATH	(sssssss d)	57 ±	5
—	B10HTT	(ssskkkd)	65 ±	1
—	ATL	(skkkkkd)	82 ±	4
C₃·S·2·77	C₃H	(kkkkkkk)	63 ±	2
C₃·S·2·77	SJL	(sssssss)	6467 ±	414
C₃·S·2·77	ATH	(ssssss d)	5879 ±	1571
C₃·S·2·77	B10HTT	(ssskkkd)	5148 ±	423
C₃·S·2·77	ATL	(skkkkkd)	4797 ±	262

[a] (C·B6·2·76) BALB/c anti-C57Bl/6; (C₃·S·2·77) C₃H anti-SJL.
[b] The letters in parentheses (k, b, s, d) refer to *H-2*-region genes *K*, *IA*, *IB*, *IJ*, *IE*, *S*, and *D*.

years cannot be stimulated by Con A supernatants at all (see below). It therefore appears that only a subpopulation of allospecific T cells can be stimulated by Con A supernatant. This population is apparently lost in cultures stimulated with spleen cells over prolonged periods of time.

TABLE 4. Effect of Lymphocyte Supernatants on Cell Proliferation

Allospecific T-cell line[a]	Stimulator cells[b]		[³H]-TdR incorporation on day 3	
B6·C·11·77	—		110 ±	1
—	BALB/c		114 ±	0.5
B6·C·11·77	BALB/c		25,125 ± 675	
B6·C·11·77	C57Bl/6 anti-BALB/c	SN	424 ±	74
B6·C·11·77	C57Bl/6	SN	351 ±	16
B6·C·11·77	C57Bl/6 PHA	SN	491 ±	143
B6·C·11·77	C57Bl/6 LPS	SN	192 ±	94
B6·C·11·77	C57Bl/6 Con A	SN	1,296 ± 256	

[a] (B6·C·11·77) C57Bl/6 anti-BALB/c.
[b] Supernatants (SN) were prepared as described by Rosenberg *et al.* (1978).

Taking advantage of the observation that allospecific T cells from relatively young mixed-lymphocyte tumor-cell cultures can be stimulated by supernatants from Con-A-stimulated spleen cells, Gillis and Smith (1977) and Nabholz et al. (1978) have established cytotoxic allospecific T-cell lines similar to the ones described herein. These lines, however, appear to differ from our lines in various aspects. They can be stimulated to proliferate by supernatant of Con-A-stimulated spleen cells, but not by spleen or tumor stimulator cells. They can be relatively easily cloned (Nabholz et al., 1978; Baker et al., 1979), which seems difficult with our lines.

2.3. Cytotoxic Potential of Allospecific T-Cell Lines

Proliferative and cytolytic activity are closely related in allospecific T-cell lines: lines that have not been stimulated for about 10 days do not show thymidine incorporation and do not kill. Activation of killing is caused only by stimulator cells able to cause cell proliferation (Dennert and Raschke, 1977). This can be seen by comparing the results referred to in Table 3 with those in Table 5: the BALB/c anti-C57Bl/6 line lyses both C57Bl/6 and HTG targets, but is not activated by HTG stimulator cells. The H-$2D^b$-coded specificities are therefore target antigens but not stimulator antigens. The C_3H anti-SJL line is activated by SJL, ATH, B10, HTT, and ATL, stimulator cells that also cause cell proliferation. Activation of cytolytic activity by entirely unrelated third-party stimu-

TABLE 5. Activation of Cytotoxic Activity by H-2-Region Genes

Allospecific T-cell line[a]	Stimulator cells	H-2 haplotype	Target[b]	Cytotoxicity (%) at 3 hr
C·B6·2·76	C57Bl/6	(bbbbbbb)	C57Bl/6	61 ± 0.5
C·B6·2·76	C57Bl/6	(bbbbbbb)	HTG	18 ± 0.5
C·B6·2·76	HTG	(ddddddb)	C57Bl/6	< 1
C·B6·2·76	HTG	(ddddddb)	HTG	< 1
C_3·S·2·77	SJL	(sssssss)	SJL	44 ± 2.3
C_3·S·2·77	ATH	(ssssssd)	SJL	42 ± 2.9
C_3·S·2·77	B10HTT	(ssskkkd)	SJL	41 ± 3.6
C_3·S·2·77	ATL	(skkkkkd)	SJL	27 ± 3.2
C_3·S·2·77	C_3H	(kkkkkkk)	SJL	< 1

[a] C·B6·2·76 (BALB/c anti-C57Bl/6) was 2.5 months in culture and C_3·S·2·77 (C_3H anti-SJL) was 3.5 months in culture at the time of this experiment.
[b] The attacker/target cell ratio was 10:1.

lator cells, which may cause cell proliferation, particularly in younger cultures (see below), has been observed. The cytolytic activity stimulated by these cells is, however, always directed against the antigenic determinants carried by the original stimulator cells (Dennert and De Rose 1976). This form of third-party stimulation of cytotoxic cells has also been observed by others using somewhat different systems (Alter *et al.*, 1976). It is possible that this third-party stimulation of cytolytic activity is caused by lymphokines secreted by a population of cells in these cultures reactive to the antigenic determinants carried by the stimulator cells.

The cytolytic activity of long-term T-killer-cell lines has never been observed to be higher than that of a mixed-lymphocyte culture after secondary or tertiary stimulation. In fact, it is a frequent observation that the cytolytic activity decreases over a period of several months and may finally disappear altogether (Dennert and De Rose, 1976; Dennert and Raschke, 1977). The reason for this is not entirely clear, but it may be that the cytolytic effector cells have only a limited potential to divide and are overgrown by the more easily propagated noncytotoxic proliferating T cells (Dennert and Raschke, 1977). Alternatively, it is possible that the cytotoxic T cells lose their cytotoxic potential on prolonged culture. Under certain circumstances, however, cytotoxic T cells may be propagated in culture for several years (Dennert, 1979).

Activated cytotoxic T cells, while showing specific killing in the absence of plant lectins, are able to lyse various kinds of target cells in their presence (Dennert and De Rose, 1976). For instance, in the presence of PHA, they will lyse not only lymphoid-tumor cells, carrying H-2 antigens to which they are not sensitized, but also syngeneic killer cells and even xenogeneic erythrocytes (Table 6). This effect of PHA may be explained by agglutination of killer cells to their targets followed by lysis of the target. It is interesting to note that PHA is also able to effect killing by allospecific killer cells that have not been stimulated (Dennert and De Rose, 1976) for at least 10 days ("quiescent" cells). A possible interpretation of this interesting finding is that "quiescent" allospecific T cells either have insufficient numbers of receptors to bind to the targets, which may be overcome by lectin agglutination, or they may lack cytolytic effector molecules that may be inducible by PHA. Similarly interesting, but also unexplained, is the finding that allospecific T-cell lines that have lost their specific cytotoxic activity (inactive lines) may be nonspecifically cytotoxic in the presence of PHA (Dennert and De Rose, 1976). These results emphasize that the effects of PHA in T-cell-mediated killing are not fully understood and that we do not know with certainty which T cells can interact with PHA in the cytotoxic reaction.

TABLE 6. Lysis of Various Targets by Killer Cells in the Presence of PHA

Allospecific T-cell line[a]	PHA[b]	Target[c]	a/t[d]	Cytotoxicity (%) at 3 hr
C·B6·9·75 (active)	−	EL4 (H-2^b)	5:1	29 ± 3
C·B6·9·75 (active)	−	P815 (H-2^d)	5:1	< 1
C·B6·9·75 (active)	−	CRBC	5:1	< 1
C·B6·9·75 (active)	−	C·B6·9·75 (H-2^d)	5:1	< 1
C·B6·9·75 (active)	+	P815 (H-2^d)	5:1	74 ± 2.0
C·B6·9·75 (active)	+	CRBC (H-2^d)	5:1	29 ± 0.1
C·B6·9·75 (active)	+	C·B6·9·75 (H-2^d)	5:1	30 ± 0.4
				at 6 hr
C·B6·9·75 (quiescent)	−	EL4 (H-2^b)	1:1	< 1
C·B6·9·75 (quiescent)	−	P815 (H-2^d)	1:1	< 1
C·B6·9·75 (quiescent)	+	EL4 (H-2^b)	1:1	25 ± 0.5
C·B6·9·75 (quiescent)	+	P815 (H-2^d)	1:1	58 ± 0.6
C·B6·9·75 (inactive)	−	EL4 (H-2^b)	1:1	< 1
C·B6·9·75 (inactive)	−	P815 (H-2^d)	1:1	< 1
C·B6·9·75 (inactive)	+	EL4 (H-2^b)	1:1	20 ± 0.4
C·B6·9·75 (inactive)	+	P815 (H-2^d)	1:1	84 ± 2.4

[a] (C·B6·9·75) BALB/c anti-C57B1/6.
[b] The final concentration was 5 μg/ml.
[c] (EL4) C57B1/6 lymphoma; (P815) DBA/2 mastocytoma; (CRBC) chicken erythrocytes.
[d] Attacker/killer-cell ratio.

2.4. Selection of Allospecific T-Cell Lines over Extended Periods of Time

The observation that there is a divergence between proliferation and cytolytic activity in allospecific T-cell lines does not mean that these cell lines are not derived from one subset of T cells. It is quite possible that the different functions such as proliferation and killing are performed by cells in different stages of development. Alternatively, it cannot be excluded that the different functions are indeed performed by different subsets of T cells in these cultures. Another complication is that even if all the cells in a particular line were derived from one subset of T cells, they may display different receptor specificities and therefore are not homogeneous when their receptors are concerned. Therefore, two avenues have been explored to distinguish among these different possibilities. One is cloning and the other is selection of lines over extended periods of time. Cloning experiments have to date been largely unsuccessful in our hands because it appears difficult to grow individual cells from microwells (unpublished results).* Successful cloning of allospecific T cells, however, has been reported by Fathman and Hengartner (1978), though the clones derived had lost their cytolytic activity. Test of these putative clones for proliferative activity showed that some of the clones could still be induced to proliferate by unrelated third-party stimulator cells, while others could not. This may either mean that these clones are not true clones or that there are receptor cross-reactivities or a high somatic mutation rate of the receptor. Since cloning was difficult with our lines, we tried to select lines over extended periods of time to find out whether lines with more limited receptor specificity could be derived. In Fig. 1, lines selected for 2.5, 5.5, and 15 months were tested for their specificity of proliferation. At 2.5 months, there is considerable stimulation by third-party cells observed. This effect could be due either to a heterogeneity in receptor specificities within the culture or to one receptor specificity that recognized cross-reacting antigens. The latter possibility appears unlikely, since in general lines selected for longer periods of time show low or no responsiveness to third-party stimulator cells (Fig. 1) (Dennert and Raschke, 1977). It is therefore possible that in the initial cultures, responder cells are stimulated that interact with antigens, which are either unique for the stimulator cells or common on other unrelated stimulator cells as well. On selection over long periods of time, only the responder cells specific for the antigenic determinants unique to the stimulator cells will survive, perhaps because their receptors have higher affinity. An alternative explanation would be that the selective pressure in these cultures for the cells responsive to the stimulator cells is small. The reason for this could be, for instance, stimulation of lymphocytes by fetal calf serum or lymphokines secreted by the lymphocytes responding to the stimulator cells. Since after 1 year of selection these lines display a receptor specificity assayed by the proliferative response that is comparable to that of isolated clones (Fathman and Hengartner, 1978), selection may be a useful substitute for cloning. But although receptor specificities may be identical in a selected line, one can never be sure that all cells in this culture are derived from one clone of cells.

One line that was selected over 3 years has been investigated in more detail (Dennert and Raschke, 1977; Dennert, 1979). The line $C \cdot C_3 \cdot 11 \cdot 75$ (BALB/c anti-C_3H) had lost its cytotoxic activity on H-2^k tumor cells such as RITL$^+$ (Table 7), but was able to lyse C_3H spleen blast targets. Mapping studies revealed that the antigens recognized in the killing reaction are most probably coded in the *IA* subregion of the

---

* Recently, cloning has been possible using conditioned media and spleen stimulator cells.

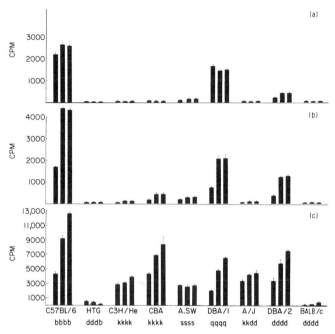

Figure 1. Results of testing of cell lines C·B6·2·75 at the age of 15 months (a), C·B6·10·75 at the age of 5.5 months (b), and C·B6·2·76 at the age of 2.5 months (c) for their proliferative response to 1000-rad-irradiated spleen cells (5 × 10⁶ cells/culture) of the various mouse strains indicated. The abbreviated haplotypes (KISD) of these mice are given. The three bars for each strain represent, from left to right, the cpm/culture for days 1, 2, and 3 (10^5 responder cells/culture). Labeling was done for 20 hr.

TABLE 7. Cytolytic Activity of Line C·C₃·11·75

Target	*H-2* haplotype	Cytotonicity (%) at 3 hr*
C₃H	*kkkkkkk*	40 ± 2.5
B10A	*kkk*dddd	43 ± 1.1
B10A (4R)	*kk*ddddd	42 ± 0.8
ATL	s*kkkkk*d	39 ± 1.1
C₃H OL	dddd*kkk*	4 ± 2.7
BALB/c	ddddddd	< 1
RITL⁺	*k*-----*k*†	< 1

* The attacker/target-cell ratio was 50:1; stimulator cells were C₃H.

† Only the serological specificities have been determined; no lymphocyte-activating determinants are present.

H-2 gene complex (Table 7). Therefore, selection of this line resulted in loss of killer cells specific for *H-2K-* and *D*-coded antigens, while killer cells specific for *IA*-region-coded antigens remained. As was to be expected, proliferation was stimulated by spleen cells carrying the IA^k antigens (Table 8). It is therefore possible that in this particular instance, the IA^k antigens provide the stimulus for both killing and cell proliferation to the same cell, which could explain the selective advantage these cells have in culture. If this were correct, one could hypothesize that *K-* and *D*-region-specific killer cells require cooperation for proliferation with *I*-region-gene-product-specific T helper cells via soluble products. It may be relevant in this regard that C·C$_3$·11·75 cells cannot be stimulated by tissue-culture supernatants from spleen cells activated by Con A (see Table 7). Therefore, this cell line appears to be refractory to stimulation by lymphokines secreted by mitogen-activated T cells.

Cell line C·C$_3$·11·75 displays another interesting function. If these cells are mixed in small numbers with B cells and sheep erythrocyte (SRBC) antigen, they are able to cause a positive allogeneic effect under certain experimental conditions (Dennert *et al.*, 1977; Waterfield *et al.*, 1979). In Fig. 2, 1.5×10^4 mitomycin-treated C·C$_3$·11·75 T lymphocytes were cultured with 5×10^5 B cells and SRBC (Waterfield *et al.*, 1979). It can be seen that a maximal humoral response is obtained with B cells carrying *IA^k*-subregion-coded antigens. It therefore appears that C·C$_3$·11·75 by interaction with *IA^k*-coded antigens on B cells can stimulate these cells in the presence of SRBC for antibody synthesis. In an

TABLE 8. Proliferative Activity of Line C·C$_3$·11·75

Responder cells[a]	Stimulator cells[b]	H-2 haplotype	[³H]-TdR incorporation on day 3
C·C$_3$·11·75	—		68 ± 13
—	BALB/c	(ddddddd)	77 ± 4
—	C$_3$HOL	(dddd*kkk*)	115 ± 3
—	C$_3$H	(*kkkkkk*)	100 ± 3
—	B10A	(*kkk*dddd)	77 ± 7
—	ATL	(s*kkkkk*d)	76 ± 3
C·C$_3$·11·75	BALB/c	(ddddddd)	1,590 ± 192
C·C$_3$·11·75	C$_3$HOL	(dddd*kkk*)	168 ± 16
C·C$_3$·11·75	C$_3$H	(*kkkkkk*)	12,138 ± 2057
C·C$_3$·11·75	B10A	(*kkk*dddd)	8,514 ± 723
C·C$_3$·11·75	ATL	(s*kkkkk*d)	5,802 ± 118
C·C$_3$·11·75	Con A SN[c]	—	137 ± 22

[a] Responder cells were 5×10^4/ml.
[b] Stimulator cells were 5×10^6/ml.
[c] Con A supernatant was prepared using BALB/c spleen cells as described by Rosenberg *et al.* (1978) and tested for its stimulatory activity on T cells from a primary mixed-lymphocyte culture.

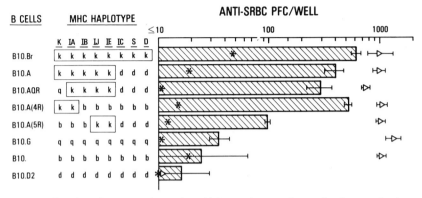

Figure 2. Results of an experiment in which varying numbers of nylon-wool-column-passed T cells from BALB/c spleen or the C·C$_3$·11·75 cell line, both mitomycin-C-treated, were added to wells containg SRBC and 5 × 10^5 B lymphocytes from the listed recombinant inbred mice. The results represent the geometric mean ± standard deviation of plaque-forming cells (PFC) activated by 1.5 × 10^4 C·C$_3$·11·75 T lymphocytes (peak antibody response) (hatched bars). Background responses of B cells alone are indicated (*). Normal BALB/c T lymphocytes routinely activated all the B cells listed except B10.D2, as would be expected (▷). However, the peak response induced with BALB/c T lymphocytes required 27-fold more cells than with the C·C$_3$·11·75 cell line. The figure represents one of three separate experiments.

attempt to elucidate the mechanism of action of these allogeneic cooperating T cells, we searched for a factor secreted by C·C$_3$·11·75 on stimulation with cells carrying IA^k-coded antigens. It was found that these T cells indeed secrete a factor that may be similar to the one previously described by Armerding and Katz (1974). The production of this factor was dependent on stimulation of C·C$_3$·11·75 cells with stimulator cells carrying IA^k-subregion genes (Waterfield et al., 1979). However, while the secretion of this factor was dependent on stimulation by specific antigen, the factor itself was nonspecific and stimulated B cells of various H-2 haplotypes (Waterfield et al., 1979). Therefore, three biological functions are induced by IA-subregion-coded antigens in this allospecific T-cell line: cytotoxicity, cell proliferation, and positive allogeneic effect.

2.5. Cell-Surface Molecules of Allospecific T-Cell Lines

One of the principal reasons to establish permanent lines of functional T cells is to study the nature and specificity of their antigen receptors. Both these questions have been dealt with in many experimental models without conclusive results. For instance, a number of reports support the contention that the T-cell receptor is related to immunoglobulin, while other experimental results do not support this possibility. Since our T-cell lines show antigen specificity, they must still continue to display specific receptors. It was therefore interesting to explore whether immunoglobulin can be found on allospecific T cells. A number of different rabbit and chicken antisera raised against mouse immunoglobulin were used for immunoprecipitation followed by analysis on polyacrylamide gels. Results showed that there is no immunoglobulin detectable on these cells (Dennert and Raschke, 1977), an observation that subsequently has been confirmed (S. Baird, unpublished results). Our failure to find immunoglobulin on these T cells of course does not prove that the T-cell receptor is not immunoglobulin, but led us to a different approach to search for it. This approach made use of the finding that cell line $C \cdot C_3 \cdot 11 \cdot 75$ cooperates with B cells for a humoral response by secreting a factor. If this factor were related to the T-cell receptor, then it should display antigen specificity. But as mentioned in the previous section, this factor did not turn out to be antigen-specific and therefore is unlikely to represent the T-cell receptor.

Allospecific cell lines carry cell-surface antigens characteristic for T cells. H-2 histocompatibility antigens and Thy-1 can be demonstrated on these cells by both quantitative absorption and direct cytotoxicity. Using immunoprecipitation and polyacrylamide gel electrophoresis, Thy-1 and T200 glycoproteins have been demonstrated (Dennert and Raschke, 1977).

3. Outlook

The possibility of establishing allospecific T-cell lines has provided us with a new tool to study T-cell functions and receptors. Since large numbers of these cells can be grown in tissue culture, both biological experiments and direct biochemical experiments aimed at isolating the T-cell receptor may now be feasible. There are, however, a number of important questions pertaining to the usefulness of these cell lines. The first is whether these lines are still representing normal cells or not. The spleen-stimulator-cell-dependent allospecific cell lines appear to have preserved most of their original functions. They proliferate only if stimulated with allogeneic spleen cells, show specific cytolytic activity, and can take part in a specific allogeneic effect. Furthermore, they do not grow in normal or immunodeficient mice (Dennert and Raschke, 1977). Therefore, they do not appear to be transformed. These findings, however, do not exclude the possibility that mutations are required for the successful establishment of allospecific T-cell lines. Cell lines dependent on Con A supernatant are different in many respects from normal T cells and spleen-stimulator-cell-dependent lines. They die within a few hours when incubated in normal media and, surprisingly, they cannot be stimulated to proliferate by either spleen or tumor stimulator cells (Dennert, unpublished results). Their cytolytic activity is often low in comparison to that of normal T killer cells (Baker *et al.,* 1979), and the specificity of their cytolytic activity has not been completely elucidated. Since chromosomal abnormalities have also been noted in these lines (Nabholz *et al.,* 1978), it appears that these T-cell lines are quite different from normal T killer cells. Nevertheless, they may be important models to study T-cell functions.

Cloning of Con-A-supernatant-dependent lines appears to be possible (Nabholz *et al.,* 1978; Baker *et al.,* 1979), while cloning of the spleen-stimulator-cell-dependent lines is difficult. This of course makes the Con-A-supernatant-dependent lines more useful for experiments in which cloned cell lines are required. Experiments under way will show whether it will after all be possible to clone well-established spleen-stimulator-cell-dependent lines. Cloned allospecific T-cell lines could be used for many interesting and important experiments. For instance, they would make it possible to answer the question whether it is really only one type of cell in $C \cdot C_3 \cdot 11 \cdot 75$ that is responsible for the functions ascribed to this line. Also, questions regarding the specificity of the T-cell receptor in the proliferative response, cytotoxic activity, and allogeneic effect can be studied only with cloned cell lines. Biochemical and serological experiments will have to be done with cloned allospecific T-cell lines aimed at finding the T-cell receptor. Many approaches for this goal could be thought of, such as dissolving the receptor from the membrane and testing it for specific binding to target antigens. Antisera or better monoclonal antibody from hybridomas specific for cell-surface antigens of allospecific T-cell lines could be prepared for the characterization of T-cell-surface antigens and antigen receptors.

In summary, allospecific T-cell lines have opened up a completely now field of experimentation and may be a most promising tool to study T-cell functions and receptors. It can be anticipated that they may be instrumental in solving the many unresolved questions involving T-cell functions in the immune system.

References

Alter, B.J., Grillot-Courvalin, C., Bach, M.L., Zier, K.S., Sondel, P.M., and Bach, F.H., 1976, Secondary cell-mediated lympholysis: Importance of H-2 LD and SD factors, *J. Exp. Med.* **143:**1005.

Andersson, L.C., and Häyry, P., 1973, Specific priming of mouse thymus-dependent lymphocytes to allogeneic cells *in vitro, Eur. J. Immunol.* **3:**595–599.

Armerding, O., and Katz, D.H., 1974, Activation of T and B lymphocytes *in vitro*. II. Biological and biochemical properties of an allogeneic effect factor (AEF) active in triggering specific B lymphocytes, *J. Exp. Med.* **140**:19.

Baker, P.E., Gillis, S., and Smith, K.A., 1979, Monoclonal cytolytic T-cell lines, *J. Exp. Med.* **149**:273–278.

Cantor, H., and Boyse, E.A., 1975, Functional subclasses of T lymphocytes bearing different Ly antigens: The generation of functionally distinct T-cell subclasses is a differentiative process independent of antigen, *J. Exp. Med.* **141**:1376.

Cerottini, J.C., Engers, H.D., MacDonald, H.R., and Brunner, K.T., 1974, Generation of cytotoxic lymphocytes *in vitro*. I. Response of normal and immune mouse spleen cells in mixed leukocyte cultures, *J. Exp. Med.* **140**:703–717.

Dennert, G., 1976, Thymus derived killer cells: Specificity of function and antigen recognition, *Transplant. Rev.* **29**:59–88.

Dennert, G., 1979, Cytolytic and proliferative activity of a permanent T killer cell line, *Nature (London)* **277**:476.

Dennert, G., and De Rose, M., 1976, Continuously proliferating T killer cells specific for H-2^b targets: Selection and characterization, *J. Immunol.* **116**:1601.

Dennert, G., and Raschke, J., 1977, Continuously proliferating allospecific T cells, lifespan and antigen receptors, *Eur. J. Immunol.* **7**:352.

Dennert, G., De Rose, M., and Allen, R.S., 1977, Failure of T cells specific for strong histocompatibility antigens to cooperate with B cells for a humoral response, *Eur. J. Immunol.* **7**:487.

Fathman, C.G., and Hengartner, H., 1978, Clones of alloreactive T cells, *Nature (London)* **272**:617–618.

Gillis, S., and Smith, K.A., 1977, Long term culture of tumor specific cytotoxic T cells, *Nature (London)* **268**:154.

Golstein, P., Svedmyr, E.A.J., and Wigrell, H., 1971, Cells mediating specific *in vitro* cytotoxicity: Detection of receptor-bearing lymphocytes, *J. Exp. Med.* **134**:1385.

Hämmerling, G.J., 1977, T lymphocyte tissue culture lines produced by cell hybridization, *Eur. J. Immunol.* **7**:743.

Köhler, G., and Milstein, C., 1976, Derivation of specific antibody-producing tissue culture tumor lines by cell fusion, *Eur. J. Immunol.* **6**:511.

MacDonald, R.H., Engers, H.D., Cerottini, J.C., and Brunner, K.T., 1974, Generation of cytotoxic lymphocytes *in vitro*. II. Effect of repeated exposure to alloantigens on the cytotoxic activity of long-term mixed leucocyte cultures, *J. Exp. Med.* **149**:718.

Nabholz, M., Engers, H.D., Collavo, D., and North, M., 1978, Cloned T-cell lines with specific cytolytic activity, *Curr. Top. Microbiol. Immunol.* **81**:176–187.

Rosenberg, S.A., Spiess, P.J., and Schwarz, S., 1978, *In vitro* growth of murine T cells. I. Production of factors necessary for T cell growth, *J. Immunol.* **121**:1946–1955.

Rubin, B., and Wigzell, H., 1973, Hapten reactive helper lymphocytes, *Nature (London)* **242**:467.

Waterfield, J.D., Dennert, G., Swain, S.L., and Dutton, R.W., 1979, Continuously proliferating allospecific T cells. I. Specificity of cooperation with allogeneic B cells in the humoral antibody response to sheep red blood cells, *J. Exp. Med.* **149**:808.

3

The Dual Specificity of Virus-Immune T Cells

Functional Indications That Virus and H-2 Molecules May Associate on the Cell Membrane

Peter C. Doherty, Jack R. Bennink, Rita B. Effros, and Mark Frankel

1. Introduction

A current obsession of cellular immunology is the definition of the T-cell receptor repertoire. Many of the questions that have been raised derive from experiments with virus systems (Doherty *et al.*, 1976a; Zinkernagel and Doherty, 1979). How do we explain the apparent dual specificity for major histocompatibility (MHC) components and for virus?

The virus models might seem, on superficial acquaintance, to constitute an unduly complex means for attempting rigorous dissection of T-cell specificity patterns. Surely, clearer analysis would be achieved by using a better-defined antigenic moiety, such as a hapten (Shearer and Schmitt-Verhulst, 1977). However, this has not proven to be the case. For instance, virus-immune effector T cells distinguish among virus-infected target cells bearing H-2K antigens that differ by, perhaps, as few as one or two amino acids (Zinkernagel, 1976; Blanden *et al.*, 1976; Brown and Nathenson, 1977). This degree of discrimination is not seen for hapten-specific lymphocytes (Forman and Klein, 1977).

The greater precision of the infectious models in this regard probably

Peter C. Doherty, Jack R. Bennink, Rita B. Effros, and Mark Frankel ● The Wistar Institute of Anatomy and Biology, Philadelphia, Pennsylvania 19104.

reflects that viral proteins are inserted, of themselves, in the plasma membrane; they do not need to be coupled to cell-surface glycoproteins using some extrinsic reagent. In fact, a substantially nonlytic virus (such as lymphocytic choriomeningitis virus or some of the exogenous oncornaviruses) probably represents the closest possible analogy to "self" that is not of host origin (Burnet and Fenner, 1949; Doherty et al., 1977a). The minor histocompatibility antigen models (Simpson and Gordon, 1977; Bevan, 1975) might be thought to constitute a more physiological situation in this regard. However, the problem here is that we know very little about the chemical nature, or even the serological identity, of most minor histocompatibility antigens. Many virus proteins are, on the other hand, extremely well characterized.

One of the best defined of all virus systems, from both the molecular and the serological aspect, is the influenza A viruses (for reviews, see Kilbourne, 1975). This chapter briefly summarizes our work with influenza, especially that concerning T-cell specificity for viral determinants. We also consider the question of specificity for *H-2*, and concentrate on experiments in which T-cell populations acutely depleted of alloreactive potential (Sprent, 1977) are stimulated with virus in irradiated, allogeneic recipients. Previously unpublished data are presented throughout.

2. The Influenza Model

2.1. Characteristics of Influenza Viruses

The influenza viruses bud from the cell surface, and utilize plasma membrane to form the mature virus particle (virion). They do not, so far as we know, incorporate any host glycoproteins. The major antigenic components of the influenza A viruses (after Kilbourne, 1975; Laver *et al.*, 1977; Schild, 1979) are discussed in the following sections.

2.1.1. The Ribonucleoprotein (RNP)

The viral genome consists of eight separate RNA segments, which readily reassort when a cell is infected with two different influenza A viruses. This has led to the generation of a range of stable, "recombinant" influenza A viruses. The RNA is associated with a series of proteins, which are antigenically cross-reactive for all influenza A viruses. There is one unconfirmed report that the RNP may be expressed on the surface of virus-infected cells (Virelizier *et al.*, 1977).

2.1.2. The Matrix (M) Protein

The M protein is a nonglycosylated structural protein that has a molecular weight of 20,000–27,000 daltons. The M protein is very similar antigenically for all influenza A viruses, but is quite different serologically from that found in the influenza B viruses. It is not known to be expressed on the surface of the virion, and antibody to M protein is not normally detected in serum after primary infection of mice with influenza viruses. However, reasonable evidence now exists that the M protein is presented on the surface of both productively (producing infectious virus) and nonproductively infected cells (Braciale, 1977b; Biddison *et al.,* 1977; Ada and Yap, 1977), and there is one experiment that indicates that it is on the cell membrane in a nonglycosylated form (Braciale, 1977b). This is intriguing, since recent findings of Lohmeyer *et al.,* (1979) show that very little M protein is synthesized in nonproductively infected cells, such as L-cell fibroblasts. This could be the reason for defective virus assembly (Lohmeyer *et al.,* 1979).

2.1.3. The Neuraminidase (N)

The N is a glycoprotein with a molecular weight of between 55,000 and 70,000 daltons, and is the minority protein on the surface of the virion, being present at much lower concentrations than the hemagglutinin (HA). The function of the N is not fully understood. However, the cleavage of neuraminic acid residues may release budded virus from the surface of the cell, since attachment appears to reflect affinity between these carbohydrate moieties and the HA. Antibody to the N may have some protective effect when people are exposed to influenza A viruses, but is much less efficient in this regard than antibody to the HA.

2.1.4. The Hemagglutinin (HA) Protein*

The HA glycoprotein is the major viral antigen presented on the surface of both the virion and the virus-infected cell, and is associated with generation of a highly protective antibody response. The HA is considered to be a trimer, the molecular weight of each subunit being about 70,000 daltons. The subunits are further divided into a heavy (45,000) and a light chain (25,000). The HA undergoes two forms of antigenic variation: (1) *Antigenic drift* appears to reflect the selection of

---

* We use the HA rather than the more usual H terminology for viral hemagglutinin throughout this chapter, to avoid confusion with the histocompatibility systems.

variant viruses in the presence of host-immune response, leading to sequential changes in the HA of epidemic viruses appearing over 7–10 years or so. Such viruses are classified in the same subtype; for instance, HAON1 viruses include PR8 (isolated in 1934) and AO/Bel (isolated in 1942), and sera raised against these two HAO molecules show extensive cross-reactivity. More rigorous analysis of cross-reactivity patterns may be made using monoclonal, hybridoma antibodies (Gerhard *et al.*, 1978). (2) *Antigenic shift* is thought to occur when an animal and a human strain of influenza virus recombine (see Section 2.1.1), thus creating a virus with virulence for man that has a completely novel HA molecule. For instance, there is absolutely no cross-neutralization between the AO (HAO) virus strains and the A2 (HA2) viruses, the latter representing new pandemic strains that swept through human populations in the late 1950's.

2.2. Specificity of Influenza-Immune T Cells

Both the primary and the secondary influenza-specific cytotoxic-T-cell responses are *H-2K-* and *H-2D*-restricted in the mouse, and *AgB*-restricted in the rat (Yap and Ada, 1977; Marshak *et al.*, 1977; Doherty *et al.*, 1978). It has been possible to examine only the secondary influenza-immune cytotoxic-T-cell response in man, and this is clearly *HLA-A-* and *HLA-B*-restricted (McMichael and Ting, 1977; McMichael, 1978; Biddison *et al.*, 1979). Furthermore, virus-specific effector T-cell function *in vivo*, measured by clearance of infectious virus from the lung, is also *H-2K-* and *H-2D*-restricted (Yap and Ada, 1978a). All influenza-immune T-cell populations studied so far thus obey rigorously the rules for MHC restriction defined previously for other viruses in murine systems (Doherty *et al.*, 1976a). Furthermore, the influenza model has provided the best evidence to date for *HLA* restriction of virus-specific cytotoxic T cells in man. Our earlier speculation (Doherty *et al.*, 1976a) that MHC restriction may serve as a general marker for cytotoxic-T-cell function has thus been supported for three separate species of mammals, using viruses that are known human pathogens.

The main reason for selecting the influenza A viruses to examine T-cell specificity was the advanced state of influenza-virus technology, especially the availability of a range of recombinant viruses. Use of these systems quickly showed that a subset of the *H-2*-restricted, virus-immune T cells was very specific for the particular influenza A virus used for immunization (Cambridge *et al.*, 1976; Effros *et al.*, 1977; Doherty *et al.*, 1977b; Ennis *et al.*, 1977a,b; Braciale, 1977a). These T cells undoubtedly recognize the viral HA, since restimulation of memory population *in vitro* with isolated HA leads to the generation of an extremely specific cytotoxic response (Zweerink *et al.*, 1977b). Indeed, one group (Ennis *et al.*, 1977a,b) claimed that the cytotoxic-T-cell response could clearly distinguish between target cells infected with A/Port Chalmers/1/1973 and A/England/42/1972, which bear HA3 antigens that are serologically very similar. However, this claim could not be substantiated by us (Fig. 1) and is not supported by later experiments from the same laboratory (Ennis *et al.*, 1978). Even so, it seems that at least some cytotoxic T cells are as discriminating as B-cells clones in distinguishing among different influenza-virus HA molecules.

There is also a further major component in the cytotoxic-T-cell response that is highly cross-reactive for all influenza A, but not for

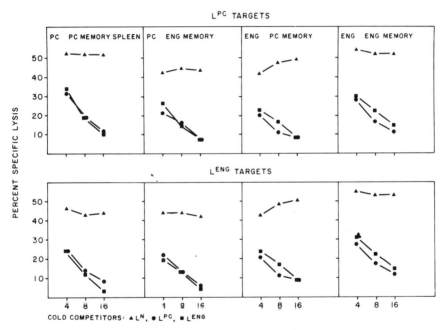

Figure 1. Results of experiments in which adult CBA/J (*H-2^k*) mice were primed intraperitoneally (Effros *et al.*, 1977) with either A/Port Chalmers/1/1973 (PC) or A/England/42/1972 (ENG). One month later, 1×10^8 memory spleen and lymph node cells from these mice were transferred intravenously (i.v.) into irradiated (950 rad) CBA/J recipients, which were then inoculated i.v. with either the homologous or the heterologous virus. This procedure stimulates both the virus (HA)-specific and the cross-reactive T-cell subsets (Doherty *et al.*, 1977b; Effros *et al.*, 1978). No evidence of any difference in specificity could be found for these two HA3N2 viruses by competitive inhibition using "cold," unlabled virus-infected L cells, interposed at ratios from 4:1 to 16:1 relative to the ^{51}Cr-labeled target cells. The results shown are for L-cell (*H-2^k*) targets infected with A/Port Chalmers/1973. The assay was incubated for 12 hr at 37°C, and results are expressed as specific ^{51}Cr release relative to the medium control (Effros *et al.*, 1978).

influenza B, viruses (Effros *et al.*, 1977; Doherty *et al.*, 1977b; Zweerink *et al.*, 1977a; Braciale, 1977a,b). These T cells could be recognizing the shared viral M protein, which is probably present on the cell surface (see Section 2.1.2). The most direct support for this idea rests in the observation (Braciale, 1977b) that inhibitors of glycosylation do not prevent the M protein from being expressed on the cell membrane, though they do suppress appearance of the viral HA, and such targets are recognized by the cross-reactive T-cell subset. Also, Reiss (1980) was able to block the cross-reactive T-cell subset with a rabbit antiserum to M protein. Most groups have had no success with such antibody blocking experiments, but this may simply reflect the quality of the reagents used (see Section 2.4).

Other possibilities are that these cross-reactive T cells may be recognizing a shared region on the viral HA—though they are not stimulated when isolated HA is used as an immunogen (Zweerink *et al.*, 1977b)—or some neoantigen complex between viral and H-2 antigen (Zinkernagel and Doherty, 1974). Whichever is the case, the existence of this cross-reactive T-cell subset offers an explanation for the heterotypic immunity between serologically different influenza A viruses described many years ago by Schulman and Kilbourne (1965) since Yap and Ada (1978b) have shown that adoptively transferred HAON1-immune T cells are quite effective in eliminating HA3N2 virus from the lung.

The existence of this cross-reactive T-cell subset is of considerable interest, since it represents a major divergence between normal cytotoxic-T-cell and serologically detectable B-cell responses. A mouse primed with, for instance, an HAON1 virus will generate a massive, secondary cytotoxic-T-cell response within 3 days of challenge with a serologically non-cross-reactive HA3N2 virus (Doherty *et al.*, 1977b). Furthermore, the early generation of these extremely potent cross-reactive T cells seems to in some way inhibit the appearance of the primary HA3-specific T-cell subset. This may simply reflect the early removal of a virus-infected stimulator population (Pang and Blanden, 1976). However, the phenomenon may be of considerable clinical interest, since all the *HLA*-restricted influenza-immune T-cell responses studied to date in man are essentially cross-reactive in character (Biddison *et al.*, 1979). This presumably reflects the operation of the secondary, cross-reactive T-cell subset, since the lymphocyte populations used in the experiments of Biddison *et al.* (1979) were from people of sufficient age to have suffered at least one attack of influenza.

The essential message emerging from the studies with influenza A viruses is that all aspects of cytotoxic-T-cell specificity encountered so far can be accounted for in terms of known viral proteins expressed on the surface of virus-infected cells. The fine specificity shown for the viral

HA molecule indicates that the T-cell recognition structure(s) are at least as discriminating as antibody molecules. The existence of the cross-reactive subset was somewhat of a surprise but cannot, at this stage, be taken as evidence for divergence of the T-cell and B-cell repertoires, since such T cells may be specific for the shared virus M protein. However, the fact that antibody to the M protein is not made during the course of primary exposure of mice to influenza (though such B-cell clones can be readily stimulated following immunization with isolated M protein in adjuvant) indicates that the requirement for potent stimulation of cytotoxic T cells and B cells may be quite different (Effros *et al.*, 1978).

2.3. Responder–Nonresponder Situations

One of the long-term questions about the nature of the strong transplantation antigens concerns the biological raison d′être for the extreme polymorphism of these systems (Burnet, 1973; Bodmer, 1972). We proposed early on (Doherty and Zinkernagel, 1975) that this could reflect an evolutionary need to prevent the emergence of virus-specific T-cell nonresponsiveness that might be widespread throughout the species. Both the existence of a duplicated system at *H-2K* and *H-2D* (*HLA-A* and -*B* in man) and the availability of a great range of alleles at each of these loci would operate to minimize the possibility of general susceptibility to a particular pathogen. It is now clear that cases of total nonresponsiveness do occur, the best-documented (for the infectious viruses) being influenza A viruses presented in the context of $H-2K^b$ and vaccinia virus at $H-2D^k$ (Doherty *et al.*, 1978; Zinkernagel *et al.*, 1978b).

The nonresponsiveness in the context of $H-2K^b$ for the influenza A viruses (Table 1) is particularly interesting, since we know that infection with any influenza A virus leads to the generation of at least two sets of virus-immune T cells (see Section 2.2): the one specific for the viral HA molecule, the other recognizing (perhaps) the M protein. Furthermore, we have now used several influenza A viruses expressing two quite distinct HA molecules, and failed to find any substantial response mapping to $H-2K^b$ (Doherty *et al.*, 1978). Most of these experiments were done with the B10.A(5R) ($H-2K^b-D^d$) recombinant, which generates potent influenza-immune cytotoxic T cells in the context of $H-2D^d$. Also, expression of the H-2K^b alloantigen is not, at least so far as can be detected by alloreactive cytotoxic T cells, modified in influenza-infected cells.

The generality of this defect for the influenza A viruses creates problems for models that seek to explain nonresponsiveness by postulating an absence of the relevant T-cell receptor repertoire (Langman,

TABLE 1. Recognizable Cytotoxic-T-Cell Response for Vaccinia Virus but Not for Influenza Virus in the Context of *H-2Kᵇ*

Virus	Immune spleen	Specific ^{51}Cr release (%) from virus-infected targets				
		B10.A(2R) K^kD^b	B10.A(5R) K^bD^d	MC57G K^bD^b	L Cell K^kD^k	P815 K^dD^d
Influenza*	B10 K^bD^b	38	3	26	5	0
Secondary	B10.A(5R) K^bD^d	10	41	2	4	24
	B10.A(2R) K^kD^b	66	7	16	72	6
	B10.Br K^kD^k	61	8	1	64	2
	B10.D2 K^dD^d	13	48	0	12	62
Primary†	(CBA × C57)Fl K^kD^k × K^bD^b	70	12	56	81	0
Vaccinia**	B10 K^bD^b	19	39	34	6	8
	B10.A(5R) K^bD^d	8	53	39	4	13
	B10.A(2R) K^kD^b	56	4	4	51	3
	B10.Br K^kD^k	55	11	3	70	1
	B10.D2 K^dD^d	10	37	1	9	36

* Immunized with HK influenza virus 5 days previously; the primary response is partially IIA-specific and partially cross-reactive (Effros *et al.*, 1977, 1978).
† The influenza-immune T cells were from mice infected with the HK (HA3N2) strain of virus, and then challenged after a further 6 weeks with PR8 (HAON1). Spleen cells were assayed 6 days later on HK-infected targets at a ratio of 100:1. The response measured is totally cross-reactive for the two viruses used (Doherty *et al.*, 1977b; Effros *et al.*, 1978).
** The vaccinia-immune T cells were from mice primed 6 days previously and were assayed on vaccinia-infected targets at a ratio of 25:1.

1978). If, for instance, the presence of a "self" receptor for *H-2Kᵇ* on a lymphocyte differentiating in thymus is considered to "preclude" (Langman, 1978) the concurrent expression of a virus-specific recognition unit on the same cell, it would not be necessary to postulate that a whole set of genes (specific for different influenza viral HA molecules and M protein, but not for vaccinia antigens) is affected. This seems extremely unlikely. The association of the phenomenon with a range of biologically similar, but antigenically distinct, viruses and virus proteins may indicate a failure of association between the *H-2Kᵇ* allele and all influenza A viruses. Some evidence exists to support this idea in the Friend virus system, in which only those *H-2* alleles that are correlated with T-cell responsiveness may be detected in disrupted virus particles (Bubbers *et al.*, 1978).

The prediction that failure to generate an appropriate "altered-self" situation results in nonresponsiveness (Doherty and Zinkernagel, 1975) may thus be fulfilled, though it could well be that the need is to present (or orient) viral and *H-2* components in close proximity rather than as a new antigenic determinant (Bevan, 1975). Variations of this model also seem to have found favor with those interested in differential responsiveness mapping to the *I* region.

2.4. Blocking Cytotoxicity with Monospecific Antisera

The lytic capacity of *H-2*-restricted effector-T-cell populations is readily blocked by treating the target cells with antisera directed against H-2 determinants (Burakoff *et al.*, 1976). However, only two groups have achieved any success in inhibiting virus-specific T cells with antisera specific for viral components (Koszinowski and Thomssen, 1975; Hale *et al.*, 1978). The general consensus (Blanden *et al.*, 1976; Zinkernagel and Doherty, 1979) is that such blocking is very difficult to achieve, a finding that has led to some speculation concerning the nature of the virus-immune T-cell repertoire. Teleologically at least, this seems rather satisfactory, since the possibility that effector T cells might be prevented from clearning virus from tissue by a concurrent antibody response would be minimized.

Both we (Effros *et al.*, 1979 and unpublished data) and Dr. T.J. Braciale (personal communication) have had no success in blocking the influenza-specific cytotoxic-T-cell response with either mouse or rabbit antisera specific for viral HA determinants. However, recent experiments using monoclonal antibodies synthesized by hybridomas produced in the laboratory of Dr. W. Gerhard (Gerhard *et al.*, 1978) clearly show that virus-specific blocking can be achieved in the influenza system. The HA-specific component of the cytotoxic-T-cell response can be almost totally inhibited by monoclonal Ig, which binds only to viral HA determinants.

Thoracic duct lymphocytes (TDL) from mice infected with the A/WSN (HAON1) strain of influenza virus are (for some reason that we do not understand) very specific for the HAO antigen, whereas spleen cells from the same mice are much more cross-reactive for targets infected with other influenza A viruses. The lytic capacity of TDL is diminished by as much as 80% by incorporating monoclonal Ig specific for HAO, while the level of cytotoxic activity in the spleen cannot be decreased by more than 40% (Effros *et al.*, 1979). A typical experiment is shown in Table 2. The concurrent presence of T cells with unpredicted specificity, such as the cross-reactive population in the influenza response, may be one reason antibody blocking has generally been difficult to achieve.

A further fascinating finding is that two monoclones specific for HAO will block the lysis of virus-infected P815 ($H-2K^d-D^d$) targets by B10.A(5R) ($H-2K^b-D^d$) immune T cells by as much as 90%, whereas lysis by BALB/G ($H-2K^d-D^b$) T cells is not decreased at all (Frankel *et al.*, 1979). The level of inhibition for BALB/c ($H-2K^d-D^d$) T cells is intermediate. Other monoclonal Ig preparations will block all three populations of cytotoxic T cells (Table 3). The implication of these findings is that influenza-immune T cells operating in the context of $H-2D^d$ may be concerned with different HAO components than lymphocytes functioning in the context of H-$2K^d$. This could reflect that there is some obligatory association between viral and H-2 antigens if T-cell binding (or lysis) is to occur (Zinkernagel and Doherty, 1974; Doherty *et al.*, 1976a), and that the viral component proximate to H-$2D^d$ is different from that involved at H-$2K^d$. An alternative explanation is that there is a difference in repertoire between the two T-cell subsets, the V gene (Eichmann, 1978; Binz and Wigzell, 1977) responsible for virus recognition in the context of H-$2D^b$ being different from that operating at H-$2K^b$.

We may be able to gain some insight into the likelihood of either possibility's being correct by determining, using mutant viruses (Gerhard and Webster, 1978) selected in the presence of a particular monoclonal Ig as immunogens, whether lysis of target cells infected with the wild-type virus is still blocked by the Ig used for immunoselection. This would imply, if blocking is still achieved, that blocking is a steric phenomenon and does not necessarily reflect precise competition between similar V-gene products expressed on B cells and T cells.

TABLE 2. Inhibition of Virus-Immune
Cytotoxic-T-Cell Effector Function with
HA-Specific Hybridoma Ascitic Fluids

Immune lymphocytes[a] (100:1)	Specific ^{51}Cr release (%) in the presence of antibody[b]					
	$H_{15}C_5{}^c$			H2/4B1		
	−	+	%I	−	+	%I
TDL	29	8	73	29	7	76
Spleen	19	12	37	19	14	26

[a] B10.D2 (K^d-D^d) mice were primed with A/WSN (HAON1) influenza virus and thoracic duct lymphocytes (TDL) were drained for 24 hr. Spleen cells were taken on day 6.

[b] The P815 (K^d-D^d) target cells were infected with A/WSN influenza virus. The cells were first held for 5 hr at 37°C to allow virus expression. Medium containing antibody was then added, followed by T cells, and the assay was incubated for 4 hr.

[c] The hybridomas used were all from BALB/c (K^d-D^d) mice, and grown in peritoneal cavities of BALB/c mice to provide ascitic fluids containing high concentrations of antibody specific for HA (Gerhard and Webster, 1978). A number of dilutions of ascitic fluid were tested, and that showing maximal inhibition (%I) is shown here. The dilutions used ranged from 1:100 to 1:2500.

TABLE 3. Inhibition of Influenza-Specific Cytotoxic-T-Cell Activity[a] by an Antibody ($H_{15}E_8$) to Viral HA in the Context of H-$2D^d$ But Not of H-$2K^d$

Immune TDL (100:1)	Target infected with A/WSN	Specific ^{51}Cr release (%)					
		$H_{15}E_8$			$H_{15}B_9$		
		−	+	%I	−	+	%I
BALB/c K^dD^d	P815 K^dD^d	51	24	53	51	20	59
B10.A(5R) K^bD^d		14	8	43	14	1	93
BALB.G K^dD^b		20	22	0	20	13	35
C57BL/6J K^bD^b	MC57G K^bD^b	23	17	27	23	16	30

[a] Mice were immunized with A/WSN (HON1) and the assay performed as described in footnote *b* to Table 2. The dilutions of ascitic fluid used ranged from 1:100 to 1:2500, the maximum level of inhibition (%I) being shown in each case.

3. Negative Selection of Alloreactive Precursors

3.1. Rationale

A central question concerning the *H-2*-restriction phenomenon is whether T cells can ever respond to virus presented in the context of H-2 antigens not encountered during the process of physiological development. The findings of Bevan and Fink (1978) and Zinkernagel (1978) with radiation chimeras indicate that apart from alloreactivity, T-cell responsiveness is totally restricted to the spectrum of H-2 determinants encountered on radiation-resistant cells in the thymus. That is, chimeras made by injecting (A × B)F$_1$ bone marrow into irradiated A recipients can respond only to virus presented in association with A but not with B. Recognition of A during the process of T-cell differentiation in thymus may be considered to "drive" mutation with resultant selection of a T-cell repertoire restricted to A (Bevan, 1977; von Boehmer *et al.,* 1978), or to select for T cells that have two distinct receptor specificities, capable of recognizing A (H-2K or H-2D antigen) and virus, respectively (Zinkernagel, 1978).

A third possibility (Doherty, 1978; Miller, 1978) is that the T-cell repertoire that would operate in the context of B is in some way suppressed, either as a result of specific deletion in the thymus or by generation of suppressor-T-cell populations restricted to B. Experimental evidence for positive (transferrable) suppression has not been forthcoming (Fink and Bevan, 1978), but the possibility of deletion cannot be discounted. It is thus legitimate to ask whether functionally mature T cells of type A can ever respond to virus presented in the context of a third alloantigen (C), which is not encountered at any stage during ontogeny.

The way to examine this is to first remove alloreactive (A anti-C) precursor lymphocytes by some depletion mechanism, and then stimulate these A lymphocytes with virus presented in the context of C. The protocol that we have used for this purpose was first developed by Ford and Atkins (1971), and has been used extensively by Sprent, Wilson, and collegues (Wilson *et al.,* 1977). Adult (A × C)F$_1$ mice are first irradiated (950 rad) and injected intravenously 24 hr later with a large number of A lymph node cells. Thoracic duct lymphoctyes (TDL) are then drained, via a cannula inserted into the cisterna chylae, from 24 to 42 hr after cell transfer. The alloreactive (A anti-C) precursors are all recruited to lymphoid tissue, and do not appear in the TDL population. These negatively selected (A$_{-c}$) T cells are then injected into a further set of irradiated (A × C)F$_1$ recipients and stimulated with virus. Spleen cells from these mice are assayed 6 days later for virus-immune cytotoxic-T-cell activity in the context of both A and C.

3.2. Responsiveness in Allogeneic Situations

The influenza model proved unsuitable for experiments of this type. The problem is that although it is possible to stimulate (*H-2K*^{k}-*D*^{k} × *H-2K*^{b}-*D*^{b})F$_1$ influenza memory-T-cell populations in both *H-2K*^{k}-*D*^{k} and *H-2K*^{b}-*D*^{b} virus-infected recipients (Bennink and Doherty, 1978a), previously unprimed lymphocytes respond only in the context of *H-2K*^{k}-*D*^{k} and not of *H-2K*^{b}-*D*^{b} when sensitized in this way (Table 4). We do not fully understand why this should be so. Though the general absence of an influenza-specific response at *H-2K*^{b} is part of the explanation, there is no obvious reason for the failure to stimulate at *H-2D*^{b} (see Section 2.3). Such problems do not limit the use of the vaccinia model (Bennink and Doherty, 1978a), so we adopted this system both for the aforestated reason and becuase we wished to compare our results with findings from chimera studies in which vaccinia virus was also the immunogen (Zinkernagel, 1978).

Only a limited number of mouse-strain combinations have been used to date in these negative-selection experiments, principally because the procedure is extremely tedious and not all *H-2* haplotypes filter reciprocally. Stimulation in the context of shared *H-2* alleles (such as *H-2D*^{d} in Table 5) may be seen when the only homology between filtered T cell and virus-infected, irradiated recipient is for the *H-2* allele with which the cytotoxic-T-cell response is identified [for instance, *H-2D*^{b} in the C57BL/6-B10.A(2R) combination (Bennink and Doherty, 1979)]. Either there is no need for *I*-region-restricted T-cell help (Zinkernagel *et al.*, 1978a) to be stimulated by house macrophages, as is the case for T–B collaboration (Sprent, 1978), or there is some form of allogeneic effect (Katz, 1972; Corley *et al.*, 1978) mediated via the irradiated (950 rad) recipient that obviates such help (Bennink and Doherty, 1978b, 1979).

The situation so far concerning specificity of negatively selected T cells can be summarized quite briefly. Lymphocytes of the H-$2K^k$-D^k or H-$2K^d$-D^d genotype cannot, after filtration and stimulation in appropriate recombinant or F mice, be induced to recognize vaccinia virus presented in the context of H-$2K^b$ (Bennink and Doherty, 1978a,b, 1979; Doherty and Bennink, 1979), though they can be stimulated with H-2^b-TNP (Wilson *et al.*, 1977). Similarly, H-$2K^b$-D^d T cells cannot be sensitized to either H-$2K^d$-vaccinia virus or H-$2D^b$-vaccinia virus (Table 5).

TABLE 4. Failure to Stimulate a Primary Influenza-Specific H-2^b-Restricted Response in Irradiated Recipient Mice

		Specific ^{51}Cr release (%) (50:1)[b]					
		L cells K^d-D^k		MC57G K^b-D^b		P815 K^d-D^d	
Source of cells transferred	950-rad recipient mice[a]	HK	N[c]	HK	N	HK	N
(CBA × C57)F$_1$	(CBA × C57)F$_1$	72	2	9	1	5	7
K^k-D^k × K^b-D^b	C57	0	3	0	0	0	2
	CBA	83	3	4	0	4	6
Unirradiated mice[d]		73	3	29	6	10	12
(CBA × C57)Fl[e]		82	3	1	1	10	3
CBA/J		15	5	26	0	9	9
C57BL/6J		10	6	4	0	84	1
B10.D2							

[a] The recipients were irradiated, injected intravenously (i.v.) with 6×10^7 spleen and lymph node cells 24 hr later, and dosed i.v. with HK (HA3N2) influenza virus after a further 3 hr. Spleen cells were assayed on day 5.

[b] Effector : target ratio.

[c] (N) Normal cells.

[d] The (CBA × C57)F$_1$ controls were given HK (HA3N2) influenza virus intraperitoneally, and had not been previously exposed to any other influenza A virus. The other controls had all been primed with one influenza A virus at least 2 months previously, and were challenged 5 days before the assay with a serologically different influenza A virus. The response measured is thus totally cross-reactive for all influenza-A-virus-infected cells (Effros *et al.*, 1977, 1978).

[e] The influenza-specific lysis (Table 5) of the MC57G target cells by (CBA × C57)F$_1$ T cells is of interest, and has also been found in three other experiments (unpublished data). The (CBA × C57)F$_1$ does not respond to influenza virus presented in the context of H-$2K^b$ (see Section 2.3), so the lysis detected here is associated with H-$2D^b$. Yet (CBA × C57)F$_1$ mice do not generate detectable cytotoxic activity specific for vaccinia virus-H-$2D^b$, though the F$_1$ lymphocytes do respond to vaccinia virus-H-$2D^b$, if stimulated in irradiated C57BL/6J recipients. Thus, the apparent rules governing level of responsiveness at H-$2D^b$ when presented with H-$2K^k$ (Zinkernagel *et al.*, 1978b) seem to vary for vaccinia and influenza virus with the (CBA × C57)F$_1$, though they are identical for the B10.A(2R) (Doherty *et al.*, 1978).

TABLE 5. Stimulation of Negatively Selected K^b-D^d T Cells in Irradiated (K^d-D^d × K^b-D^b)F$_1$ Recipients[a]

	5RSV K^bD^d		HTGSV K^dD^b		2RSV K^kD^b		MC57G K^bD^b		BALB/c K^dD^d	
E:T[b]	Vacc.	N	Vacc.	N	Vacc.	N	Vacc.	N	Vacc.	N
20:1	44	0	1213		0	0	49	0	66	0
40:1	46	0	2019		01	4	70	11	64	0

[a] The B10.A(5R) T cells were first filtered through 950-rad (BALB/c × C57)F$_1$ mice, and then stimulated with vaccinia virus in a further set of irradiated (BALB/c × C57)F$_1$ recipients. Spleen cells were assayed 6 days later on virus-infected (Vacc.) and normal (N) target cells.
[b] (E : T) Effector : target ratio.

However, negatively selected T cells from H-$2K^d$-D^d and H-$2K^b$-D^b mice can be stimulated to mediate strong cytotoxicity for vaccinia-infected targets expressing H-$2K^k$-D^k. One experiment is shown in Table 6. In other experiments, filtered BALB/c and B10.D2 T cells have been primed in A/J and B10.A mice, and C57BL/6J T cells in B10.A(4R) recipients. We do not yet know whether this "aberrant" response (Doherty and Bennink, 1979) to H-$2K^k$-vaccinia virus can be induced in irradiated recipients that do not share at least one H-2 allele (mapping to H-$2D$) (Bennink and Doherty, 1979) with the T-cell population. Even so, it is quite clear that lymphocytes can, at least in this case, be sensitized to vaccinia virus presented in the context of an H-2 allele not encountered in the thymus (Doherty and Bennink, 1979; Bennink and Doherty, 1979). There is also one experiment that indicates that H-$2K^d$-D^d T cells can be primed to H-$2K^s$ vaccinia virus (Doherty and Bennink, 1979), but this has not been repeated.

The capacity of H-2^d and H-2^b T cells to recognize vaccinia virus presented in the context of H-$2K^k$ has been interpreted as reflecting two possible alternative mechanisms (Doherty and Bennink, 1979; Bennink and Doherty, 1979). One postulate is that a T cell with receptor units for self H-2 and for neoantigen (X) may, because the two recognition components can be made proximate or assembled into one large binding site, be used in an "aberrant" way to interact with an antigenic entity formed by association between vaccinia virus and H-$2K^k$. The alternative idea is that a vaccinia-virus-H-$2K^k$ "altered-self" complex is recognized via a highly conserved, alloreactive T-cell repertoire (Jerne, 1971; Bellgrau and Wilson, 1979), being common to BALB/c and C57BL/6 mice that differ for both H-2 type and for non-H-2 genetic background.

A further set of experiments that need to be done is to find whether H-2^b and H-2^d T cells can also be sensitized to influenza virus, or Sendai virus, presented in the context of H-$2K^k$. We would (if the "aberrant" stimulation of cytotoxic T cells turns out to be generally true for all viruses encountered in association with H-$2K^k$) probably need to abandon the concepts discussed above and consider that virus-specific T cells expressing a second, "physiological" receptor with higher affinity for H-$2K^k$ than for H-$2K^b$ or for H-$2D^b$ exist in H-2^b mice.

4. General Discussion

The dual specificity of H-2-restricted virus-immune T cells shows evidence of considerable precision, both for virus and for H-2. We have discussed specificity for H-2 at some length previously, and have speculated that the "self"-restricted T cell may be using a binding site (perhaps encoded by a single V_H gene) (Binz and Wigzell, 1977) from the alloreactive repertoire for this purpose (Doherty et al., 1976b; Zinkernagel and Doherty, 1977). The great specificity for viral HA demonstrated in the influenza model (see Section 2.2) must influence us toward the viewpoint that viral antigen is also seen as a distinct entity, again, perhaps, via a V_H gene shared with the B-cell repertoire. Thus, for

TABLE 6. Sensitization of Negatively Selected K^d-D^d T Cells to K^k-Vaccinia Virus[a]

| | Specific ^{51}Cr release (%) (20:1) | | | | | |
| | L cell K^kD^k | | BALB/c K^dD^d | | MC57G K^bD^b | |
Cells	Vacc.	N	Vacc.	N	Vacc.	N
BALB/c T cells[a] stimulated in 950-rad (C3H × DBA/2)F₁ recipients	49	21	32	6	0	19
950-rad (C3H × DBA/2)F₁[b]	0	0	0	0	—	—
Unirradiated controls (primed 6 days previously)						
BALB/c	9	9	32	4	8	4
(C3H × DBA/2)F₁	46	10	27	4	17	11
C57BL/6J	19	30	4	16	74	26

[a] The BALB/c T cells were filtered through 950-rad (C3H × DBA/2)F₁ mice, and 1.5×10^7 TDL were stimulated for 6 days with vaccinia virus in a further set of irradiated recipients.

[b] These mice were irradiated and injected with vaccinia virus, but were not given TDL.

reasons of specificity alone, we are inclined toward the viewpoint that the self-restricted T-cell recognition reflects the operation of two distinct genetic elements, with affinity for H-2 antigen and viral components, respectively. It is obvious, however, that these two recognition units are in some way functionally linked, a necessity that has been the subject of much speculation (Doherty *et al.*, 1976b; Zinkernagel and Doherty, 1977; Langman, 1978; Blanden and Ada, 1978; Zinkernagel, 1978). Does this also require that there be an association between viral and H-2 antigen?

A central question to be dealt with concerns the lack of response associated with *H-2K*^{b} for all influenza A viruses tested so far, but not for vaccinia virus or for Sendai virus (see Section 2.3). Thus, there is a general defect in capacity to recognize both a variety of HA molecules and the component recognized by the cross-reactive T-cell subset. The difference between the viral HA molecules may be even greater than that for different H-2 molecules. For instance, there is absolutely no serological cross-reactivity between HAO and HA3. This seems to make extremely unlikely the idea that there is a defect in T-cell repertoire [failure to express concurrently the antiviral and anti-self receptor units (see Section 2.3)]. The problem can, however, be approached from the viewpoint that there is a failure of association between virus and H-2 antigen. The emphasis of this argument depends essentially on the nature of the cross-reactive (influenza-A-specific but not HA-specific) response, which we have not yet resolved.

One possiblility is that the cross-reactive T cells may be recognizing a highly conserved region of the viral HA, which may be serologically "silent." Arguments against this idea are that the conserved regions of influenza A and B HA are as similar as, for instance, HAO and HA3 (see Laver *et al.*, 1977), but there is T-cell cross-reactivity only in the latter case. Also, stimulating memory T cells with isolated HA induces generation only of HA-specific cytotoxic activity (Zweerink *et al.*, 1977b). This could, however, reflect incorrect orientation of the HA molecule when supplied in a form extrinsic to the stimulator cell. The HA molecules and H-2 could be considered to make a constant association, during the normal process of virus synthesis and budding, which would then be recognized by the cross-reactive T-cell subset. The same associative event would also bring the unique determinants of HA sufficiently close to the H-2 molecule for recognition by the HA-specific subset to occur. The general failure in response to influenza A virus associated with *H-2K*^{b} could thus reflect absence of one associative interaction. The fact that monoclonal Ig (see Section 2.4) specific for influenza HA determinants blocks the virus-specific, but not the cross-reactive, T-cell subset could simply reflect the distance between the two viral determinants on the HA molecule.

The alternative idea, that the cross-reactive T-cell subset recognizes the viral M protein, requires the adoption of a somewhat different concept. The argument here would be that there is a defect in the capacity of the H-2 molecule to associate with the virus as a whole. Perhaps, as may be the case in the Friend virus model (Bubbers *et al.,* 1978), the H-2 molecule needs to be incorporated into the virus particle before any viral component can be seen in an *H-2*-restricted way.

The antibody blocking experiments (see Section 2.4) also provide some indication that there may need to be an association between viral HA and H-2. The fact that at least one monoclonal Ig specific for viral HA blocks HAO-specific cytotoxic-T-cell activity in the context of *H-2D^d*, but not of *H-2K^d*, may reflect that the point of association (and thus the proximity of the relevant determinants) of the HA and H-2 determinants differs for the K^d and D^d molecules. The alternative is that there is a difference in the HA-specific T-cell repertoires for lymphocytes operating at *K*-end and *D*-end.

The fact that the negatively selected *H-2K^d-D^d* and *H-2K^b-D^b* T cells can be induced to recognize vaccinia virus presented in the context of *H-2K^k* (see Section 3.2) also tends toward the idea that the virus and the H-2 may be associated. Either *H-2K^k*-vaccinia virus is seen as an alloantigen or a compound receptor specific for self (*H-2^b* or *H-2^d*) and some other antigenic determinant may interact in an "aberrant" way with an *H-2K^k*-vaccinia virus complex (Doherty and Bennink, 1979). The latter form of interaction may be considered to occur only if the two recognition units, on the one hand, and the virus and H-2, on the other, can be made proximate. However, the possibility that this phenomenon is not restricted to vaccinia virus, and may thus reflect cross-reactivity on the part of some "self"-recognition structure, is yet to be investigated (see Section 3.2).

The situation at present is thus not totally unlike that in late 1975, when we first reviewed the *H-2* restriction of virus-immune T cells (Doherty *et al.,* 1976a), though the field has moved very rapidly since then. Many phenomena can best be explained by postulating that there needs to be an association, however transient or tenuous, between virus and H-2 molecules. Whether this reflects solely the biochemical natures of the molecules themselves, the need for the virus particle and H-2 to associate in some general way, or the capacity of the cytotoxic T cells to reorient separate structures on the target-cell membrane is far from clear. For instance, does the differential blocking (see above) of HA-specific cytotoxic-T-cell function with monoclonal antiviral Ig reflect binding near the point of association between virus and H-2, or that virus with bound Ig cannot be brought into apposition with the H-2?

Many of our concepts may be too rigidly stated. We must bear in mind that we are considering interactions between cell surfaces, probably mediated via a number of repeated recognition units that may be quite mobile in the plasma membrane. The rules that govern enzyme–substrate reactions, or antigen–antibody reactions, thus need to be transposed to this seemingly more gross context. There is probably validity in both the "altered-self" and the "dual-recognition" concept. Either could operate in a particular circumstance. The problem may be more etymological than immunological, being as much a concern of cell-surface geographers (Bourguignon *et al.,* 1978) as of biochemists.

5. Summary

The experiments described herein address the question of dual specificity of cytotoxic T cells for virus and for H-2. Influenza-immune T cells may distinguish between viral hemagglutinin (HA) and H-2 molecules with a discriminatory capacity at least equivalent to that found for B cells. However, there are also other influenza-immune T-cell subsets that, though *H-2*-restricted, were not predicted from our knowledge of antibody response in this disease. It is thus surprising that general low or nonresponsiveness is recognized for all influenza A viruses presented in the context of a particular *H-2* allele (*H-2K^b*), even though the viral HA molecules may differ from each other to the extent that there is absolutely no serological cross-reactivity between them. Effector-T-cell function specific for the influenza HA can be blocked with monoclonal Ig directed against the HA molecule. Furthermore, at least one of these Ig preparations greatly inhibits HA-specific cytotoxic T-cell activity in the context of *H-2D^d* but not of *H-2K^d*. The problem of T-cell specificity for H-2 is approached using negative-selection protocols to allow stimulation (with vaccinia virus) of lymphocyte populations acutely depleted of alloreactive capacity in the context of H-2 antigens not encountered during ontogeny. Both *H-2K^b-D^b* and *H-2K^d-D^d* T cells can be sensitized to *H-2K^k*-vaccinia virus, but the converse does not occur. Possible implications of these experiments for models of T-cell recognition are discussed.

NOTE ADDED IN PROOF. Two important sets of experiments have been done since this article was written. Studies with monoclonal antibodies which bind to the influenza virus matrix (M) protein have failed to confirm that there are significant amounts of M protein on the surface of the virus-infected cell (Gerhard *et al.,* 1980). This could either reflect that the monoclonal Ig populations tested recognize determinants on the M protein that are embedded in the plasma membrane, or that the specificity of the antiserum used for the original studies is suspect. The latter seems more likely to be true. Evidence that the HA molecule is recognized by the cross-reactive T-cell subset is now available from the experiments of Koszinowski *et al.* (1980), who found that target cells sensitized with isolated HA incorporated into liposomes were readily lysed by the heterospecific cytotoxic T lymphocytes (CTL). Thus, it now seems very likely that the cross-reactive CTL are recognizing the viral HA molecule.

ACKNOWLEDGMENTS. We thank Dr. Walter Gerhard for advice and criticism. The experiments with antibody blocking would not have been possible without the marvelous technology that he has developed for the analysis of the influenza A viruses. These studies were supported by U.S. Public Health Service grants AI 14162, AI 13989, CA 20833, and NS 11036, and by the National Multiple Sclerosis Society.

References

Ada G.L., and Yap, K.L., 1977, Matrix protein expressed at the surface of cells infected with influenza viruses, *Immunochemistry* **14**:643.

Bellgrau, D., and Wilson, D.B., 1979, Immunological studies of T-cell receptors. II. Limited polymorphism of idiotypic determinants on T-cell receptors specific for major histocompatibility complex alloantigens, *J. Exp. Med.* **149**:234.

Bennink, J., and Doherty, P.C., 1978a, T-cell populations specifically depleted of alloreactive potential cannot be induced to lyse H-2-different virus-infected target cells, *J. Exp. Med.* **148**:128.

Bennink, J., and Doherty, P.C., 1978b, Different rules govern help for cytotoxic T cells and for B cells, *Nature (London)* **276**:829.

Bennink, J., and Doherty, P.C., 1979, Reciprocal stimulation of negatively selected, high-responder and low-responder T cells in virus-infected recipients, *Proc. Natl. Acad. Sci. U.S.A.* **76**:3482.

Bevan, M.J., 1975, Interaction antigens detected by cytotoxic T cells with the major histocompatibility complex as modifier, *Nature (London)* **256**:419.

Bevan, M.J., 1977, In a radiation chimera, host H-2 antigens determine immune responsiveness of donor cytotoxic cells, *Nature (London)* **269**:417.

Bevan, M.J., and Fink, P.J., 1978, The influence of thymus H-2 antigens on the specificity of maturing killer and helper cells, *Immunol. Rev.* **42**:3.

Biddison, W.E., Doherty, P.C., and Webster, R.G., 1977, Antibody to influenza virus matrix protein detects a common antigen on the surface of cells infected with A influenza viruses, *J. Exp. Med.* **146**:690.

Biddison, W.E., Shaw, S., and Nelson, D.L., 1979, Virus specificity of human influenza virus immune cytotoxic T cells, *J. Immunol.* **122**:660.

Binz, H., and Wigzell, H., 1977, Antigen-binding, idiotypic T-lymphocyte receptors, in: *Contemporary Topics in Immunobiology,* Vol. 7, *T Cells* (O. Stutman, ed.), pp. 113–177, Plenum Press, New York.

Blanden, R.V., and Ada, G.L., 1978, A dual recognition model for cytotoxic T cells based on thymic selection of precursors with low affinity for self H-2 antigens, *Scand. J. Immunol.* **7**:181.

Blanden, R.V., Hapel, A.J., and Jackson, D.C., 1976, Mode of action of Ir genes and the nature of T cell receptors for antigen, *Immunochemistry* **13**:179.

Bodmer, W.F., 1972, Evolutionary significance of the HLA system, *Nature (London)* **237**:139.

Bourguignon, L.Y.W., Hyman, R., Trowbridge, I., and Singer, S.J., 1978, Participation of histocompatibility antigens in capping of molecularly independent cell surface components by their specific antibodies, *Proc. Natl. Acad. Sci. U.S.A.* **75**:2406.

Braciale, T., 1977a, Immunologic recognition of influenza virus-infected cells. I. Generation of a virus-strain specific and a cross-reactive subpopulation of cytotoxic T cells in the response to type A influenza viruses of different subtypes, *Cell. Immunol.* **33**:423.

Braciale, T., 1977b, Immunologic recognition of influenza virus-infected cells. II. Expression of influenza A matrix protein on the cell surface and its role in recognition by cross-reactive cytotoxic T cells, *J. Exp. Med.* **146**:673.

Brown, J.L., and Nathenson, S.G., 1977, Structural differences between parent and mutant H-2K glycoproteins from two H-2K gene mutants: B6-C-H-2^{ba} (HZ1) and B6-H2^{bd} (M505), *J. Immunol.* **118**:98.

Bubbers, J.E., Chen, S., and Lilly, F., 1978, Nonrandon inclusion of H-2K and H-2D antigens in Friend virus particles from mice of various strains, *J. Exp. Med.* **147**:340.

Burakoff, S.J., Germain, R.N., Dorf, M.E., and Benacerraf, B., 1976, Inhibition of cell-mediated cytolysis of trinitrophenyl-derivatized target cells by alloantisera directed to the products of the K and D loci of the H-2 complex, *Proc. Natl. Acad. Sci. U.S.A.* **73**:625.

Burnet, F.M., 1973, Multiple polymorphism in relation to histocompatibility antigens, *Nature (London)* **245**:359.

Burnet, F.M., and Fenner, F.J., 1949, The production of antibodies, Monograph, Walter and Eliza Hall Institute, Melbourne, MacMillan.

Cambridge, G., MacKenzie, J.S., and Keast, D., 1976, Cell-mediated immune response to influenza virus infection in mice, *Infect. Immunol.* **13**:36.

Corley, R.B., Kindred, B., and Lefkovits, I., 1978, Positive and negative allogeneic effects mediated by MLR-primed lymphocytes: Quantitation by limiting dilution analysis, *J. Immunol.* **121**:1082.

Doherty, P.C., 1978, Cell-mediated immunity to viruses and intracellular bacteria, in: *Clinics in Rheumatic Diseases,* Vol. 4 (N.J. Zvaifler, ed.), pp. 549–563, Saunders, London.

Doherty, P.C., and Bennink, J.R., 1979, Vaccinia-specific cytotoxic T cell responses in the context of H-2 antigen not encountered in thymus may reflect aberrant recognition of a virus-H-2 complex, *J. Exp. Med.* **149**:150.

Doherty, P.C., and Zinkernagel, R.M., 1975, A biological role for the major histocompatibility antigens, *Lancet* **1**:1406.

Doherty, P.C., Blanden, R.V., and Zinkernagel, R.M., 1976a, Specificity of virus-immune effector T cells for H-2K and H-2D compatible interactions: Implications for H-antigen diversity, *Transplant. Rev.* **29**:89.

Doherty, P.C., Gotze, D., Trinchieri, G., and Zinkernagel, R.M., 1976b, Models for recognition of virally modified cells by immune thymus derived lymphocytes, *Immunogenetics* **3**:517.

Doherty, P.C., Effros, R.B., and Bennink, J.R., 1977a, Cell-mediated immunity in virus infections: Influenza virus and the problem of self–non-self discrimination, *Perspect. Virol.* **10**:73.

Doherty, P.C., Effros, R.B., and Bennink, J.R., 1977b, Heterogeneity of cytotoxic responses of thymus-derived lymphocytes after immunization with influenza virus, *Proc. Natl. Acad. Sci. U.S.A.* **74**:1209.

Doherty, P.C., Biddison, W.E., Bennink, J.R., and Knowles, B.B., 1978, Cytotoxic T-cell responses in mice infected with influenza and vaccinia viruses may vary in magnitude with H-2 genotype, *J. Exp. Med.* **148**:534.

Effros, R.B., Doherty, P.C., Gerhard, W., and Bennink, J. R., 1977, Generation of both cross-reactive and virus-specific T-cell populations after immunization with serologically distinct influenza A viruses, *J. Exp. Med.* **145**:557.

Effros, R.B., Bennink, J.R., and Doherty, P.C., 1978, Characteristics of secondary cytotoxic T cell responses in mice infected with influenza A viruses, *Cell. Immunol.* **36**:345.

Effros, R.B., Frankel, M.E., Gerhard, W., and Doherty, P.C., 1979, Inhibition of influenza immune T cell effector function by virus-specific hybridoma antibody, *J. Immunol.* **123**:1343.

Eichmann, K., 1978, Expression and function of idiotypes on lymphocytes, *Adv. Immunol.* **26**:195.

Ennis, F.A., Martin, W.J., Verbonitz, M.W., and Butchko, G.M., 1977a, Specificity studies on cytotoxic thymus-derived lymphocytes reactive with influenza virus-infected cells: Evidence for dual recognition of H-2 and viral hemagglutinin antigens, *Proc. Natl. Acad. Sci. U.S.A.* **74**:3006.

Ennis, F.A., Martin, W.J., and Verbonitz, M.W., 1977b, Hemagglutinin specific cytotoxic T cell response during influenza infection, *J. Exp. Med.* **146**:893.

Ennis, F.A., Wells, M.A., Butchko, G.M., and Albrecht, P., 1978, Evidence that cytotoxic T cells are part of the host's response to influenza pneumonia, *J. Exp. Med.* **148**:1241.

Fink, P.J., and Bevan, M.J., 1978, H-2 antigens of the thymus determine lymphocyte specificity, *J. Exp. Med.* **148**:766.

Ford, W.L., and Atkins, R.C., 1971, Specific unresponsiveness of recirculating lymphocytes after exposure to histocompatibility antigens in F_1 hybrid rats, *Nature (London) New Biol.* **234**:178.

Forman, J., and Klein, J., 1977, Immunogenetic analysis of H-2 mutations. VI. Crossreacting in cell-mediated lympholysis between TNP-modified cells from H-2 mutant strains, *Immunogenetics* **4**:183.

Frankel, M.F., Effros, R.B., Doherty, P.C., and Gerhard, W., 1979, Indications of a differential association between influenza virus hemagglutinin and two H-2 molecules *J. Immunol.* **123**:2438.

Gerhard, W., and Webster, R.G., 1978, Antigenic drift in influenza A viruses. I. Selection and characterization of antigenic variants of A/PR/8/34 (HON1) influenza virus with monoclonal antibodies *I Exp. Med.* **148**;383.

Gerhard, W., Croce, C.M., Lopes, D.W., and Koprowski, H., 1978, Repertoire of antiviral antibodies expressed by somatic cell hybrids, *Proc. Natl. Acad. Sci. U.S.A.* **75**:1510.

Gerhard, W., Yewdell, J., Frankel, M.E., Lopes, A.D., and Staudt, L., 1980, Monoclonal antibodies against influenza virus, in: *Monoclonal Antibodies* (R.H. Kennett, T.J. Mckearn, and K.B. Bechtol, eds.), p. 317, Plenum Press, New York.

Hale, V.H., Witte, O.N., Baltimore, D., and Eisen, H.N., 1978, Vesicular stomatitis virus glycoprotein is necessary for H-2 restricted lysis of infected cells by cytotoxic T lymphocytes, *Proc. Natl. Acad. Sci. U.S.A.* **75**:970.

Jerne, N.K., 1971, The somatic generation of immune recognition, *Eur. J. Immunol.* **1**:1.

Katz, D.H., 1972, The allogeneic effect on immune responses: Model for regulatory influences of T lymphocytes on the immune system, *Transplant. Rev.* **12**:141.

Kilbourne, E.D., 1975, Epidemiology of influenza, in: *The Influenza Viruses and Influenza* (E.D. Kilbourne, ed.), p. 483, Academic Press, New York.

Koszinowski, U., and Thomssen, R., 1975, Target cell-dependent T cell-mediated lysis of vaccinia virus-infected cells, *Eur. J. Immunol.* **5**:245.

Koszinowski, U.H., Allen, H., Gething, M.J., Waterfield, M.D., and Klenk, H.D., 1980, Recognition of viral glycoproteins by influenza A-specific cross-reactive cytotoxic T lymphocytes, *J. Exp. Med.* **151**:945.

Langman, R.E., 1978, The role of the major histocompatibility complex in immunity: A new concept in the functioning of a cell-mediated immune system, *Rev. Physiol. Biochem. Pharmacol.* **81**:1.

Laver, W.G., Bachmayer, H., and Weil, R. (eds.), 1977, *The Influenza Virus Hemagglutinin, Topics in Infectious Diseases,* Vol. 3, Springer-Verlag, Vienna.

Lohmeyer, J., Talens, L.T., and Klenk, H.-D., 1979, Biosynthesis of the influenza virus envelope in abortive infection, *J. Gen. Virol.* **42**:73.

Marshak, A., Doherty, P.C., and Wilson, D.B., 1977, The control of specificity of cytotoxic T lymphocytes by the major histocompatibility complex (Ag-B) in rats and identification of a new alloantigen system showing no Ag-B restriction, *J. Exp. Med.* **146**:1773.

McMichael, A., 1978, HLA restriction of human cytotoxic T lymphocytes specific for influenza virus: Poor recognition of virus associated with HLA A2, *J. Exp. Med.* **148**:1458.

McMichael, A.J., and Ting, A., 1977, HLA restriction of cell-mediated lysis of influenza virus-infected human cells, *Nature (London)* **270**:524.

Miller, J.F.A.P., 1978, Restriction imposed on T lymphocyte reactivities by the major histocompatibility complex: Implications for T cell repertoire selection, *Immunol. Rev.* **42**:76.

Pang, T., and Blanden, R.V., 1976, Regulation of the T cell response to ectromelia virus infection. I. Feedback suppression by effector T cells, *J. Exp. Med.* **143**:469.

Reiss, C.S., and Schulman, J.L., 1980, Influenza virus M protein expression on infected cells is responsible for cross-reactive recognition by cytotoxic thymus derived lymphocytes, *Infect. Immunol.* **29**:719.

Schild, G.C., 1979 (ed.), Influenza, *Br. Med. Bull.,* Vol. 35.

Schulman, J.L., and Kilbourne, E.D., 1965, Induction of partial specific heterotypic immunity in mice by a single infection with influenza A virus, *J. Bacteriol.* **89**:170.

Shearer, G.M., and Schmitt-Verhulst, A.M., 1977, Major histocompatibility complex restricted cell-mediated immunity, *Adv. Immunol.* **25**:55.

Simpson, E., and Gordon, R.D., 1977, Responsiveness to HY antigen Ir gene complementation and target cell specificity, *Immunol. Rev.* **35**:59.

Sprent, J., 1977, Recirculating lymphocytes, in: *The Lymphocyte: Structure and Function* (J.J. Marchalonis, ed.), p. 43, Marcel Decker, New York.

Sprent, J., 1978, Role of the H-2 complex in introduction of T helper cells *in vivo.* I. Antigen-specific selection of donor T cells to sheep erythrocytes in irradiated mice dependent upon sharing of H-2 determinants between donor and host, *J. Exp. Med.* **148**:478.

Virelizier, J.L., Allison, A.C., Oxford, J.S., and Schild, G.C., 1977, Early appearance of ribonucleoprotein antigen on surface of influenza virus-infected cells, *Nature (London)* **266**:52.

von Boehmer, H., Haas, W., and Jerne, N.K., 1978, Major histocompatibility complex-linked immune-responsiveness is acquired by lymphocytes of low-responder mice differentiating in thymus of high-responder mice, *Proc. Natl. Acad. Sci. U.S.A.* **75**:2439.

Wilson, D.B., Lindahl, K.F., Wilson, D.H., and Sprent, J., 1977, The generation of killer cells to trinitrophenyl-modified allogeneic targets by lymphocyte populations negatively selected to strong alloantigens, *J. Exp. Med.* **146**:361.

Yap, K.L., and Ada, G.L., 1977, Cytotoxic T cells specific for influenza virus-infected target cells, *Immunology* **32**:151.

Yap, K.L., and Ada, G. L., 1978a, The recovery of mice from influenza virus infection: Adoptive transfer of immunity with immune T lymphocytes, *Scand. J. Immunol.* **7**:389.

Yap, K.L., and Ada, G.L., 1978b, The recovery of mice from influenza A virus infection: Adoptive transfer of immunity with influenza virus specific cytotoxic T lymphocytes recognizing a common virion antigen, *Scand. J. Immunol.* **8**:413.

Zinkernagel, R.M., 1976, Virus specific T cell-mediated cytotoxicity across the H-2 barrier to "virus-altered alloantigen," *Nature (London)* **261**:139.

Zinkernagel, R.M., 1978, Thymus and lymphohemopoietic cells: Their role in T cell maturation in selection of T cells' H-2 restrictions-specificity and in H-2-linked Ir gene control, *Immunol. Rev.* **42**:224.

Zinkernagel, R.M., and Doherty, P.C., 1974, Activity of sensitized thymus derived lymphocytes in lymphocytic choriomeningitis reflects immunological surveillance against altered self components, *Nature (London)* **251**:547.

Zinkernagel, R.M., and Doherty, P.C., 1977, The concept that surveillance of self is mediated via the same set of genes that determines recognition of allogeneic cells, *Cold Spring Harbor Symp. Quant. Biol.* **41**:505.

Zinkernagel, R.M., and Doherty, P.C., 1979, MHC restricted cytotoxic T cells: Studies on the biological role of polymorphic major transplantation antigens determining T cell restriction-specificity function and responsiveness, *Adv. Immunol.* **27**:51.

Zinkernagel, R.M., Althage, A., Cooper, S., Kreeb, G., Klein, P.A., Sefton, B., Flaherty, L., Stimpfling, J., Shreffler, D., and Klein, J., 1978a, Ir genes in H-2 regulate generation of anti-viral cytotoxic T cells: Mapping to K or D and dominance of unresponsiveness, *J. Exp. Med.* **148**:592.

Zinkernagel, R.M., Callahan, G.N., Althage, A., Cooper, A., Steilein, J.W., and Klein, J., 1978b, The lymphoreticular system in triggering virus-plus-self-specific cytotoxic T cells: Evidence for T help, *J. Exp. Med.* **147**:879.

Zweerink, H.J., Courtneidge, S.A., Skehel, J.J., Crumpton, M.J., and Askonas, B.A., 1977a, Cytotoxic T cells kill influenza virus-infected cells but do not distinguish between serologically distinct A viruses, *Nature (London)* **267**:354.

Zweerink, H.J., Askonas, B.A., Millican, D., Courtneidge, S.A., and Skehel, J.J., 1977b, Cytotoxic T cells to type A influenza virus: Viral hemagglutinin induces A-strain specificity while infected cells confer cross-reactive cytotoxicity, *Eur. J. Immunol.* **7**:630.

4

Hapten Recognition by Cytotoxic T Cells
The Modifying Influence of the Major Histocompatibility Complex

Christopher S. Henney, Zuhair K. Ballas, and Keiko Ozato

1. Introduction

The observation by Shearer (1974) that cytotoxic lymphocytes could be generated against hapten-modified surfaces of syngeneic cells has served as the platform from which many recent studies on the specificity of recognition by effector T cells have been launched. Shearer's observations have had a twofold impact: (1) they provided, for the first time, the possibility of raising cytotoxic T lymphocytes (CTL) against a defined hapten; and (2) they revealed that lysis of haptenated cells was restricted by the major histocompatibility complex (MHC), in that in murine systems, the effector and haptenated target cell had to share $H\text{-}2K$ and/ or $H\text{-}2D$ haplotypes for lysis to occur (Shearer, 1974; Forman *et al.*, 1977a,b). This MHC restriction of hapten-specific T killer cells is widely regarded as analogous to similar restriction that exists for cytotoxic cells directed against viral antigens (Zinkernagel and Doherty, 1974), minor histocompatability antigens (Bevan, 1975), and H-Y antigens (Gordon *et al.*, 1975).

The studies to be described herein were initiated in an attempt to define the fine specificity of recognition by MHC-restricted CTL directed

Christopher S. Henney, Zuhair K. Ballas, and Keiko Ozato • Basic Immunology Program, Fred Hutchinson Cancer Research Center, Seattle, Washington 98104.   Dr. Ozato's present address is: Immunology Branch, National Cancer Institute, Bethesda, Maryland 20014.

against the haptens dinitrophenol (DNP) and trinitrophenol (TNP). In particular, we were interested in asking whether products of the MHC gene complex on the surface of the target cell needed to be chemically modified by hapten for the cell to be susceptible to attack, or, alternatively, whether the hapten and MHC gene products could be separately presented on the cell surface. This is clearly one way of addressing the issue of whether effector T cell–target cell interactions involve the separate, "dual" recognition of hapten and MHC product(s) or the simple recognition of altered "self" determinants. Answers to this question are, of course, of fundamental importance in defining the nature of antigen recognition by T cells.

The experimental approaches we chose to employ were twofold: (1) to introduce hapten onto the cell surface by cell fusion with haptenated liposomes (Ozato *et al.*, 1978) and (2) to incubate unmodified target cells with haptenated proteins, and thus to display hapten on the cell surface in the form of passively adsorbed protein (Schmitt-Verhulst *et al.*, 1978). These approaches, both of which lead to hapten display on the cell surface without chemical modification of MHC products, allow one to ask, furthermore, whether the "triggering" of cytotoxic cell differentiation in primary cultures has different antigenic requirements than those that must be displayed on the target cell for it to be susceptible to attack by differentiated effector cells.

2. Materials and Methods

2.1. Preparation of Liposomes

In preparing the liposomes, 2 mg chicken egg yolk phosphatidylcholine (EYPC) or 2 mg dipalmitoylphosphatidylcholine (DPPC) (Calbiochem, San Diego, California) dissolved in chloroform–methanol (2:1) were mixed with 10% (wt./wt.) phosphatidylethanolamine (PE) in glass tubes. The solvent was removed under nitrogen, and 2 ml Hanks' balanced salt solution (HBSS) was added to the dried lipid. The mixtures were allowed to stand for 10 min at room temperature (45°C for DPPC liposomes), vigorously vortexed for 3 min, and subjected to ultrasonication (Sonifier, Heat Systems Ultrasonic Model 75-D, Plainview, New York) for 10 min at 4 watts. Sonication was performed in ice for EYPC liposomes and at 40–45°C for DPPC liposomes.

Dinitrophenylated liposomes (Six *et al.*, 1973; Yasuda *et al.*, 1977) were formed with dinitrophenylaminocaproylphosphatidylethanolamine (DNP-Cap-PE) or dinitrophenylphosphatidylethanolamine (DNP-PE) (both obtained from Avanti Biochemicals, Birmingham, Alabama) in place of PE. Trinitrophenylated liposomes were prepared by incubating unsubstituted liposomes [2 mg lipids/ml phosphate-buffered saline (PBS)] with 10 mM 2,4,6-trinitrobenzene sulfonic acid (TNBS) at 37°C for 30 min at pH 8.5. Unreacted TNBS was removed by passing 1 ml of the liposome suspension through a Sephadex G-75 column (9 × 500 mm) equilibrated with PBS at pH 7.4.

Liposome uptake by P815 mastocytoma cells was studied with dinitrophenylated liposomes comprised of either EYPC or DPPC and containing trace amounts of [³H]dioleyl phosphatidylcholine (PC) or [³H]-DPPC, respectively. In this experiment, 2×10^5 cells were incubated with 0.5 ml liposome dispersion containing 0.25 mg lipids in 12 × 75 mm glass tubes for 60 min at either 37 or 0°C. After incubation, cells were washed three times with PBS, transferred to new tubes, and then solubilized in 10% Triton X-100. The specific activity of the liposomes employed was $8-10 \times 10^3$ cpm/μg lipid. Further details of the liposome preparation and of the uptake assay are described elsewhere (Ozato *et al.*, 1978; Huang *et al.*, 1978).

2.2. Preparation of Haptenated Bovine Serum Albumin

Bovine serum albumin [BSA (Fraction V, Sigma, St. Louis, Missouri)], 40 mg, was mixed with equal amounts of sodium carbonate and 2,4-dinitrobenzene sulfonic acid [(DNBS) Eastman Kodak, Rochester, New York] in 2 ml distilled water and incubated at 37°C overnight in the dark. Spectrophotometric analysis (Little and Eisen, 1967) revealed that such reaction conditions yielded approximately 19 mol DNP/mol BSA.

TNP-proteins were prepared by dissolving the proteins [bovine, γ-globulin (BGG), BSA, human serum albumin (HSA), and keyhole limpet hemocyanin (KLH)] in 0.4 M borate buffer pH 9.0 at an initial concentration of 20 mg/ml. The resulting solution was mixed with equal volumes of 40 mM TNBS dissolved in the same buffer. The reaction was carried out overnight at 37°C and then dialyzed exhaustively against PBS, pH 7.4, at 4°C in the dark. Calculations of TNP derivatization were based on the value of 1.54×10^4 as the molar extinction coefficient of TNP-lysine at 348 nm. Reactions as described usually resulted in substitution of 40–50 mol/mol for BGG and HSA and 30–40 mol/mol for BSA. For preparation of HSA preparations bearing a variety of substitutions, the reaction was carried out as described above except that decreasing concentrations of TNBS (down to 1 mM) were added to a constant (20 mg/ml) concentration of HSA.

2.3. Purified Anti-DNP Antibody

Rabbit anti-DNP antiserum was prepared by hyperimmunization (four intramuscular injections of 1 mg each in complete Freund's adjuvant at 2-week intervals) with maximally substituted dinitrophenylated KLH (50–100 mol/mol). Specific anti-DNP antibody was obtained by passing the antiserum (20 ml) through an immunoabsorbent column (9 × 230 mm) prepared with Sepharose 2B coupled with DNP-HSA. After extensive washing with borate-buffered saline, pH 8.0, antibody was eluted with glycine-HCl buffer, pH 3.0. The eluted material, after neutralization with a Tris-HCl buffer, pH 8.0, was concentrated, dialyzed against PBS, pH 7.4, and stored at $-20°C$. The preparation has been previously described (Ozato and Henney, 1978b).

2.4. [^{125}I]-Anti-DNP Antibody

The anti-DNP antibody prepared as described above was labeled with ^{125}I by the method of Hunter and Greenwood (1962). In this procedure, 75 μg antibody protein in 25 μl HBSS was reacted with 2 mCi "carrier-free" Na^{125}I (New England Nuclear, Boston, Massachusetts). The mixture was diluted in 1 ml PBS containing 4 mg/ml KI and 50 mg/ml BSA and the ^{125}I-labeled protein eluted from a Sephadex G-25 column (9 × 600 mm) equilibrated with PBS, pH 7.5, and containing 2% BSA.

2.5. Membrane-Vesicle Preparation

Membrane-vesicle preparations from spleen cells were prepared according to the method of Svehag and Schilling (1973). Spleen cell suspensions, freed of erythrocytes by incubation with 0.84% NH_4Cl, were treated with 10 mM TNBS at 37°C for 10 min, suspended in 2 ml HBSS, and sonicated (4 watts, 4 min) in an ethanol–ice bath. The materials so produced were centrifuged at 1100 g for 10 min at 8°C to remove nuclei and mitochondria. Supernatants were subjected to ultracentrifugation (Beckman Instruments, Palo Alto, California, Model L2-65B) at 140,000 g for 60 min at 4°C. The resulting pellets were dissolved in PBS containing 1 mM Ca^{2+}, and 1 mM Mg^{2+}, and were resonicated for 1 min at 0°C. A similar preparation was prepared from nonhaptenated spleen cells. All samples were estimated for protein content by the method of Lowry *et al.* (1951) and were stored at $-20°C$ before use.

2.6. Binding of [^{125}I]-Anti-DNP Antibody to Haptenated Cells

^{125}I-anti-DNP antibody was diluted in RPMI 1640 (GIBCO, Grand Island, New York) containing 1% BSA and 100 μg/ml heated (63°C, 20 min) human γ-globulin. Cells treated with various reagents to induce DNP display were transferred into glass tubes (2 × 10^5 cells/tube), incubated at 4°C for 40 min with 400 μl of the aforementioned antibody, and then washed extensively. The specific activity of the antibody preparation used was 20–40 × 10^4 cpm/μg anti-DNP antibody.

2.7. C-Mediated and K-Cell-Mediated Cytolysis

P815 cells (2 × 10^6) were prelabeled by incubation (30 min, 37°C) with Na$_2$^{51}CrO$_4$ (New England Nuclear) and haptenated by the procedures described above. After extensive washing, 2 × 10^4 cells in 100 μl were transferred to a U-bottomed microtiter plate (Linbro Scientific, Hamden, Connecticut) and incubated with various concentrations of purified anti-DNP antibody diluted in RPMI 1640 containing 10% fetal calf serum (FCS) for 10 min at room temperature. Fresh rabbit serum (100 μl diluted to 12% in the medium described above) or human peripheral lymphocytes (4 × 10^5 cells in 100 μl) were then added to assess C-mediated or K-cell-mediated cytolysis, respectively. For the C-mediated assay, cells were further incubated for 40 min at 37°C; for K-cell-mediated lysis, cells were incubated for 4 hr at 37°C. The percentage of specific lysis was calculated as follows:

$$\text{Specific lysis (\%)} = \frac{A - N}{T - N} \times 100$$

where A is the ^{51}Cr released in the presence of antibody, T is the total lysis obtained by freezing and thawing target cells through two cycles, and N is the ^{51}Cr released in the absence of antibody.

2.8. Generation of Hapten-Specific Cytotoxic Responses.

Primary hapten-specific cytotoxic cells were generated *in vitro* according to the method of Shearer (1974). To achieve this, 10^7 mouse spleen cells (DBA/2, C57BL/6, AKR, and CBA strains obtained from Jackson Laboratory, Bar Harbor, Maine) were treated with 15 mM DNBS in HBSS, pH 7.8, for 30 min, 37°C, or with 10 mM TNBS for 10 min in PBS, pH 7.4, at 37°C. Treated cells were washed three times with RPMI 1640, and 2 × 10^6 cells were used to stimulate 10^7 responder spleen cells in 2 ml RPMI 1640 containing 10% FCS, 5×10^{-5} M 2-mercaptoethanol, and supplemented with 40 μg/ml of gentamycin (Schering Corp., Kenilworth, New Jersey). Cultures were carried out in 17×100 mm plastic tubes (Falcon Plastics, Oxnard, California) for 5 days at 37°C in an atmosphere of 5% CO_2 and humidified air. In some experiments, 7×10^6 mouse spleen cells (CBA or C57BL/6 strain) were incubated either with soluble protein or TNP-protein antigens at 100 μg/ml or with 2×10^6 syngeneic spleen cells treated with varying concentrations of TNBS (as indicated in Section 3.2) in 2-ml volume in 24-well culture plates (Linbro Chemical Company, New Haven, Connecticut). At the end of culture, cells were harvested, and viability was assessed by erythrocin B exclusion. Such populations were used as effector cells in cytotoxicity assays.

2.9. T-Cell Mediated Cytolytic Assays

P815 mastocytoma cells (H-2^d) and EL4 lymphoma cells (H-2^b) maintained in ascites form in DBA/2 and C57BL/6 mice, respectively, were used as target cells for evaluating cytotoxic responses. In some of the studies, as noted, targets were also prepared from mouse spleen cells stimulated with lipopolysaccharide [(LPS) Difco Labs, Detroit, Michigan] at a final concentration of 10 μg/ml for 3 days. All target cells were labeled with $Na_2{}^{51}CrO_4$. Some were then treated with either 15 mM DNBS (30 min, 37°C in HBSS, pH 7.8) or 10 mM TNBS (10 min, 37°C, PBS, pH 7.4). When target cells bearing TNP-proteins were used, spleen cell "blasts" were labeled with $Na_2{}^{51}CrO_4$, then incubated with the TNP-proteins at a cell density of 10^6/ml and a final TNP-protein concentration of 1 mg/ml for 90 min at 37°C. The target cells were placed in V-bottomed microtiter plates, and various concentrations of effector lymphocytes were added. The cultures were incubated at 37°C for 4 hr, the plates were centrifuged briefly, and an aliquot of the supernatant was then collected and assessed for radioactivity by gamma ray spectrometry. Cytolysis was estimated according to the following formula:

$$\text{Cytolysis } (\%) = \frac{A - N}{T - N} \times 100$$

where A is the ^{51}Cr release in the presence of effector cells, N is the ^{51}Cr release in the presence of normal lymphocytes, and T is the total lysis obtained after two cycles of freezing and thawing.

3. Results

3.1. Hapten Presentation on Target Cells after Direct Chemical Modification and after Interaction with Dinitrophenylated Liposomes and Dinitrophenylated Protein

P815 mastocytoma cells were incubated with DNP-containing liposomes of varying composition, and the display of cell-surface-associated hapten was then assessed both by [^{125}I]-anti-DNP antibody binding and by measuring the susceptibility of the cells to lysis by complement and by human K cells in the presence of anti-DNP antibody. Two types of liposomes were used in such studies: those composed of egg yolk phosphatidylcholine (EYPC) and those containing dipalmitoylphosphatidylcholine (DPPC). In both cases, the liposomes additionally contained 10% (wt./wt.) of either phosphatidylethanolamine (PE) or the haptenated derivative DNP-caproylphosphatidylethanolamine (DNP-Cap-PE). To encourage optimal liposome–cell interactions, we made use of previous observations (Huang *et al.,* 1978) and incubated EYPC liposomes with the cells at 37°C and DPPC liposomes at 0°C.

The amount of hapten transferred to the P815 cell surface following incubation with liposomes was quantitatively compared with that elicited by direct dinitrophenylation of the cell surface [using 2,4-dinitrobenzene sulfonic acid (DNBS)] and with that obtained by incubation of the cells with dinitrophenylated bovine serum albumin (DNP-BSA).

Incubation with DNP-liposomes of either composition resulted in efficient hapten transfer to P815 cells as indicated by [^{125}I]-anti-DNP-antibody-binding criteria and by enhanced susceptibility of the cells to complement and to K-cell-mediated cytolysis in the presence of anti-DNP antibody (data for DPPC-containing liposomes are shown in Table 1). By each of these criteria, the degree of hapten transfer to the tumor cell surface was greater following incubation with DNP-bearing liposomes than was observed, under the experimental conditions employed, for direct surface modification (15 mM DNBS, 30 min, 37°C) or following incubation with DNP-BSA (1 mg/ml, 90 min, 37°C). Hapten transfer to P815 cells was observed with both EYPC and DPPC liposomes at concentrations between 0.5 and 2.0 mg lipid/ml. Concentrations of liposomes above 3.0 mg/ml impaired cell viability.

The association of dinitrophenylated liposomes with P815 cells was further studied using ^{3}H-labeled liposomes. Following incubation of P815 cells (2×10^5/ml) with 1 mg/ml DNP-Cap-PE-EYPC (60 min, 37°C), the cell-associated lipid was 1.5 pg/cell (9.6×10^7 DNP molecules/cell). Over the same incubation period at 0°C, using DPPC liposomes, 2.6 pg lipid/

TABLE 1. Hapten Presentation on P815 Cells Following
Incubation with Haptenated Proteins and Haptenated
Liposomes[a]

Treatment of cells	[125I]-anti-DNP antibody bound (cpm × 10^{-2}/ 2 × 10^5 cells)	Specific lysis (%) by anti-DNP antibody and:	
		Complement	K cells
Untreated	51 ± 4	2.0	3.0
DNP-liposomes	855 ± 18	29.0	19.0
Liposomes (unhaptenated)	48 ± 3	0.5	0.1
DNP-BSA	91 ± 5	11.0	14.0
BSA	47 ± 2	2.0	1.0
DNBS	107 ± 9	10.0	11.0

[a] Data amended from Ozato and Henney (1978). In this experiment, 2 × 10^5 P815 cells were incubated with DNBS (15mM, 30 min, 37°), with DNP-BSA or BSA (1 mg/ml, 90 min, 37°C), or with 1 mg/ml liposomes (30 min, 37°C). Two sets of liposomes were used with equivalent results: those composed of EYPC and 10% (wt./wt.) PE and those composed of DPPC and 10% PE. To obtain DNP-liposomes, DNP-Cap-PE was substituted for PE. The data shown are for PE-DPPC and DNP-Cap-PE-DPPC. The specific activity of the [125I]-anti-DNP antibody used was 25 × 10^4 cpm/μg antibody. The anti-DNP antibody concentration used for lysis by rabbit complement was 25 μg/ml; that for K-cell-mediated lysis, 8 μg/ml.

cell (16.6 × 10^7 DNP molecules/cell) was measured. Under similar experimental conditions, DBA/2 mouse splenocytes took up approximately 20% of the amount of liposomes that became associated with P815 cells, a value similar to that we have previously obtained with human lymphocytes (Ozato et al., 1978).

The persistence of hapten delivered to the P815 cell surface following incubation with DNP-liposomes was then assessed. Mastocytoma cells were incubated with DNP-Cap-PE-EYPC (or the corresponding DPPC liposomes) for 60 min at 37°C (0°C for DPPC) and the lysis by anti-DNP antibody and rabbit complement measured using a portion of the cells. The remainder of the cells were incubated at either 0 or 37°C for periods up to 3 hr and the susceptibility to complement lysis reassessed. As can be seen in Table 2, there was little decrease in the amount of 51Cr released in the presence of complement after the 3-hr incubation period, suggesting that the DNP transferred to the cell surface following interaction with liposomes was not transiently expressed. Indeed, in further studies, not shown, P815 cells incubated with DNBS or DNP-BSA and then cultured for a further 3 hr often showed a considerable decrease in their susceptibility to C attack; P815 cells preincubated with DNP-liposomes showed no such decline. In these same studies, we have observed that lymphocytes incubated with DNP-bearing liposomes also

TABLE 2. Persistence of DNP Determinants on Target Cells[a]

| | ^{51}Cr release (%) by anti-DNP+C | | |
| | | After 3 hr at: | |
Hapten transferred by:	Immediately	0°C	37°C
Untreated	2	2	2
DNP-liposomes	21	22	18
DNP-protein	10	7	6
DNBS	10	6	4

[a] DNP hapten was transferred to P815 cells (as in Table 1), and susceptibility to lysis by anti-DNP antibody in the presence of rabbit complement was assessed either immediately or after 3 hr at 0 or 37°C.

displayed hapten for prolonged (> 6-hr) periods (Ozato and Henney, 1978).

Since hapten-bearing lipids, in the form of liposomes, could be used to transfer hapten to the surface of both lymphocytes and mastocytoma cells, and since the hapten thereby transferred was accessible for a period of at least several hours, we asked whether such cells could elicit a hapten-specific cytotoxic response in syngeneic spleen cell cultures.

3.2. Generation of a Primary Hapten-Specific Cytotoxic Response *in Vitro* Using a Variety of Hapten-Bearing Stimulator Cells

Normal DBA/2 spleen cells were incubated with DNP- (or TNP-) liposomes containing either EYPC or DPPC and 10% (wt./wt.) of the appropriate PE (see Section 2.1). For this step, 10^7 spleen cells in 0.5 ml Hanks' balanced salt solution were incubated with 0.01, 0.05, 0.1, 0.5, 1, or 2 mg lipid/ml; the cells were then washed and 2×10^6 cells added to 10^7 normal DBA/2 spleen cells. The cells were cocultured for 5 days at 37°C, and the cytotoxic activity generated was assessed using syngeneic P815 or allogeneic, EL4, cells modified with DNBS [or 2,4,6-trinitrobenzene sulfonic acid (TNBS)]. As controls for these experiments, DBA/2 spleen cells directly modified by treatment with 15 mM DNBS (30 min, 37°C) [or with 10 mM TNBS (30 min, 37°C)] were used as stimulator cells. Furthermore, DBA/2 spleen cells incubated with 0.5–2 mg/ml DNP-BSA [or 0.5–1.5 mg/ml trinitrophenylated (TNP)-BSA] at 37°C for 90 min were also assessed for their ability to stimulate a hapten-specific cytotoxic response.

Typical results from these studies are shown in Fig. 1. Using stimulator cells that had been directly chemically modified, demonstrable cytotoxic responses were seen over the concentration range 0.1–15 mM TNBS and 10–20 mM DNBS, the optimal concentration varying with the mouse strain employed. The responses to TNBS-modified cells were usually greater than to DNBS-modified cells. In both cases, the cytotoxicity elicited was hapten-specific and showed a strong syngeneic preference, both points as previously described (Shearer, 1974; Forman, 1977). Thus, cells raised against TNBS-treated stimulator cells lysed TNBS-modified targets effectively, but caused no significant lysis of DNBS-modified targets and vice versa. Further, DBA/2 effector cells lysed haptenated P815 cells but did not kill haptenated EL4 cells (Fig.

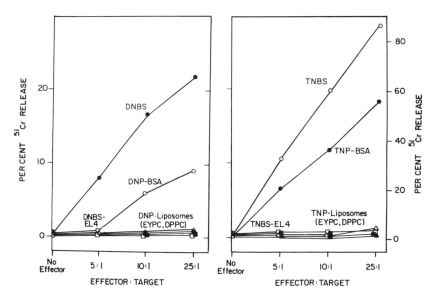

Figure 1. Attempts to raise CTL responses against stimulator cells incubated with haptenated liposomes and haptenated proteins. *Left:* DNP response. DBA/2 spleen cells were stimulated with syngeneic lymphocytes treated with 15 mM DNBS for 30 min; with lymphocytes incubated for 90 min at 37°C with 1 mg/ml DNP-BSA, or with syngeneic lymphocytes incubated with 0.5 mg/ml liposomes for 1 hr at 0°C (DPPC-liposomes) or 37°C (EYPC-liposomes). *Right:* TNP response. As for DNP response, except that 10 mM TNBS for 10 min and corresponding TNP-liposomes and TNP-BSA (0.5 mg/ml) were used. All cultures were terminated after 5 days and the cytotoxic response toward DNBS- or TNBS-treated P815 cells assessed in a 4-hr assay. In the experiment shown, the percentage of spontaneous release was 1.5%/hr for both DNP and TNP P815 target cells. As specificty controls, allogeneic EL4 target cells modified with TNBS or DNBS in a manner identical to that used for P815 cells were employed. The percentage of spontaneous release from these target cells was in the range of 2–4%/hr. From Ozato and Henney (1978), with permission of the Williams and Wilkins Co.

1), whereas C57BL/6 effectors lysed haptenated EL4 cells effectively, but lysed haptenated P815 cells to a much lesser extent (data not shown).

In these studies, spleen cells incubated with TNP-BSA elicited a significant cytotoxic response in both strains (DBA/2 and C57BL/6), confirming the recent observations of Schmitt-Verhulst *et al.* (1978). Furthermore, cells incubated with DNP-BSA were also capable of eliciting a hapten-specific cytotoxic response with a preference for syngeneic target cells. This response was, in these strains, always significantly less than that observed with DNBS-treated cells and was more readily demonstrated using DBA/2 responder cells than with C57BL/6 cells. As will be demonstrated later, much greater reactivity was induced by haptenated proteins when they were tested with the CBA and AKR strains. In our more recent studies using TNP-proteins, we have observed only weak cytotoxic activity in DBA/2 and C57BL/6 spleen-cell populations (Table 3) (also unpublished observations of Ballas and Henney, 1979). Indeed, strong cytotoxic responses to haptenated proteins have been routinely observed only in mice of the $H\text{-}2^k$ haplotype. Detailed studies in these strains of mice are shown in Table 3. The data shown are in keeping with those described in Fig. 2 and with the observations of Schmitt-Verhulst *et al.* (1978) that CTL induced by haptenated proteins are both hapten-specific and MHC-restricted.

In contrast to the stimulatory capacity of spleen cells incubated with haptenated proteins, cells incubated with haptenated liposomes uniformly failed to elicit cytotoxicity. This was true of EYPC- and DPPC-containing liposomes bearing either TNP or DNP haptens and covered a large range of liposome concentrations. The results using DBA/2 cells are shown in Fig. 1; similar findings have also been made using C57BL/6 spleen cells. In other studies, we have used liposomes in which DNP was coupled directly to PE without a caproic acid "spacer." Cells treated with such liposomes bore DNP but did not elicit hapten-specific cytotoxic responses (data not shown). In other studies, we have exposed DBA/2 spleen cells to haptenated liposomes at daily intervals throughout a 5-day culture period without inducing demonstrable cytotoxic responses.

3.3. Target Cells "Haptenated" by Various Procedures: Their Susceptibility to Lysis by *H-2*-Restricted, Hapten-Specific Cytotoxic T Lymphocytes

Although cells incubated with hapten-bearing liposomes did not stimulate hapten-specific cytotoxic responses, we considered it possible that such cells could serve as targets for hapten-specific cytotoxic T lymphocytes (CTL). To test this hypothesis, P815 cells were "haptenated," as previously, either by direct surface modification using DNBS (or

TABLE 3. Induction and Specificity of Cytotoxic Cells Generated by Stimulation with Haptenated Proteins[a]

		Specific cytolysis (%) of spleen cells							
		H-2^k				H-2^d		H-2^b	
Responder	Stimulator	AKR	TNBS AKR	CBA	TNBS CBA	DBA/2	TNBS DBA/2	C57BL/6	TNBS C57BL/6
CBA	TNBS-CBA	4	75	0	90	0	0	0	7
	TNP-HSA	—	—	0	66	—	—	0	0
	TNP-BGG	2	51	3	43	0	5	—	—
AKR	TNBS-AKR	0	95	0	97	0	11	—	—
	TNP-BGG	0	29	0	27	0	0	—	—
C57BL/6	TNBS-C57BL/6	—	—	0	19	—	—	2	58
	TNP-HSA	—	—	0	0	—	—	0	25

[a] Spleen-cell suspensions were prepared and cultured with the indicated TNP-protein at final concentrations of 100 μg/ml or at 2:1 ratios with irradiated syngeneic spleen cells treated with 1.0 mM TNBS for 10 min at 37°C. After 5 days, the cultures were harvested, washed, and incubated with ^{51}Cr-labeled targets at an effector/target-cell ratio of 20 : 1 for 4 hr. The target cells were incubated with 10 μg/ml LPS for 3 days prior to ^{51}Cr labeling.

TNBS), by incubation with DNP- (or TNP-) BSA, or by incubation with hapten-bearing liposomes composed of EYPC or DPPC. The lysis of these cells by CTL obtained by culturing DBA/2 spleen cells with syngeneic DNBS- (or TNBS-) modified spleen cells, was then measured. The results are shown in Fig. 2. As can be seen, target cells incubated with haptenated BSA became susceptible to cytotoxic attack. The concentrations of haptenated BSA necessary to render target cells susceptible to hapten-specific cytotoxic attack were of the same order ($\approx$ 1 mg/ml DNP-BSA; 300–500 μg/ml TNP-BSA) as those needed to stimulate killer-cell production in primary cultures.

In contrast to what was seen with target cells bearing haptenated proteins, target cells incubated with haptenated liposomes (range 0.01–2 mg lipids/ml) were insusceptible to lysis by either DNP- or TNP-specific killer cells. The replacement of DNP-Cap-PE by DNP-PE did not change this negative result. It was considered possible that spleen cells treated with hapten-bearing liposomes might generate killer cells with a specificity restricted to liposome-treated target cells. This possiblity was explored extensively, using a variety of liposome preparations, but no evidence in support of the contention has been obtained.

In an attempt to explore the fine specificity of the CTL induced following incubation with TNP-proteins, we asked whether such cells could lyse targets bearing haptenated proteins other than those used to elicit the cytotoxic response. In this approach, we were interested in asking whether CTL recognized hapten only in the context of the protein "backbone" used for sensitization, as Benacerraf and Gell (1959) had classically shown to be the case for another T-cell-mediated phenomenon:

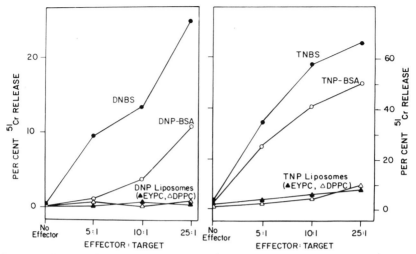

Figure 2. Susceptibility of haptenated target cells to syngeneic hapten-specific cytotoxic cells. *Left:* Anti-DNP response. *Right:* Anti-TNP response. ^{51}Cr-labeled P815 target cells were treated with various haptenic reagents, and their susceptibility to hapten-specific CTL of DBA/2 origin raised against DNBS- (or TNBS-) spleen cells was assessed in a 4-hr ^{51}Cr-release assay. Liposome treatment of tumor cells was carried out as described for lymphoyctes (see the Fig. 1 caption), using a concentration of 0.5 mg lipid/ml. Treatment of P815 cells with haptenated BSA (90 min, 37°C) was carried out at a concentration of 1 mg/ml for DNP-BSA and 0.5 mg/ml for TNP-BSA. From Ozato and Henney (1978), with permission of the Williams and Wilkins Co.

delayed hypersensitivity. The results shown in Table 4 clearly demonstrate that the CTL induced were hapten-specific. No evidence was obtained for the concept that recognition involved a component of the protein backbone on which the hapten was presented. Thus, as can be seen in Table 4, cytotoxic cells induced by TNP–human serum albumin (HSA) lysed target cells bearing TNP–bovine γ globulin (BGG), and TNP–keyhole limpet hemocyanin (KLH) in addition to those cells bearing homologous hapten–protein conjugates. Furthermore, cells induced by hapten–protein conjugates did not lyse cells incubated with unsubstituted protein (Ballas, unpublished observations).

In an attempt to define the optimal hapten concentration required for sensitization with haptenated proteins, and to ask whether this density was also optimal for susceptibility to attack by differentiated effector cells, the following experiments were designed. HSA preparations displaying a range of hapten substitutions (20–40 mol/mol) were used to induce CTL from CBA spleen-cell populations. The cells thus induced were assayed against lipopolysaccharide (LPS)-induced CBA

TABLE 4. Generation of Cytotoxic T Cells by Haptenated Proteins[a]

CBA spleen cells stimulated with	Specific lysis (%) of CBA spleen-cell "blasts" treated by incubation with:				
	Medium	TNBS	TNP-HSA	TNP-BGG	TNP-KLH
TNBS	0	86.5	68.3	55.8	66.3
TNP-HSA	0	51.1	51.9	37.0	47.8
HSA	0	0	0.7	1.9	0
TNP-BGG	0.3	45.1	48.6	23.8	35.8
BGG	2.5	0	0	2.0	0
TNP-KLH	3.1	65.9	58.8	42.6	65.4
KLH	6.0	0	0	4.7	0

[a] Culture was carried out as in Table 3 using 100 μg/ml of stimulating protein. Targets were labeled with ^{51}Cr and then treated with 1.0 mM TNBS for 10 min at 37°C or with the indicated proteins (at a final concentration of 1 mg/ml) for 90 min at 37°C. Data presented are from a 4-hr assay using an effector/target-cell ratio of 10:1.

blast cells that had been previously incubated with the same protein preparations used to induce the effector cells. Target cells incubated with proteins ranging in hapten substitution from 20 to 40 mol/mol showed little difference serologically in the amount of hapten they displayed (Table 5). Interestingly, however, cells displaying TNP-$_{20}$HSA were not susceptible to lysis, nor did they stimulate killer-cell production. In contrast, the same protein substituted above 30 TNP mol/mol was both an efficient initiator of cytotoxic cells and, when displayed on the target-cell surface, was an adequate target for attack (Table 5). We have carried out a number of studies of this type; in no case did we observe a

TABLE 5. Complement-Mediated and T-Cell-Mediated Lysis of Haptenated Target Cells[a]

CBA spleen cells stimulated with	Lysis by anti-TNP antibody and complement	Specific lysis (%) of CBA spleen-cell blasts treated by incubation with:			
		TNBS	TNP$_{40}$-HSA	TNP$_{30}$-HSA	TNP$_{20}$-HSA
Medium	1.3	1.5	2.0	3.0	3.4
TNBS	73.1	65.8	32.1	27.4	6.9
TNP$_{40}$-HSA	74.0	53.7	30.8	23.4	5.1
TNP$_{30}$-HSA	72.6	41.5	24.0	25.6	6.3
TNP$_{20}$-HSA	54.7	9.7	4.8	5.5	5.6

[a] CBA spleen cells were incubated for 5 days with 100 μg haptenated HSA or with TNBS-treated CBA spleen cells. The subscript number indicates the degree of substitution of the proteins used, in mole/mole. The data presented are from a 4-hr cytotoxicity assay carried out on day 5 of culture using ^{51}Cr-labeled LPS-induced "blast" cells of CBA spleens that had been incubated (90 min, 37°C) with 1 mg/ml of the indicated protein, or with 10 mM TNBS. The effector-cell/target-cell ratio was 10:1. The ability of anti-TNP antibody, in the presence of complement, to lyse the same target cells is also recorded.

haptenated protein that could elicit cytotoxic-cell production but not serve to "sensitize" a target cell for lytic attack.

3.4. Attempts to Inhibit Hapten-Specific Cytolysis with Haptenated Cells

It was considered possible that the failure of hapten-specific CTL to lyse target cells incubated with liposomes might reflect, not a deficiency in antigenicity of the target cells, but either an insusceptibility of the cells to lysis, perhaps because of altered membrane lipid composition, or an improper presentation of hapten on the cell surface. The antigenicity of the liposome-treated target cells was thus assessed in an alternative manner, by measuring their ability to inhibit the lysis of DNBS- (or TNBS-) treated target cells by cytotoxic cells of appropriate anti-hapten specificity. A typical experiment employing DNP-specific CTL is shown in Fig. 3. It can be seen that the lysis of DNBS-modified target cells was inhibited by homologous cells and by cells incubated with DNP-BSA. In contrast, cells incubated with DNP-bearing liposomes caused no greater inhibition than that seen with unsubstituted P815 cells. Thus, cells incubated with hapten-bearing liposomes do not appear to be recognized by hapten-specific CTL. One explanation of the data shown in Fig. 3 is that liposome-treated target cells become intrinsically insusceptible to CTL attack. To address this issue, the following experiments were devised: ^{51}Cr-P815 cells were incubated with liposomes of varying composition, with or without hapten, and the susceptibility to lysis by allogeneic CTL, directed against H-2 antigens of the target cell, was then assessed. No difference in the cytolysis of P815 cells was observed following liposome treatment, indicating that cells treated with the liposome preparations used in these studies were not intrinsically resistant to T-cell-mediated lysis (Ozato and Henney, 1978).

These findings were underlined by further experiments. Since cells exposed to hapten-bearing liposomes were not themselves capable of inducing cytotoxic responses in spleen-cell populations, we asked whether cells treated with liposomes could stimulate CTL production when subsequently treated with DNBS. Alternatively, we questioned whether the stimulatory activity of cells treated with DNBS persisted when the cells were subsequently treated with DNP-bearing liposomes. These experiments were pursued with both EYPC and DPPC liposomes containing DNP-Cap-PE with similar results. Cultures in which stimulator cells were pretreated with DNP-liposomes before DNBS treatment showed a level of cytotoxic activity similar to that seen with controls treated with DNBS alone. The specificity of the cytotoxic response was also not affected by exposure of the stimulator cells to liposomes. Thus,

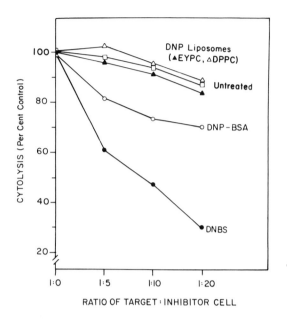

Figure 3. Inhibition of DNP-specific cytotoxicity by target cells bearing DNP. Untreated P815 cells or cells bearing DNP following exposure to DNP-liposomes (1 mg/ml, 60 min, 37°C), to DNP-BSA (1 mg/ml, 90 min, 37°C), or to DNBS (15 mM, 30 min, 37°C) were used to inhibit the cytolysis of DNBS-treated [^{51}Cr]-P815 cells by cytotoxic cells of DBA/2 origin that displayed DNP specificity. CTL were raised by coculturing 10^7 DBA/2 spleen cells for 5 days with 2×10^6 DNBS-treated DBA/2 spleen cells. In the experiment shown, cytolysis was measured in a 4-hr ^{51}Cr-release assay at an effector target-cell ratio of 50:1. The specific cytotoxic activity in the absence of inhibitor cells was 28.7%, the spontaneous release of ^{51}Cr in the absence of effector cells was 6.2%. From Ozato and Henney (1978), with permission of the Williams and Wilkens Co.

exposure of cells to liposomes did not interfere with the subsequent ability of these populations to stimulate hapten-specific CTL responses following DNBS treatment. Furthermore, incubation of DNBS-treated cells with DNP-liposomes was without effect on their ability to elicit production of hapten-specific CTL (Ozato and Henney, 1978b).

The observation that CTL could be inhibited by target cells bearing haptenated proteins was studied in further detail. As can be seen in Fig. 4, the lysis of TNP-HSA-bearing target cells by CBA killer cells induced by TNP-HSA was inhibited equally well by CBA blast cells bearing TNP-HSA, TNP-KLH, or TNP-BGG as by blast cells directly haptenated by treatment with TNBS. When killer cells were induced with TNBS-treated syngeneic spleen cells, however, the inhibition profile by various haptenated cells depended on the amount of TNBS used for "priming"

Figure 4. Inhibition of effector cells induced by TNP-HSA by target cells bearing
various TNP-proteins. Untreated CBA
spleen cells (LPS blasts) or CBA spleen
cells incubated with 1.0 mM TNBS (10 min,
37°C) or with 1 mg/ml (90 min, 37°C) of
TNP-HSA, TNP-KLH, or TNP-BGG were
used to inhibit lysis of ^{51}Cr-labeled CBA
spleen cells (LPS blasts) incubated with
TNP-HSA (1 mg/ml) for 90 min at 37°C.
CTL were CBA spleen cells incubated with
soluble TNP-HSA at a final concentration
of 100 μg/ml for 5 days. The experiment
shown is a 4-hr ^{51}Cr-release assay at an

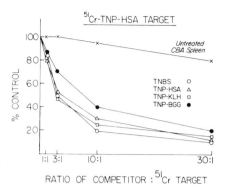

effector target-cell ratio of 10:1. The percentage of specific cytolysis in the absence of
competitors was 45.4%. Spontaneous release of ^{51}Cr targets was 25%.

(Fig. 5). Thus, killer cells induced by 1 mM TNBS were inhibited more
readily by 1-mM-TNBS-treated inhibitor cells than by cells treated with
0.1 mM TNBS (Fig. 5A). Cells bearing haptenated proteins behaved like
those cells treated with low doses of TNBS. In contrast, when killer
cells were raised to 0.1-mM-TNBS-treated cells and tested on target cells
treated with this amount of TNBS, comparable inhibition was observed
with 0.1- and 1.0-mM-TNBS-treated cells and with cells bearing haptenated protein (Fig. 5B). One interpretation of these observations is that at
the higher concentrations of TNBS, a greater diversity of effector-cell
clones is generated than is induced when lower doses of TNBS or TNP
proteins are used.

4. Discussion

In the studies presented herein, we have explored the ability of
MHC-restricted hapten-specific T cells to interact with target cells that
have been haptenated by three different procedures: fusion with haptenated liposomes, direct chemical modification with nitrobenzoic acids,
and incubation with nitrophenylated proteins. We will first consider the
cells "haptenated" by fusion with DNP- (and TNP-) bearing liposomes.

Hapten-bearing liposomes composed of both EYPC and DPPC were
found to interact with a variety of cells and to be capable of transferring
hapten to the cell surface (see Table 1) (see also Ozato et al., 1978). The
hapten thus conferred was readily accessible on the cell surface, as
shown by anti-DNP-antibody-binding studies and by the resulting sus-

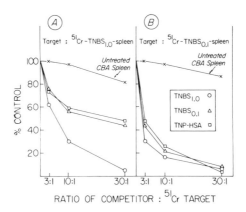

Figure 5. Untreated CBA spleen cells (LPS blasts) or cells treated with 1.0 mM TNBS (10 min, 37°C), 0.1 mM TNBS (10 min, 37°C), or TNP-HSA (1 mg/ml for 90 min, 37°C) were used to inhibit lysis of ^{51}Cr-labeled CBA spleen cells incubated with 1.0 mM TNBS (A) or 0.1 mM TNBS (B). CTL were CBA spleen cells incubated with TNBS-modified (1.0 mM TNBS for 10 min, 37°C) syngeneic spleen cells in a 5-day culture. The experiment shown is a 4-hr ^{51}Cr-release assay at an effector target-cell ratio of 5:1 (A) or 10:1 (B). The percentage of specific cytolysis in the absence of competitors was 61.6% (A) and 46.5% (B). Spntaneous release of ^{51}Cr targets was less than 30%.

ceptibility of the cell to complement and to K-cell-mediated lysis in the presence of anti-DNP antibody (Table 1). Indeed, under optimal conditions, it was possible to confer a higher density of hapten by interaction of P815 mastocytoma cells with DNP-bearing liposomes than was possible by direct chemical modification of the cell surface using DNBS. In addition, we observed that hapten transferred to the cell surface via interaction with liposomes remained exposed for longer periods than that introduced by treatment with DNBS (see Table 2).

Despite the ready display of cell-surface hapten, cells modified by liposome interaction failed to stimulate hapten-specific cytotoxic responses *in vitro* (see Fig. 1). This finding emphasizes that the presence of hapten *per se* is an insufficient requirement for "triggering" the precursors of cytotoxic cells. Furthermore, cells "haptenated" via interaction with liposomes were not susceptible to the action of hapten-specific CTL (see Fig. 2), nor did they competitively inhibit the lysis of target cells that had been modified by treatment with DNBS (or TNBS) (see Fig. 3). By all these criteria, cells haptenated via liposome interaction were not "recognized" by hapten-specific effector T cells. Indeed, liposome-treated cells behaved like unsubstituted cells in that they induced hapten-specific CTL only following treatment with DNBS (Ozato and Henney, 1978).

In other studies, we observed that cells that had interacted with haptenated liposomes also failed to stimulate the differentiation of syngeneic "memory" cell populations into cytotoxic cells (Ozato and Henney, 1978). In this context, it is useful to point out that cells that had interacted with liposomes were capable of stimulating both primary and secondary responses to alloantigens, so that the overall antigenicity of the cells (and, indeed, their susceptibility to cytotoxic attack by alloimmune CTL) was not affected by their assimilation of exogenous lipid. It is, however, conceivable that liposomes became associated to a lesser extent with alloantigen-presenting (stimulator) cells than with other lymphocytes in the spleen-cell pool.

The studies reported in Tables 4 and 5 and in Figs. 4 and 5 make several interesting points with respect to the use of haptenated proteins to induce CTL formation.

1. There was no evidence that the protein backbone contributed to the specificity of the response engendered. Thus, CTL induced by TNP-HSA lyse, with equivalent efficiency, cells bearing TNP coupled to KLH and to BSA (Table 4).

2. We have examined a variety of serum proteins; all, when haptenated, were capable of stimulating CTL formation. There was, then, no evidence that the phenomenon described was restricted by the proteins used to "present" hapten.

3. There seemed to be a "threshold" of substition of the various proteins below which they did not serve as appropriate antigenic matrices for hapten presentation. Thus, when HSA was substituted to differing extents with TNP, only hapten concentrations equal to or greater than 30 mol/mol elicited hapten-specific cytotoxic effectors and rendered cells susceptible to lysis (Table 4). Hapten concentrations below this were not efficient, even though they often rendered cells equally susceptible to lysis by complement and anti-TNP. The "threshold" substitution for TNP varied with the different proteins employed.

The observations that haptens transferred to the cell surface via interactions with liposomes were not reactive with hapten-specific CTL parallel closely a recent report by Henkart et al. (1977). These investigators found that TNP coupled to a stearoyl dextran and then bound to mouse spleen cells was similarly "unrecognized" by T effector cells. These findings led them to suggest that the H-2 restriction of TNP-specific CTL, and their inability to lyse cells bearing TNP-dextran, were linked, and the the effector cell was directed against, and required on the target cell, hapten-modified H-2 antigen. This conclusion has also been reached by Forman et al. (1977a,b), using a biochemical approach. These investigators observed that target cells treated with increasing amounts of TNBS became able to stimulate hapten-specific CTL and to serve as targets only when they exhibited MHC-encoded products that could be precipitated by anti-TNP antibody. These studies together with our own findings using haptenated liposomes seem to lend credence to a "single-receptor" model for hapten recognition by T effector cells. This concept, however, seems to be at odds with the findings that di- (and tri-) nitrophenylated proteins can stimulate CTL production and that cells incubated with haptenated proteins can serve as targets for hapten-specific CTL (see Figs. 1–5) (Schmitt-Verhulst *et al.*, 1978; Ozato and Henney, 1978).

One could use several arguments in attempting to "marry" the two conflicting arms of these data. A prominent consideration would be that transhaptenation from protein to cell-surface components might be responsible for the effects noted. This is unlikely, since the protein preparations used were haptenated covalently under conditions in which the substitution was primarily with ϵ-NH_2 groups of lysine. Indeed, in a careful study addressed to this point, Schmitt-Verhulst *et al.* (1978) established that the hapten present on the TNP-BSA preparations used to "sensitize" target cells did not dissociate or cause trinitrophenylation of other cell-surface components. Thus, it appears unlikely that the ability of haptenated proteins to induce CTL formation and to render target cells susceptible to the action of such cells is due to a secondary haptenation of MHC products.

It is possible that the contrasting findings obtained employing haptenated liposomes and haptenated proteins to induce CTL formation can be reconciled by proposing that T cells cannot recognize hapten in a lipophilic environment, but require that the hapten be presented in association with protein. If so, there still seems to be a stringent requirement for presenting the hapten on a protein matrix. Thus, even though incubation with TNP[20]-HSA rendered cells susceptible to lysis by anti-TNP and complement, this procedure did not render the cells susceptible to lysis by hapten-specific CTL (see Table 4). This is reminiscent of the findings of Forman *et al.* (1977a,b) that there was a "threshold" concentration of TNBS needed to induce cells capable of stimulating CTL production. Hence it seems clear that two criteria have to be met for hapten to be recognized by cytotoxic T cells:

1. The hapten needs to be presented on the cell surface in association with a protein.
2. A critical hapten density is necessary irrespective of whether the protein substituted is an integral component of the cell membrane (as in TNBS) or is passively inserted.

While both MHC products and hapten need to be presented to the T cell, the studies with TNP proteins argue that they do not have to be present on the same molecule. Nevertheless, there appear to be some stringent structural relationships between hapten and H-2 antigens, for the mere presence of hapten on the surface of a cell of appropriate *H-2* haplotype is not sufficient either to trigger CTL formation or to serve as a target for hapten-specific CTL. It is possible that highly substituted proteins show an increased tendency to interact with MHC gene products in some way. Clearly, more studies on the interrelationship between haptenated proteins and the H-2 antigens of cells with which they are incubated are called for.

ACKNOWLEDGMENTS. Some of these studies were initiated in the Department of Medicine, Johns Hopkins University Medical School. This work was supported by grants Al 15383 and Al 15384 from the National Institute of Allergy and Infectious Disease.

References

Benacerraf, B., and Gell, P.G., 1959, Studies on hypersensitivity. III. The relation between delayed reactivity to the picryl group of conjugates and contact sensitivity, *Immunology* 2:219.

Bevan, M.J., 1975, The major histocompatibility complex determines susceptibility to cytotoxic T cells directed against minor histocompatibility antigens, *J. Exp. Med.* 142:1349.

Forman, J., 1977, Cytotoxic T cells distinguish between trinitrophenyl- and dinitrophenyl-modified syngeneic cells, *J. Exp. Med.* 146:600.

Forman, J., Vitetta, E.S., Hart, D.A., and Klein, J., 1977a, Relationship between trinitrophenyl and H-2 antigens on trinitrophenyl-modified spleen cells. I. H-2 antigens on cells treated with trinitrobenzene sulfonic acid are derivatized, *J. Immunol* 118:797.

Forman, J., Vitetta, E.S., and Hart, D.A., 1977b, Relationship between derivatization of H-2 antigens with trinitrophenyl and the ability of trinitrophenyl-modified cells to react functionally in the CML assay, *J. Immunol.* 118:803.

Gordon, R.D., Simpson, E., and Samelson, L.E., 1975, *In vitro* cell-mediated immune responses to the male specific (H-Y) antigen in mice, *J. Exp. Med.* 142:1108.

Henkart, P.A., Schmitt-Verhulst, A.M., and Shearer, G.M., 1977, Specificity of cytotoxic effector cells directed against trinitrobenzene sulfonate-modified syngeneic cells: Failure to recognize cell surface-bound trinitrophenyl dextran, *J. Exp. Med.* 146:1068.

Huang, L., Ozato, K., and Pagano, R.E., 1978, Interactions of phospholipid vesicles with murine lymphocytes. I. Vesicle–cell absorption and fusion as alternate pathways of uptake, *Membrane Biochem.* 1:1.

Hunter, W.W., and Greenwood, F.C., 1962, Preparation of iodine-131 labelled human growth hormone of high specific activity, *Nature (London)* 194:495.

Little, J.R., and Eisen, H.N., 1967, Preparation of immunogenic 2,4-dinitrophenyl and

2,4,6-trinitrophenyl proteins, in: *Methods in Immunolgy and Immunochemistry* (C.A. Williams and M.W. Chase, eds.), Vol. 1, p. 128, Academic Press, New York.

Lowry, O.H., Rosebrough, N.J., Farr, L.A., and Randall, R.J., 1951, Protein measurement with Folin phenol reagents, *J. Biol. Chem.* **193**:265.

Ozato, K., Ziegler, H.K., and Henney, C.S., 1978, Liposomes as model membrane systems for immune attack. I. Transfer of antigenic determinants to lymphocyte membranes following interactions with hapten bearing liposomes, *J. Immunol.* **121**:1376.

Ozato, K., and Henney, C.S., 1978, Studies on lymphocyte-mediated cytolysis. XII. Hapten transferred to cell surfaces by interaction with liposomes is recognized by antibody but not by hapten-specific H-2 restricted cytotoxic T cells, *J. Immunol.* **121**:2405.

Rollinghoff, M., Starzinski-Powitz, A., Pfizenmaier, K., and Wagner, H., 1977, Cyclophosphamide-sensitive T lymphocytes suppress the *in vivo* generation of antigen-specific cytotoxic T lymphocytes, *J. Exp. Med.* **145**:455.

Schmitt-Verhulst, A.M., Pettinelli, C.B., Henkart, P.A., Lunney, J.K., and Shearer, G., 1978, H-2 restricted cytotoxic effectors generated *in vitro* by the addition of trinitrophenyl-conjugated soluble proteins. *J. Exp. Med.* **147**:352.

Shearer, G.M., 1974, Cell mediated cytotoxicity to trinitrophenyl-modified syngeneic lymphocytes, *Eur. J. Immunol.* **4**:527.

Six, H.R., Uemura, K., and Kinsky, C.S., 1973, Effect of immunoglobulin class and affinity on the initiation of complement dependent damage to liposomal model membranes sensitized with dinitrophenylated phospholipids, *Biochemistry* **13**:4003.

Svehag, S.E., and Schilling, W., 1973, Solubilization of species-specific antigens and murine alloantigens by pulsed high frequency sonic energy, *Scand. J. Immunol.* **2**:115.

Yasuda, T., Dancey, G.F., and Kinsky, S.C., 1977, Immunogenicity of liposomal model membranes in mice: Dependence on phospholipid composition, *Proc. Natl. Acad. Sci. U.S.A.* **74**:1234.

Zinkernagel, R.M., and Doherty, P.C., 1974, Restriction of *in vitro* T cell-mediated cytotoxicity in lymphocytic choriomeningitis within a syngeneic or semiallogeneic system, *Nature (London)* **248**:701.

5

New Thoughts on the Control of Self-Recognition, Cell Interactions, and Immune Responsiveness by Major Histocompatibility Complex Genes

David H. Katz

1. Introduction

It is abundantly clear that our perceptions about the major histocompatibility complex (MHC) have changed quite substantially during the 1970's. No longer does the term histocompatibility connote merely identities, similarities, or differences among tissue-transplantation antigens inherited by each individual member of a given species. Now, that term stands for a polymorphic family of genes and molecules the biological functions of which appear to play central roles in governing cell differentiation, cell–cell recognition, quality as well as quantity of immunological responsiveness, and probably a variety of other functions that have yet to be discovered. The realization that the biological importance of the MHC is broader than had initially been apparent has generated considerable excitement, a flurry of basic research endeavors, and an increasingly voluminous literature that becomes more and more difficult to keep track of and, at times, to understand. As can be expected, much of the literature, particularly recently, tends to be a bit repetitious in terms of both experimental approach and interpretation of data, a situation that seems to be inevitable whenever a given area of science is highly popular and pursued by large numbers of investigators.

David H. Katz • Department of Cellular and Developmental Immunology, Scripps Clinic and Research Foundation, La Jolla, California 92037.

In view of this problem, this chapter was purposely prepared with its main goal being to share some new thinking, supported in part by new data, on some rather well-worn topics pertaining to involvement of MHC genes and molecules in immunological responses. Only for purposes of orienting the reader will previous work and concepts be reviewed, and this will be done as briefly as possible.

2. Self-Recognition and Cell–Cell Interactions

One of the important advances in our fundamental understanding of MHC control of the immune system has been the realization that when immune responses require cell–cell interactions for proper development and control, such interactions occur most efficiently between partner cells that are genetically identical in certain key regions of the MHC. These genetic restrictions were first described in studies of interactions between regulatory (i.e., helper) T lymphocytes and B-lymphocyte precursors of antibody-secreting cells (Kindred and Shreffler, 1972; Katz et al., 1973a,b) and in cooperative T lymphocyte–macrophage interactions (Rosenthal and Shevach, 1973). Subsequently, similar restrictions were found to exist in the most efficient lysis of target cells by specific cytotoxic T lymphocytes (CTL) or killer cells (Shearer, 1974; Zinkernagel and Doherty, 1974a; Koszinowski and Ertl, 1975; Bevan, 1975; Gordon et al., 1975). Genetic mapping studies documented that gene(s) controlling T–B cell interactions are located in the *I* region of the mouse *H-2* complex (Katz et al., 1975), a remarkable association with the same region containing *Ir* genes (see below) and also the genes encoding cell-surface macromolecules known to be the most potent alloantigens in stimulating the development of mixed-lymphocyte reactions (MLRS) (Bach et al., 1972). The genes involved in the CTL–target cell interactions have been mapped in the *K* and *D* regions of the *H-2* complex (Schmitt-Verhulst and Shearer, 1975; Blanden et al., 1975), the regions initially recognized to contain genes encoding the classic serologically defined transplantation antigens.

Essentially two major concepts have evolved to explain the MHC-linked genetic restrictions on cell interactions. The first hypothesis, which stemmed from analysis of such restrictions in T–B cell interactions, considered that interactions among various cell types in the immune system are mediated by cell-interaction (CI) molecules located on the cell surface, at least some of which are encoded by MHC genes (i.e., *I*-region genes in this case), and which are quite distinct from the lymphocyte receptors specific for conventional antigens (Katz et al., 1973a,b; Katz and Benacerraf, 1975). The CI-molecule concept therefore emphasizes a dual-recognition mechanism that involves at least two distinct molecular interactions in lymphocyte activation, one utilizing antigen-specific receptors and the second consisting of reactions between the relevant CI structures and their corresponding receptors. The second major concept, derived primarily from studies in the CTL systems, considered that T lymphocytes have receptors that recognize, not antigen alone, but antigen in some form of association with MHC-gene products on cell-surface membranes; this concept of "altered-self" (Zinkernagel and Doherty, 1974b) recognition by T lymphocytes has subsequently been modified in various ways, but all versions still differ substantially from the CI-molecule concept in predicting the existence of a *single* receptor on T cells simultaneously recognizing modified determinants on the cell surface. To date, no definitive proof has been obtained to establish which of these two models is correct.

These two very distinct hypotheses concerning the basis of MHC restrictions on cellular interactions among components of the immune system place such genetic restrictions in very different biological perspectives. Single-recognition mechanisms, such as the altered-self model, limit the biological connotations of these genetic restrictions to the immune system. The CI-molecule concept of dual recognition, on the other hand, suggests the existence of a mechanism for highly specific *self-recognition* that aside from its obvious importance for proper cell communication in the immune system where it was first discovered and analyzed provides a general mechanism for control of effective cell interactions in nonimmunological organ systems as well. Moreover, delineation of the mechanisms responsible for conserving self-recognition and, alternatively, understanding processes that potentially disturb it (and the consequences of such disturbances to the individual) could open an important avenue toward elucidating crucial events in normal and abnormal cell differentiation in eukaryotic organisms. In many ways, therefore, what we have been studying as a curious phenomenon in the immune system may have substantial biological implications.

3. Concept of Adaptive Differentiation

The validity of the CI-molecule concept as an appropriate interpretation of the basis for genetic restrictions in T–B cell interactions came under question amid the reports of other investigators who failed to find similar restrictions in different systems in which T–B cell cooperative responses were analyzed. Particularly important were those studies performed with cells obtained from bone marrow chimeras. Studies were made with lymphocytes obtained from bone marrow chimeric mice that had been prepared by reconstituting lethally irradiated $(A \times B)$ F_1 recipients with a mixture of bone marrow cells derived from each of the respective parents, A and B. In such circumstances, T lymphocytes that were originally derived from donors of different H-2 haplotypes (i.e., parent A and parent B), but had differentiated within a mutual host F_1 environment, were found to be independently capable of interacting effectively with B cells derived from conventional donors of the opposite parental type (von Boehmer et al., 1975).

Since the parental A and B lymphoid populations of such chimeras were mutually tolerant of one another (i.e., unable to exert reciprocal alloreactivity), the question arose as to whether the *failure* of partner cells derived from nontolerant histoincompatible donors to interact effectively might be due to some type of inhibitory influences resulting from subtle alloreactivity between such cells. However, this seemed untenable for a number of reasons discussed more fully elsewhere (Katz, 1976, 1977a,b; Katz and Benacerraf, 1976).

It became necessary, therefore, to address the paradox that consisted of (1) the striking degree of MHC-linked genetic restrictions imposed on effective T–B cell interactions; (2) the absence of demonstrable suppressive influences to explain such genetic restrictions; and (3) the seemingly contradictory data obtained with T- and B-lymphocyte populations derived from bone marrow chimeras. These paradoxical observations seemed to be most logically explained by a concept of *adaptive differentiation* of lymphoid-cell precursors (Katz, 1976, 1977a,b; Katz and Benacerraf, 1976; Katz et al., 1976). We proposed that the process of stem-cell differentiation is critically regulated by histocompatibility molecules on cell surfaces, and that such differentiation is "adaptive" to the environment in which it takes place. This concept, in brief, predicted that (1) during early differentiation, lymphoid-cell precursors "learn" the relevant compatibilities required of them for *effective* cell–cell interactions; and (2) moreover, this learning process is dictated by the MHC phenotype of the environment in which such differentiation takes place.

Our first experiments designed to address this possibility yielded results that were indeed consistent with the hypothesis (Katz, 1976; Katz and Benacerraf, 1976). Subsequently, a number of studies by different investigators, using both conventional animals and (primarily) artificially constructed bone marrow chimeras, have demonstrated that lymphocytes do indeed undergo adaptive differentiation. This has been shown in the case of T lymphocytes destined to become CTL (Bevan, 1977; Zinkernagel et al., 1978a,b) as well as regulatory T cells responsible for providing helper function (Katz et al., 1978; Sprent, 1978; Kappler and Marrack, 1978). In addition, Zinkernagel et al. (1978a,b) and Fink and

Bevan (1978) have provided evidence that the primary stages of adaptive differentiation of T-cell precursors of CTL take place within the thymic microenvironment. The situation is a bit less clear in the case of helper T lymphocytes, which, in some cases, have appeared to be influenced to a similar extent by the thymus (Waldmann et al., 1979; Bevan and Fink, 1978), whereas our own studies have revealed that the thymus exerts only partial influence on the learning process undergone by helper T cells, and that a significant extrathymic influence is also crucial for T cells of this category (Katz et al., 1979).

Additionally, our own studies have emphasized the fact that B lymphocytes also undergo similar processes of adaptive differentiation in both conventional (Katz, 1976; Katz and Benacerraf, 1976) and bone marrow chimera (Katz et al., 1978) animal models. The significance of the findings made with B lymphocytes to the whole issue pertaining to single vs. dual recognition models cannot be overemphasized. Thus, quite unlike the situation with T cells—in which the argument can be made that T lymphocytes that manifest restrictions of one type or another could be reflecting their receptor specificities for antigen-plus-"self" (Zinkernagel and Doherty, 1974b)—this argument does not easily explain the findings on a B-cell adaptation; indeed, B-cell adaptive differentiation is almost exclusively explainable by a dual-recognition, i.e., CI-molecule, model.

The available evidence, therefore, supports the likelihood that adaptive differentiation normally dictates the phenotypic expression of preferential cell–cell interactions among components of the immune system. We have recently developed a theoretical model to explain how adaptive differentiation of lymphocytes may occur during normal development. This model has been described elsewhere (Katz, 1980) and will be summarized here only by the following seven statements.

1. All cell interactions within an individual member of the species are interactions of *self-recognition*. These self-recognition processes are mediated through cell-surface cell-interaction (CI) molecules [defined in (4) below].

2. Each individual member of a species possesses the genotypic library for *all* CI-molecule specificities expressed in the species. This library spans not only many different specificities but also a whole spectrum (i.e., from low to high) of binding affinities between the two interacting molecules.

3. One of the earliest and most important decisions in morphogenesis is which CI phenotype will be worn by the background environment. Once this decision has been made, by whatever mechanism, the phenotype of self-reactivity characteristic of that individual is firmly established.

4. CI molecules are defined as follows: in any interaction between two partner cells, at least one of the two CI molecules is a product of MHC gene(s); the second molecule may either be an MHC-gene product or a product of a non-MHC gene; i.e., it could be, in part, encoded by a V gene. Thus, in any set of two interacting CI molecules, one molecule can be considered to be the ligand (hereafter termed $CI_{A,B, \text{ or } C}$), whereas the second molecule may be considered to be the specific receptor for that ligand (hereafter termed $\alpha CI_{A,B, \text{ or } C}$).

5. Determined by the CI phenotype of the environment, differentiating lymphocytes undergo a process of *selection* that involves deletion or abortion of cells with high-affinity receptors for native (i.e., self-) CI molecules; this deletion process is accompanied by a corollary process in which cells with low-to-moderate-affinity receptors for native CI molecules predominantly emerge. These cells then constitute the functional interacting populations involved in self-regulating further differentiation and responsiveness.

6. A concomitant selection process occurs among the cells bearing receptors for CI molecules expressed predominantly in other individual members of the species (i.e., nonself). In these cases, cells with high-affinity receptors predominate, whereas low-to-moderate-affinity nonself cells are eliminated. The latter cells can serve no useful function in the inappropriate environment and, without this selection mechanism, might proliferate uncontrollably.

7. On the basis of the aforementioned points, all cell interactions within a species, even those occurring between cells from *different* individual members of the species, are interactions of *self-recognition*. They differ only in the binding affinities of interactions; i.e., those occurring among partner cells involved in physiological responses within the same individual are of low to moderate affinity, while those occurring between cells from different individuals are of high affinity. These high-affinity reactions are most probably those that we have classically termed *alloreactions*.

With this summary of our thinking on these issues as a background, I would now like to focus the subsequent discussion on how our model addresses certain important issues that are still unexplained.

4. Relevance of the Proposed Mechanisms of Adaptive Differentiation to Certain Unresolved Immunological Puzzles

Any theoretical framework constructed to explain differentiation events in the immune system must take into account at least certain of the major unresolved questions. Foremost among many in our field are the interrelated issues of recognition mechanisms in general, T-cell recognition in particular, and the nature and function of MHC-linked immune-response *(Ir)* genes. It is on these three indisputably intertwined points that the remainder of this discussion will focus. These issues have been addressed in recent hypothetical papers by several other investigators who have been directly working in the pertinent areas (Janeway *et al.,* 1976; Benacerraf, 1978; Schwartz, 1978), and naturally there are some areas of overlap as well as clear differences among the various opinions (as will be pointed out below).

5. Recognition Mechanisms in the Immune System

The only undebatable point concerning questions of immunological recognition mechanisms is that B lymphocytes have Ig molecules on their surface membranes that are specifically capable of binding antigenic determinants. The exact molecular nature of corresponding antigen-binding receptors on T cells has not yet been delineated, although substantial evidence supports the likelihood that at least certain of these receptors on T cells have antigen-combining sites encoded by the same heavy-chain *V* genes used by B cells for synthesis of their Ig receptors (Binz and Wigzell, 1977a,b; Krawinkel *et al.,* 1977).

The controversial points are as follows: (1) Are recognition events in the immune system singular or dualistic in nature? (2) Are T cells unique in their clear dependency on reacting with MHC-gene products, in addition to non-MHC antigens (by whatever mechanism), to be properly activated, or is this a more general requirement including B cells as well? (3) Why are so many cells within a given individual capable of reacting to nonself alloantigens?

To summarize briefly our own thinking on these points:

1. We favor the possibility that there are two recognition systems that operate in concert with one another for purposes of cell triggering, i.e., one receptor for MHC (i.e., CI) molecules on partner cells, and a second receptor for non-MHC (i.e., conventional) antigens; these receptors coexist, *but as separate entities,* on each individual lymphocyte. The alternative possibility, namely, that a single receptor binds to a "complex antigenic determinant" comprised of antigenic fragments associated with self-MHC determinants, seems unlikely to us for reasons given in detail elsewhere (Katz, 1976, 1977a,b). Nevertheless, formal proof for one or the other of these two possibilities is still lacking.

2. Although the greatest experimental emphasis thus far has been placed on T-cell functions and the genetic restrictions imposed thereon, this alone does not provide a very strong argument against a more

general requirement for other cells, notably B lymphocytes (but not to exclude macrophages), to also recognize and react with CI molecules on interacting partner cells in order to consummate the purpose of the interaction. Indeed, as mentioned above, we have obtained data that speak strongly in favor of this possibility (Katz, 1976; Katz and Benacerraf, 1976; Katz et al., 1978).

In other words, we believe that B lymphocytes, like T cells, have two independent recognition mechanisms, one of which is directed toward self-CI molecules. Hence, when partner cells (i.e., T and B lymphocytes) interact with one another, we envisage a two-way bridge being created by the binding of each cell to the other via their respective αCI receptors and the corresponding CI target molecules recognized by such receptors; this is in addition to the binding of antigenic determinants by antigen-specific receptors on each cell. Likewise, we believe that just as macrophages exert selective pressures on T cells during antigen-induced responses, they exert comparable selective pressures on B cells via similar MHC-linked recognition events (i.e., recognition of macrophage CI molecules by αCI receptors on B cells). T cells can likewise exert such selective pressures on one another and on B cells, and vice versa.

3. The existence of relatively large numbers of alloreactive cells has been one of the most perplexing issues in transplantation biology. As discussed in detail elsewhere (Katz, 1980), the adaptive-differentiation model summarized above provides an explanation for the high frequency of cells that appear to be alloreactive when appropriately manipulated experimentally, and also suggests an important function they may play as regulatory cells within their native environment, i.e., to provide an important "brake" to minimize replication of cells bearing the corresponding nonself-CI molecules. The proposed importance of this regulatory surveillance mechanism provokes the logical question of what provides an analogous brake for growth of low-to-moderate-affinity αCI$_A$-type cells in individual A. This brake is inherent in the sophisticated regulatory feedback control mechanisms that constitute the normal operation of the immune system of individual A; indeed, it is conceivable that A-type cells performing negative regulatory functions that limit or ablate any given response may do so by binding to target CI molecules with combining sites higher than usual affinity.

The aspect of our thinking with respect to differences in affinity being a crucial point of distinction between interactions with self (low)- vs. nonself (high)-CI specificities is in agreement with a model proposed recently by Janeway et al. (1976). Where our reasoning differs fundamentally from theirs is that we believe that low-affinity receptors for self-

CI molecules and high-affinity receptors capable of reacting with nonself-CI molecules exist on *separate* cells altogether. Janeway *et al.* (1976) have proposed that the same receptor that binds to self with low affinity is capable of binding with high affinity to certain nonself-MHC antigens. If this were so, it would become difficult to account for the fact that there are B lymphocytes capable of producing alloantibodies specific for nonself-MHC antigens (including Ia antigens); such alloantibodies that would have high affinity for nonself would likewise have the capacity to bind to self with low affinity, a situation of potential danger to the individual because of the likely interference with normal physiological cell interactions that would result from the presence of such antibodies.

Our thinking also agrees with that of Janeway *et al.* (1976) in considering that the antiidiotype antibodies directed against alloantigen receptors in the rat, which have been analyzed so extensively and well by Binz and Wigzell (1977a,b), are actually recognizing idiotypes on the second of two receptors on T cells; in our terminology, the Binz–Wigzell antiidiotypic antibodies are reacting with high-affinity αCI receptors. If the model proposed here is, in principle, correct, we would further state that it should be possible to induce antibodies capable of reacting with low-affinity αCI receptors for self-CI molecules. Such anti-αCI antibodies would be capable of blocking physiological cell–cell interactions. Recent experiments in our laboratory, which are presented below, are most readily interpretable in the context of such an anti-αCI response playing a natural regulatory role in certain immune responses.

6. Some Current Thoughts on *Ir* Genes

The *Ir* genes, located in the *I* region of the mouse *H-2* complex, have clearly been found to be quite specific in terms of the responses over which their control is exerted. This, together with the fact that most responses controlled by *Ir* genes involve the participation of T cells, prompted the speculation that *Ir* genes encode antigen-receptor molecules on T lymphocytes (Benacerraf and McDevitt, 1972). It now appears that this is not the case.

Before we discuss our own thinking on this issue, it is pertinent to analyze other recent speculations concerning *Ir*-gene function. Although several examples could be cited, we believe that two of these, proposed by investigators who have devoted considerable energy to this problem, are of particular interest and attractiveness. Thus, Benacerraf (1978) has recently made an elegant statement of the case in favor of *Ir*-gene function being located at the level of macrophage antigen presentation, a notion originally proposed by Rosenthal, Shevach, Paul, and their colleagues (Rosenthal and Shevach, 1973; Paul *et al.*, 1977; Rosenthal, 1978; Schwartz, 1978). Benacerraf (1978) further formalized such notions by stating that the products of *Ir* genes, present on the surface membrane of the macrophage, could have combining-site activity capable of reacting with defined sequences of a limited number of amino acids (i.e., 3 or 4) within the structure of a larger macromolecule; the consequence of this reaction between *Ir*-gene product and a given amino acid sequence would be a highly specific display of the resulting complex formed between the exogenous antigen and the macrophage-bound *Ir*-gene product. This complex would then be recognized specifically by T cells with receptors consisting of combining sites of corresponding specificity for a given complex. This model therefore postulates that the T cell sees antigen oriented in a unique structural way by virtue of its reaction with the *Ir*-gene products; although the implied suggestion is that such recognition occurs via a *single* receptor entity, a dual-recognition model is not altogether ruled out.

The attractiveness of this model is that it accounts for the exquisite specificity of *Ir*-gene function without demanding an extraordinarily large number of distinct *Ir* genes. Thus, Benacerraf (1978) has beautifully explained the possibility that specificity differences could be accounted for by imagining that a limited number of *Ir* genes, each capable of reacting with a defined sequence of 3 or 4 amino acids, could display a highly diverse antigenic universe depending on differences in the way that each complex macromolecule would subsequently become oriented on the macrophage surface membrane after reacting with the *Ir*-gene product(s). Uniqueness, therefore, would be more a property of the inherent structural attributes of the exogenous antigen than of any enormous number of individual *Ir* genes. This model also accounts for most of the work demonstrating the level of control by *Ir* genes in terms of macrophage–T cell interactions and the like.

The second model, recently proposed by Schwartz (1978), also considers that T cells see antigen in the form of a complex developed by associations with *Ir*-gene products on the macrophage surface via a single receptor for this "complex antigenic determinant" (CAD). Schwartz goes further in proposing that self-antigens associate with *Ir*-gene products and during the early course of ontogeny, potentially reactive T cells for such self-CADs are deleted during the process of tolerance induction. Nonself-antigens also must interact with *Ir*-gene products to form CADs that are then necessarily recognized by T cells with corresponding receptor specificity. *Ir*-gene defects are thereby explained as reflecting those situations in which a CAD formed between a nonself-antigen and *Ir*-gene product exhibits sufficient mimicry with the self-CAD; since T cells capable of recognizing self-CAD have been deleted, any CAD of sufficient mimicry will naturally fail to elicit a response. This model likewise accounts for many observations made recently, particularly those that focused on the relationship of *Ir*-gene function to macrophage antigen presentation.

However, neither of these models adequately accounts for several observations that appear to be central to all these issues.

Let us first consider the allogeneic effect, the descriptive term given to the biological consequences of a transient transplantation reaction whereby one cell population provides differentiation signals to a target-cell population as a result of reacting with such target cells via specific allorecognition (see Katz, 1977b, Chapter XI). It is pertinent that the allogeneic effect represents precisely the circumstance in which a reaction with MHC-encoded target molecules (i.e., *I*-region molecules), concomitant in time with the exposure of the target cell to its relevant antigenic determinants, results in the delivery of stimulatory signals to such target cells that drive them onward along the pathway of differentiation. Since the alloreactive cells that mediate this effect need not exhibit any relationship to the non-MHC antigen employed, it is clear that the pertinent recognition necessary for the triggering events is that concerned with the MHC-encoded cell-surface target molecules. This exemplifies, therefore, the occurrence of two independent recognition events, i.e., one directed to CI-molecule determinants and the other directed to non-MHC antigens, capable of triggering lymphocytes. Clearly, there is no obvious relationship between such triggering events and the need for complex antigenic determinants, of the type described above, in such circumstances.

Perhaps more important is the fact that several experimental situations have been used to demonstrate the ability of an appropriately timed allogeneic effect to overcome *Ir*-gene defects. On the one hand, it has been possible to demonstrate the capacity of an allogeneic effect to permit nonresponder mice to make IgG (as well as IgM) antibody responses to a synthetic antigen under *Ir*-gene control (Ordal and Grumet, 1972). In this instance, the allogeneic effect provided a necessary stimulus to target B cells, thereby replacing a normal interaction step missing in such circumstances. More recently, we have used the allogeneic effect as a mechanism for stimulating the induction of (responder × nonresponder) F_1 helper T cells capable of effectively interacting with nonresponder B cells, in studies that will be summarized below.

7. Some New Observations on *Ir*-Gene Mechanisms

If *Ir* genes do not encode the combining site(s) of antigen-specific T-cell receptors, what role is served by these genes? We believe that an important clue to the answer to this question is the concomitant location in the *I* region of the *Ir* genes and the genes responsible for (1) effective cell–cell communication among different lymphoid cells and (2) encoding determinants that are strong stimulants of alloreactivity in MLRS. We further believe that the answer is, in fact, quite simple: *Ir genes encode CI molecules*.

Experimental support for this interpretation was obtained several years ago. We reported then that T cells from (responder × nonresponder) F₁ hybrids primed to the synthetic terpolymer L-glutamic acid-L-lysine-L-tyrosine (GLT), responses to which are governed by *H-2* linked *Ir-GLT* genes, were restricted in their ability to provide GLT-specific help for 2,4-dinitrophenyl (DNP)-primed B cells from the respective parental mice in response to DNP-GLT (Katz *et al.*, 1973c). Thus, such F₁ T cells were able to provide normal helper activity for DNP-specific B cells from responder, but not from nonresponder, donor mice. This finding contrasted sharply with the indiscriminant ability of F₁ T cells to interact effectively with partner B cells from *either* parent when the carrier antigen employed was not one to which responses were governed by a known *Ir* gene. This observation has subsequently been confirmed by others in studies conducted in mice (Pierce, 1977; Press and McDevitt, 1977) and guinea pigs (Yamashita and Shevach, 1978).

These observations were interpreted as an indication that in heterozygous individuals, independent subpopulations of interacting T lymphocytes existed, one each corresponding to the respective parental type (Katz *et al.*, 1973c). Hence, we envisaged that stimulation of a (responder × nonresponder) F₁ T cell population by GLT would sensitize only the population of T cells able to recognize and react with the functional cell-interaction (CI) phenotype of the responder parent; F₁ T cells corresponding to the nonresponder parent CI phenotype would not be stimulated by GLT. This situation would therefore be manifested as defective ability of F₁ T cells to interact with nonresponder B cells irrespective of the antigen specificity of the latter. This original interpretation (Katz *et al.*, 1973c) has been reinforced by the subsequent demonstrations of the existence of independent F₁ T-cell subpopulations reactive with each respective parental CI phenotype (Skidmore and Katz, 1977; Paul *et al.*, 1977; Miller and Vadas, 1977; Thomas and Shevach, 1978; McDougal and Cort, 1978; Swierkosz *et al.*, 1978).

Quite recently, we have designed experiments to determine whether the normally restricted cooperating phenotype of (responder × nonresponder) F₁ T cells specific for GLT could be experimentally manipulated to express a different cooperating phenotype. Specifically, we were interested in generating GLT-specific F₁ T cells that might now express cooperative helper activity for nonresponder B cells. These studies have demonstrated that the usually restricted cooperating phenotype of (responder × nonresponder) F_1 T cells *can* be changed by inducing an allogeneic effect during the priming of such F_1 mice (Katz *et al.*, 1979). The experimental data presented below confirm this point.

CAF$_1$ T cells obtained from mice primed to GLT, either in the absence of any allogeneic effect or in the presence of an allogeneic effect induced by one or the other parental cell type, display the pattern of cooperative helper activity for DNP-primed B cells from either A/J, BALB/c, or CAF$_1$ donor mice that is depicted in Figs. 1 and 2. The only pertinent difference between the two experiments illustrated in these figures is that 5×10^6 B cells and 10×10^6 helper T cells were transferred

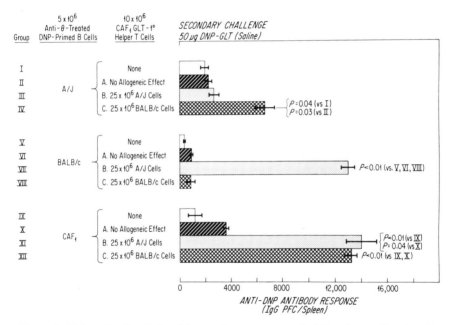

Figure 1. Helper-T-cell activity of (responder × nonresponder) F_1 spleen cells primed to GLT under the influence of an allogeneic effect. Irradiated (675 rads) CAF$_1$ recipient mice were injected intravenously (i.v.) with 5×10^6 DNP-primed B cells from either A/J, BALB/c, or CAF$_1$ donors, either in the absence of helper cells or together with 10×10^6 spleen cells taken from F_1 mice primed to GLT either alone (50 μg GLT in CFA followed 10 days later by a second injection of 50 μg in saline) or under the influence of an allogeneic effect induced by i.v. injection (on day 10 after initial immunization with GLT) of 25×10^6 spleen cells from parental A/J or BALB/c donors; spleens were removed from such donor mice 7 days after the second injection of GLT. All recipients were challenged with 50 μg DNP-GLT in saline. The data are presented as geometric mean levels of individual IgG DNP-specific plaque-forming cells/spleen of groups of 5 mice each assayed on day 7 after cell transfer and secondary challenge. Horizontal brackets represent standard errors, and relevant P values depicting statistically significant differences are indicated alongside the corresponding bracket.

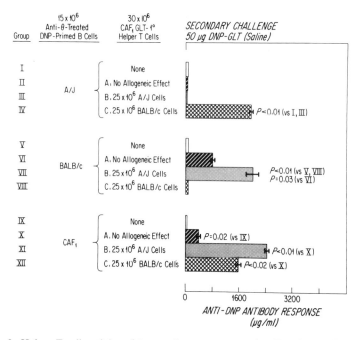

Figure 2. Helper-T-cell activity of (responder × nonresponder) F_1 spleen cells primed to GLT under the influence of an allogeneic effect. The same protocol as described in Fig. 1 was employed, with the only difference being the numbers of transferred B and T cells given to each recipient mouse. The data are presented as geometric mean levels of serum anti-DNP antibodies of individual mice in groups of 5 mice each bled on day 7 after cell transfer and secondary challenge. Horizontal brackets represent the range of standard errors, and relevant P values of statistically significant differences are indicated.

in one experiment (Fig. 1), while 15×10^6 B cells and 30×10^6 helper T cells were transferred in the other (Fig. 2).

What these experiments have revealed is that CAF_1 helper T cells primed to GLT in the absence of an allogeneic effect provide no help for B cells from A/J mice and variable levels of help for B cells from BALB/c or CAF_1 donor mice depending on the numbers of GLT helper T cells transferred. Note, for example, that 10×10^6 F_1 helper T cells provided only marginal help for F_1, and even less for BALB/c, B cells (Fig. 1), while significant levels of helper activity were observed in both cases when 30×10^6 GLT-primed F_1 cells were transferred (Fig. 2).

The remarkable findings are those pertaining to the patterns of F_1 helper activity, for the various B cells, that were generated under the influence of allogeneic effects induced by one or the other parental cell type. First, note that F_1 helper T cells generated under the influence of an allogeneic effect induced by either A/J or BALB/c parental cells were clearly and significantly enhanced in their levels of cooperative activity for B cells derived from F_1 donors (Figs. 1 and 2, groups XI and XII). This pattern of indiscriminately enhanced F_1 helper-T-cell activity as manifested with F_1 B cells did not hold true when such F_1 T cells were assayed for their ability to help nonresponder A/J or responder BALB/c parental B cells. Thus, F_1 T cells generated under the influence of an allogeneic effect induced by parental BALB/c cells were clearly capable of providing GLT-specific help for nonresponder A/J B cells (group IV), but were unable to provide detectable help for responder BALB/c cells (group VIII). Conversely, F_1 T cells generated during an allogeneic effect induced by parental A/J cells did not display effective helper activity for nonresponder A/J B cells (group III), while exhibiting significantly enhanced helper activity for responder BALB/c B cells (group VII).

These studies make two important points: (1) First, the usually restricted phenotype of (responder × nonresponder) F_1 T cells, which typically is permissive only for providing cooperative helper activity for B cells of responder type, but not of nonresponder type, *can* be changed by inducing an allogeneic effect during the priming of such F_1 mice. This is true *provided the allogeneic effect is induced by cells derived from the opposite, i.e.,* responder, parental type. (2) Actually, the ultimate cooperating phenotype of GLT-primed F_1 helper T cells is differentially and reciprocally directed toward B cells of one parental type or the other depending on which parental donor cells are used for inducing the allogeneic effect that takes place during the priming regimen. Thus, F_1 T cells primed to GLT under the influence of an allogeneic effect induced by parental BALB/c cells now provide effective help for nonresponder A/J B cells, but do not do so for responder BALB/c B cells, and vice versa. On the other hand, F_1 T cells primed to GLT under the influence of an allogeneic effect induced by either parental cell type display significantly enhanced levels of helper activity for B cells derived from F_1 donors.

The fact that the allogeneic effect induces such exquisite discriminatory helper activities when F_1 T cells are assayed on parental B cells, but loses this discriminatory aspect when F_1 B cells serve as the partner B cells in the assay, is perhaps the most pertinent aspect of these findings with respect to understanding the regulatory events that these data reflect. Parenthetically, the results with F_1 B cells provide additional arguments against any significant contribution made by contaminating parental B cells that may be carried over in the final assay system, but this possibility has been more directly circumvented as described elsewhere (Katz *et al.,* 1979).

We believe that these results illustrate the consequences of two interdependent events that are schematically illustrated in Fig. 3: First,

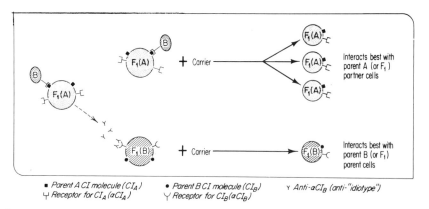

Figure 3. Influence of parental-cell-induced allogeneic effect on differentiation of F_1 lymphocytes. See the text for explanation.

the allogeneic effect induced by one parental cell type exerts powerful stimulatory signals that substantially augment the normal differentiation signals induced by immunization with antigen alone; this has been amply documented to occur in many previous studies (see Katz, 1977b, Chapter XI). The consequences of such stimulatory signals are reflected in the significant enhancement of GLT-specific helper-T-cell activity provided to B cells from F_1 responder and nonresponder donors. Of particular note is the capacity of the allogeneic effect, induced by responder cells, to draw out permissiveness of F_1 cells in providing GLT-specific help to the nonresponder B cells. Thus, the allogeneic effect has obviously provided the necessary stimulus, in addition to antigen, to encourage the differentiation of the subset of nonresponder T cells capable of interacting with DNP-primed nonresponder B cells.

The fact that the allogeneic effect was effective in inducing GLT-specific helper T cells, presumably of the "nonresponder-type" subset, must be viewed with serious consideration in the context of the afore-mentioned speculations that *Ir*-gene products react specifically with antigenic determinants at the level of the macrophage to orient and display the relevant determinants for recognition by T cells of corre-sponding specificity. It is difficult to envisage, for example, how an allogeneic effect could circumvent an *absolute* requirement for *Ir*-gene-controlled antigen display by macrophages. Rather, these data seem to argue against any such absolute requirement for macrophage presentation and tend to favor the possibility that the allogeneic effect permits the development of GLT-specific F_1 helper cells capable of interacting with nonresponder B cells by either (1) direct stimulation of the "nonrespon-der-type" subset of F_1 GLT-specific T cells to differentiate into effective helper cells or (2) elimination of some type of inherent suppressive mechanism that normally blocks development of GLT-specific helper T cells capable of cooperating with nonresponder B cells.

The second of the two interdependent events, and by far the more difficult to address, pertains to the explanation for the very striking discriminatory aspects of helper activities when F_1 T cells primed to antigen under influence of an allogeneic effect are assayed on *parental* B cells. Obviously, no direct evidence is available at present to permit conclusions concerning this aspect of the data. Nevertheless, we consider it possible that aside from the stimulatory consequences of the allogeneic effect in inducing helper-T-cell function as discussed above, a second consequence may be the stimulation of an F_1 response against certain of its own receptors that self-recognize native CI determinants (αCI). Thus, as illustrated in Fig. 3, when parental *B* cells induce an allogeneic effect in an $(A \times B)$ F_1, the response within the F_1 would be directed against self-receptors for *B*-type CI molecules (anti-αCI$_B$), and vice versa. These types of anti-"idiotype" responses against self-recognizing receptors would be capable of preventing development of helper T cells belonging to the corresponding parental-type T-cell subpopulation without adversely affecting the development of helper cells corresponding to the opposite parental-type T-cell subpopulation.

If studies currently in progress demonstrate anti-αCI reactions to be the mechanism responsible for the data just described, then one wonders what relationship such anti-αCI responses might have to the whole picture portrayed by *Ir* genes and the specificity they appear to display for the antigens under their control.

Let us now return to the premise stated at the outset of this section, namely, that *Ir* genes encode CI molecules. If *Ir* genes are actually *CI* genes and if CI molecules are distinct entities from antigen-specific receptors, how then do *Ir* genes exert such apparent specificity for antigen in responses over which they display control? In the context of the model being proposed here, there are three possible answers to this question depending on whether *Ir* genes encode molecules serving as (1) αCI receptors (at least in part), alone; (2) target CI molecules themselves; or (3) both αCI receptors and target CI molecules. These possibilities will be considered separately below.

If *Ir* genes encode αCI receptor molecules alone, either in part or whole, then it must be assumed that the affiliation of specific antigen-binding receptors on a given lymphocyte and the αCI receptor expressed by that same cell is somehow linked, either genetically or epigenetically, within a given individual of the species. Nevertheless, such affiliations could be initially random within the species at large. As discussed above, during the process of adaptive differentiation within a given individual, high-affinity αCI cells that are reactive with self-CI molecules of that individual's environment are deleted. It follows, then, that among the populations of deleted high-affinity cells would exist a certain fraction of the V-gene repertoire for non-MHC antigens; this fraction of the repertoire would therefore be functionally silent. Thus, if the antigen receptor for X happened to be affiliated consistently with a high-affinity αCI$_A$ receptor molecule within the environment of individual A, then functional deletion of such high-affinity αCI$_A$ cells would concomitantly be phenotypically displayed as an inability to develop responses to antigen X. Since abortion of high-affinity αCI$_A$ cells merely implies *functional* deletion of their CI-molecule-binding capability, such cells could still be present in the population. In this case, they would display their antigen-specific receptors capable of binding X but be impotent with respect to cooperating with partner cells to make an appropriate response; this is consistent with experimental observations (Dunham *et al.*, 1972; Hämmerling *et al.*, 1973).

If *Ir* genes encode target CI molecules, rather than αCI receptors, how can their apparent specificity for antigen be envisaged? Here again, the assumptions mentioned above with regard to the affiliation between antigen-specific receptors and αCI receptors on the same cell still pertain. However, an additional mechanism for *Ir*-gene-linked unresponsiveness now enters the equation. Let us assume that in individual A, there is heterogeneity among CI$_A$ that we can denote CI$_{A1, A2, A3, etc.}$; for each CI$_A$ specificity, there will be corresponding αCI$_A$ receptors, i.e., αCI$_{A1}$, αCI$_{A2}$, αCI$_{A3}$, and so on, each of which will be affiliated with certain antigen-specific receptors. Let us further assume that the *Ir-GLT* gene encodes, in nonresponder individual A, CI$_{A1}$ molecules; specificity of *Ir*-gene function in this case reflects an affiliation on the same cells of anti-GLT receptors with αCI$_{A1}$ receptors. Anything that prevents the reaction αCI$_{A1} \rightarrow$ CI$_{A1}$ would be manifested as specific unresponsiveness to GLT, for example, something analogous to an anti-αCI$_{A1}$ idiotype reaction, as suggested above. Perhaps a nonresponder individual displays that phenotype because, for some reason, αCI$_{A1}$ is particularly effective in eliciting a strong (and early) anti-αCI$_{A1}$ reaction that, in turn, blunts any possible response to GLT from developing.

These two possible mechanisms by which *Ir* genes may function are by no means mutually exclusive. It is pertinent to emphasize the fact that although in both circumstances the phenotypic effect is displayed as poor responsiveness or nonresponsiveness, there is no defect in *Ir*-gene expression *per se* but rather the consequence of the expression of the relevant *Ir* gene. Moreover, if both mechanisms are valid, one can easily understand how *Ir*-gene complementation can occur in certain circumstances when responder F$_1$ hybrids are derived from two nonresponder parental strains; in such cases, one nonresponder parent would be so as a result of one of these mechanisms, and vice versa. In those situations in which nonresponsiveness may reflect the third possibility mentioned above—namely that Ir genes encode both αCI receptors and target CI molecules—and in which both mechanisms just discussed operate simultaneously to result in nonresponsiveness, one would not expect to find a suitable complementing nonresponder partner strain to give rise to a responding F_1 hybrid.

This definition of Ir genes also explains why it is easier to find Ir-gene defects in highly inbred individuals and more difficult to detect such defects as population heterozygosity increases. It seems likely that as heterozygosity increases, so would heterogeneity of CI-molecule specificities possessed by any one individual. This, in turn, would increase the likelihood that loss of a given αCI-molecule-binding cell (either by deletion because of high affinity or because of anti-αCI reactions), with concomitant loss of responsiveness to the antigen for which specific receptors were affiliated on the same cell, might be compensated by the association of receptors for the same antigen on cells possessing a different αCI specificity. Finally, consistent with this reasoning is the experimental finding that tetraparental bone marrow chimeras constructed from bone marrow populations of nonresponder and responder parent origins fail to manifest cooperative activity between the responder T cell and nonresponder B cell (Press and McDevitt, 1977).

8. Conclusions

The process of adaptive differentiation is one in which highly effective selective mechanisms are initiated by contact between developing cells and the normal cell-interaction (CI) molecules predominantly expressed in the surrounding environment. These selective mechanisms involve self-recognition and result in functional deletion of clones of cells that possess high-affinity receptors for CI molecules that are predominantly expressed in the environment. The consequence of this process is to shift the affinity spectrum of self-recognition toward the lower end, where cells possessing such low-to-moderate-affinity αCI molecules and their corresponding receptors are then capable of engaging in functional interactions necessary for development and maintenance of the system.

A second consequence is that cells with self-recognition capabilities for all the other CI molecules in the species express such CI-molecule receptors but, in the absence of environmental selection, are shifted toward the higher end of the affinity spectrum of CI-binding capabilities. These cells may play a very important functional role in a surveillance mechanism that operates to eliminate the majority of low-to-moderate-affinity cells of the same CI specificity that have no useful function in the inappropriate environment in which they find themselves. Because of their high-affinity binding capacity for CI molecules of other individual members of the species, certain of these cells manifest alloaggressive responses in mixed-lymphocyte reactions and other transplantation reactions.

Although the precise nature of the molecular interactions involved in these processes has yet to be defined, it seems clear that these interactions must occur to a very great extent by direct cell contact. For several years, we have stressed the fact that self-recognition appears to be a fundamental biological process concerned with control of many types of developmental and differentiation events. In this chapter, we have presented some new thoughts on possible mechanisms of self-recognition and regulatory interactions in the immune system. In particular, new speculations concerning *Ir* genes and the manner in which they function have been discussed in light of recent experimental observations as presented here. Clearly, only time and sophisticated molecular approaches to these issues will ultimately sort out the correct answers.

ACKNOWLEDGMENTS. I am grateful to all of my colleagues for their participation in the studies in our laboratory which have contributed to the notions presented here. Anthea Hugus and Keith Dunn provided excellent assistance in preparation of the manuscript. Our work was supported by NIH Grants 13781, 13874, and RRO-5514 and Grant 1-549 from The National Foundation-March of Dimes. This is publication number 101 from the Department of Cellular and Developmental Immunology and publication number 1725 from the Immunology Departments, Scripps Clinic and Research Foundation, La Jolla, California.

References

Bach, F.H., Widmer, M.B., Bach, M.L., and Klein, J., 1972, Serologically defined and lymphocyte-defined components of the major histocompatibility complex in the mouse, *J. Exp. Med.* **136**:1430.

Benacerraf, B., 1978, A hypothesis to relate the specificity of T lymphocytes and the activity of I region-specific *Ir* genes in macrophages and B lymphocytes, *J. Immunol.* **120**:1809.

Benacerraf, B., and McDevitt, H.O., 1972, Histocompatibility-linked immune response genes, *Science* **175**:273.

Bevan, M.J., 1975, The major histocompatibility complex determines susceptibility to cytotoxic T cells directed against minor histocompatibility antigens, *J. Exp. Med.* **142**:1349.

Bevan, M.J., 1977, In a radiation chimaera, host H-2 antigens determine immune responsiveness of donor cytotoxic cells, *Nature (London)* **269**:417.

Bevan, M.J., and Fink, P.J., 1978, The influence of thymus H-2 antigens on the specificity of maturing killer and helper cells, *Immunol. Rev.* **42**:3.

Binz, H., and Wigzell, H., 1977a, Antigen-binding, idiotypic T-lymphocyte receptors, in: *Contemporary Topics in Immunobiology* (O. Stutman, ed.), p. 113, Plenum Press, New York.

Binz, H., and Wigzell, H., 1977b, Antigen-binding, idiotypic receptors from T lymphocytes: An analysis of their biochemistry, genetics, and use as immunogens to produce specific immune tolerance, in: *Origins of Lymphocyte Diversity, Cold Spring Harbor Symp. Quant. Biol.* **41**:275.

Blanden, R.V., Doherty, P.C., Dunlop, M.B.C., Gardner, I.D., and Zinkernagel, R.M., 1975, Genes required for cytotoxicity against virus-infected target cells in *K* and *D* regions of H-2 complex, *Nature (London)* **254**:269.

Dunham, E.K., Unanue, E.R., and Benacerraf, B., 1972, Antigen binding and capping by lymphocytes of genetic nonresponder mice, *J. Exp. Med.* **136**:403.

Fink, P.J., and Bevan, M.J., 1978, H-2 antigens of the thymus determine lymphocyte specificity, *J. Exp. Med.* **148**:766.

Gordon, R.D., Simpson, E., and Samelson, L.E., 1975, *In vitro* cell-mediated immune responses to the male specific (H-Y) antigen in mice, *J. Exp. Med.* **142**:1108.

Hämmerling, G.J., Masuda, T., and McDevitt, H.O., 1973, Genetic control of the immune response: Frequency and characteristics of antigen-binding cells in high and low responder mice, *J. Exp. Med.* **137**:1180.

Janeway, C.A., Jr., Wigzell, H., and Binz, H., 1976, Two different V_H gene products make up the T-cell receptors, *Scand. J. Immunol.* **5**:993.

Kappler, J.W., and Marrack, P., 1978, The role of H-2 linked genes in helper T-cell function. IV. Importance of T-cell genotype and host environment in *I*-region and *Ir* gene expression, *J. Exp. Med.* **148**:1510.

Katz, D.H., 1976, The role of the histocompatibility gene complex in lymphocyte differentiation, in *Proceedings of the First International Symposium on the Immunobiology of Bone Marrow Transplantation, Transplant. Proc.* **8**:405.

Katz, D.H., 1977a, The role of the histocompatibility gene complex in lymphocyte differentiation, in: *Origins of Lymphocyte Diversity, Cold Spring Harbor Symp. Quant. Biol.* **41**:611.

Katz, D.H., 1977b, *Lymphocyte Differentiation, Recognition, and Regulation*, Academic Press, New York.

Katz, D.H., 1980, Adaptive differentiation of lymphocytes: Theoretical implications for mechanisms of cell–cell recognition and regulation of immune responses, *Adv. Immunol.* **29**:137.

Katz, D.H., and Benacerraf, B., 1975, Hypothesis: The function and interrelationships of T cell receptors, Ir genes and other histocompatibility gene products, *Transplant. Rev.* **22**:175.

Katz, D.H., and Benacerraf, B., 1976, Genetic control of lymphocyte interactions and differentiation, in *The Role of Products of the Histocompatibility Gene Complex in Immune Responses* (D.H. Katz and B. Benacerraf, eds.), p. 355, Academic Press, New York.

Katz, D.H., Hamaoka, T., and Benacerraf, B., 1973a, Cell interactions between histoincompatible T and B lymphocytes. II. Failure of physiologic cooperative interactions between T and B lymphocytes from allogeneic donor strains in humoral responses to hapten–protein conjugates, *J. Exp. Med.* **137**:1405.

Katz, D.H., Hamaoka, T., Dorf, M.E., and Benacerraf, B., 1973b, Cell interactions between histoincompatible T and B lymphocytes. III. Demonstration that the H-2 gene complex determines successful physiologic lymphocyte interactions, *Proc. Natl. Acad. Sci. U.S.A.* **70**:2624.

Katz, D.H., Hamaoka, T., Dorf, M.E., Maurer, P.H., and Benacerraf, B., 1973c, Cell interactions between histoincompatible T and B lymphocytes. IV. Involvement of the immune response *(Ir)* gene in the control of lymphocyte interactions in responses controlled by the gene, *J. Exp. Med.* **138**:734.

Katz, D.H., Graves, M., Dorf, M.E., DiMuzio, H., and Benacerraf, B., 1975, Cell interactions between histoincompatible T and B lymphocytes. VII. Cooperative responses between lymphocytes are controlled by genes in the *I* region of the *H-2* complex, *J. Exp. Med.* **141**:263.

Katz, D.H., Chiorazzi, N., McDonald, J., and Katz, L.R., 1976, Cell interactions between histoincompatible T and B lymphocytes. IX. The failure of histoincompatible cells is not due to suppression and cannot be circumvented by carrier-priming T cells with allogeneic macrophages, *J. Immunol.* **117**:1853.

Katz, D.H., Skidmore, B.J., Katz, L.R., and Bogowitz, C.A., 1978, Adaptive differentiation of murine lymphocytes. I. Both T and B lymphocytes differentiating in $F_1 \rightarrow$ parental chimeras manifest preferential cooperative activity for partner lymphocytes derived from the same parental type corresponding to the chimeric host, *J. Exp. Med.* **148**:727.

Katz, D.H., Katz, L.R., Bogowitz, C.A., and Maurer, P.H., 1979, Adaptive differentiation of murine lymphocytes. II. (Responder × nonresponder) F_1 cells can be taught to preferentially help nonresponder, rather than responder, B cells, *J. Exp. Med.* **150**:20.

Kindred, B., and Shreffler, D.C., 1972, H-2 dependence of co-operation between T and B cells *in vivo*, *J. Immunol.* **109**:940.

Koszinowski, U., and Ertl, H., 1975, Lysis mediated by T cells and restricted by H-2 antigen of target cells infected with vaccinia virus, *Nature (London)* **255**:552.

Krawinkel, U., Cramer, M., Berek, C., Hämmerling, G., Black, S.J., Rajewsky, K., and Eichmann, K., 1977, On the structure of the T-cell receptor for antigen, in: *Origins of Lymphocyte Diversity, Cold Spring Harbor Symp. Quant. Biol.* **41**:285.

McDougal, J.S., and Cort, S.P., 1978, Generation of T helper cells *in vitro*. IV. F_1 T helper cells primed with antigen-pulsed parental macrophages are genetically restricted in their antigen-specific helper activity, *J. Immunol.* **120**:445.

Miller, J.F.A.P., and Vadas, M.A., 1977, The major histocompatibility complex: Influence on immune reactivity and T-lymphocyte activation, *Scand. J. Immunol.* **6**:771.

Ordal, J.C., and Grumet, F.C., 1972, Genetic control of the immune response: The effect of graft-*versus*-host reaction on the antibody responses to poly-L(Tyr,Glu)-poly-D,L-Ala--poly-L-Lys in nonresponder mice, *J. Exp. Med.* **136**:1195.

Paul, W.E., Shevach, E.M., Thomas, D.W., Pickeral, S.F., and Rosenthal, A.S., 1977, Genetic restriction in T-lymphocyte activation by antigen-pulsed peritoneal exudate cells, in: *Origins of Lymphocyte Diversity, Cold Spring Harbor Symp. Quant. Biol.* **41**:571.

Pierce, S.K., 1977, Recognition restrictions in lymphocyte collaborative interactions in IgG_1 antibody responses, in: *Immune System: Genetics and Regulation* (E.E. Sercarz, L.A. Herzenberg, and C.F. Fox, eds.), p. 447, Academic Press, New York.

Press, J.L., and McDevitt, H.O., 1977, Allotype-specific analysis of anti-(Tyr,Glu)-Ala-Lys antibodies produced by Ir-IA high and low responder chimeric mice, *J. Exp. Med.* **146**:1815.

Rosenthal, A.S., 1978, Determinant selection and macrophage function in genetic control of the immune response, *Immunol. Rev.* **40**:136.

Rosenthal, A.S., and Shevach, E.M., 1973, Function of macrophages in antigen recognition by guinea pig T lymphocytes. I. Requirement for histocompatible macrophages and lymphocytes, *J. Exp. Med.* **138:**1194.

Schmitt-Verhulst, A.-M., and Shearer, G.M., 1975, Bifunctional major histocompatibility-linked genetic regulation of cell-mediated lympholysis to trinitrophenyl-modified autologous lymphocytes, *J. Exp. Med.* **142:**914.

Schwartz, R.H., 1978, A clonal deletion model for Ir gene control of the immune responses, *Scand. J. Immunol.* **7:**3.

Shearer, G.M., 1974, Cell-mediated cytotoxicity to trinitrophenyl-modified syngeneic lymphocytes, *Eur. J. Immunol.* **4:**527.

Skidmore, B.J., and Katz, D.H., 1977, Haplotype preference in lymphocyte differentiation. I. Development of haplotype-specific helper and suppressor activities in F_1 hybrid activated T cell populations, *J. Immunol.* **119:**694.

Sprent, J., 1978, Restricted helper function of $F_1 \rightarrow$ parent bone marrow chimeras controlled by K-end of H-2 complex, *J. Exp. Med.* **147:**1838.

Swierkosz, J.E., Rock, K., Marrack, P., and Kappler, J.W., 1978, The role of *H-2*-linked genes in helper T-cell function. II. Isolation on antigen-pulsed macrophages of two separate populations of F_1 helper T cells each specific for antigen and one set of parental *H-2* products, *J. Exp. Med.* **147:**554.

Thomas, D.W., and Shevach, E.M., 1978, Nature of the antigenic complex recognized by T lymphocytes. V. Genetic predisposition of independent F_1 T cell subpopulations responsive to antigen-pulsed parental macrophages, *J. Immunol.* **120:**445.

von Boehmer, H., Hudson, L., and Sprent, J., 1975, Collaboration of histoincompatible T and B lymphocytes using cells from tetraparental bone marrow chimeras, *J. Exp. Med.* **142:**989.

Waldmann, H., Pope, H., Bettles, C., and Davies, A.J.S., 1979, The influence of thymus on the development of MHC restrictions exhibited by T-helper cells, *Nature (London)* **277:**137.

Yamashita, U., and Shevach, E.M., 1978, The histocompatibility restrictions on macrophage T-helper cell interaction determine the histocompatibility restrictions on T-helper cell B-cell interactions, *J. Exp. Med.* **148:**1171.

Zinkernagel, R.M., and Doherty, P.C., 1974a, Restriction of *in vitro* T cell-mediated cytotoxicity in lymphocytic chorimeningitis within a syngeneic or semiallogeneic system, *Nature (London)* **248:**701.

Zinkernagel, R.M., and Doherty, P.C., 1974b, Immunological surveillance against altered self components by sensitised T lymphocytes in lymphocytic choriomeningitis, *Nature (London)* **251:**547.

Zinkernagel, R.M., Callahan, G.N., Althage, A., Cooper, S., Klein, P.A., and Klein, J., 1978a, On the thymus in the differentiation of "H-2 self-recognition" by T cells: Evidence for dual recognition, *J. Exp. Med.* **147:**882.

Zinkernagel, R.M., Callahan, G.N., Althage, A., Cooper, S., Streilein, J.W., and Klein, J., 1978b, The lymphoreticular system in triggering virus plus self-specific cytotoxic T cells: Evidence for T help, *J. Exp. Med.* **147:**897.

6

The Role of Cell-Surface Antigens in Progressive Tumor Growth (Immunological Surveillance Re-revisited)

Lionel A. Manson

There has been a massive effort mounted during the last decade to understand malignancy in immunobiological terms. One cannot say at present that there exists a consensus among workers in the field of tumor immunology as to the role, if any, that the immune systems of the host play in the emergence and expansion of a malignant clone to form a visible tumor that can then continue to grow, metastasize, and kill the host. The current status of knowledge in the field has been most succinctly stated by Möller and Möller (1979). They have summarized the evidence that supports the assumption that most if not all tumors are clonal in origin, and reviewed our understanding, or lack thereof, of the role of the immune system in progressive tumor growth. Their discussion revolves around the postulate that the role of the T-cell system is immunological surveillance, and that the emergence of a tumor is due to its failure. They conclude that this postulate is untenable in its present form. They have described the assumptions inherent in the theory as follows: "The only chance for tumors to appear is either when the T cell system has failed or when tumors possess very weak TSTA which are not efficiently recognized."

Lionel A. Manson • The Wistar Institute of Anatomy and Biology, Philadelphia, Pennsylvania 19104.

In this essay, I would like to propose a third possibility that might rejuvenate the theory, but in a considerably modified form.

We have been studying the host–tumor interactions of a number of mouse lymphomas and thymomas. All the tumors are compatible with the host of origin: i.e., the inoculation of as few as 100 cells intraperitoneally or subcutaneously leads to the appearance several weeks later of a massive tumor. Most of our studies were carried out with two carcinogen-induced tumors, the L-5178Y thymoma and the P815Y mastocytoma, growing in their host of origin, the DBA/2 mouse. I will concentrate on the data collected during the past several years with these two tumor systems.

In the earlier studies, it was shown that these two tumors were immunologically cross-reactive (Goldstein and Manson, 1975: Manson *et al.*, 1975), and to the present day there is no immunological test that differentiates between the two. They are, however, quite different in behavior in tissue culture and thus can be relatively easily identified. It was also found that each contained a strong tumor-associated transplantation antigen (TATA). DBA/2 mice could be immunized by mitomycin-C-treated cells or by a cell-free membrane preparation of the tumor cells, the microsomal lipoproteins (MLP). After immunization, mice would reject a challenge of 500 cells, and once having rejected this challenge were resistant to a further challenge of 1×10^5 cells. Such resistant mice remain immune to further challenges for many months. In this study, we also observed that one could not induce a primary cell-mediated T-cell lympholytic response in DBA/2 spleen cultures *in vitro;* however, one could induce large amounts of such "killer" cells in cultures of DBA/2 spleen cells obtained from immunized DBA/2 mice. The killer cells so induced would kill L-5178Y or P815Y, but not L-1210, another DBA/2 leukemia, or EL-4, a C57BL/6 thymoma.

Since it was observed that the L-5178Y contained a TATA, efforts were made to obtain an antiserum to this antigen in the syngeneic host. After multiple immunizations, antibody was detected in immunized mice, using cultured cells as the solid phase in a radioimmunoassay (RIA) (Goldstein *et al.*, 1973) and ^{125}I-labeled L-5178Y MLP in an immunoprecipitation test (Manson *et al.*, 1975). This antibody was not cytolytic for the tumor cells in the presence of rabbit or guinea pig complement.

In continuing studies with the L-5178Y lymphoma, Goldstein (1976) has made a number of interesting and important observations. He studied the immunological status of the L-5178Y-tumor-bearing mouse, asking the question whether an immunological suppression, either specific or nonspecific, was responsible for the emergence of the L-5178Y tumor from very small inocula. Using a variety of *in vivo* and *in vitro* tests to evaluate the capacities of the spleens of tumor-bearing mice to mount both cell-mediated and humoral responses during progressive tumor growth, he concluded that as long as the tumor load in the animal was less than 5×10^7 cells per animal, spleen cells appeared to be immunologically normal. When the tumor load exceeded 5×10^7 cells per animal, the spleens of such animals were impaired in responding to test antigens. As has been noted, DBA/2 spleen cells do not develop a primary T-killer-cell response in *in vitro* culture, but spleen cells from immunized animals will. In his studies, spleen cells obtained from mice with a tumor load of less than 5×10^7 cells per animal behaved as though they were immunologically naïve, and would not develop T killer cells in culture, even though they would respond to allogeneic cells with a primary response. Antibody was not detected either in the serum or in the ascitic fluid of the tumor-bearing mouse in the RIA. It was thus concluded that the growing ascites did not impress itself immunologically on the immune-response systems of the host during the critical period of clonal expansion from 10^3 cells to 5×10^7 cells. Also, it was clear that immunosuppression was not operative during this period of time.

During this time, Biddison and Palmer were investigating the progressive growth of the P815Y ascitic tumor in the DBA/2 mouse (Biddison and Palmer, 1977; Biddison *et al.*, 1977). Since no immune response has been found either in the serum or in the spleens of the tumor-bearer, methods were developed for determining whether an immune response was detectable *in situ* in the expanding tumor mass itself. The data that have been published deal with the studies that were carried out with respect to the cell-mediated immune responses observable in the tumor mass. First, as was found in L-5178Y studies, no T-cell responses were detectable in the spleens or lymph nodes of the tumor-bearing mouse. To study the tumor mass itself, Biddison and Palmer (1977) separated the ascitic tumor mass on a Sta-put gradient. The slowest-sedimenting fraction appeared to be essentially small host lymphocytes, whereas the largest cells appeared to be P815Y. Several interesting observations were made. At 10 days after the intraperitoneal inoculation of 1000 P815Y cells, host lymphocytes could be separated from the ascitic mass that contained T-killer-cell activity toward P815Y. Unlike the T-killer-cell activity that is found in immunized DBA/2 spleen-cell cultures, which do *not* kill EL4 (an *H-2^b* lymphoma), the ascitic, primary T killer cells were *not H-2 restricted*. In Table 1 are shown the cell lines and the strains of their hosts of origin tested to date that are sensitive to these killer cells in a 4-hr ^{51}Cr-release assay (Thorn *et al.*, 1974). These T killer cells are not totally cross-reactive, since two DBA/2 and two A strain cell lines are not killed. In this respect, they behave in an *H-2*-unrestricted fashion, much unlike virus-induced cytotoxic T cells (see Chapters 3 and 8). They do, however, resemble allogeneic killer T cells, which, by definition, are

TABLE 1. Sensitivity of Murine Cell Lines to DBA/2-Anti-P815Y Killer Cells

Line	Strain of origin	*H-2* type	Characteristic	Sensitivity
P815Y	DBA/2	*d*	Methylcholanthrene-induced mastocytoma	+
L-5178Y	DBA/2	*d*	Methylcholanthrene-induced lymphoma	+
GM86	DBA/2	*d*	Friend-virus-induced leukemia	+
EL4	C57BL/6	*b*	Dimethylbenzanthracene-induced lymphoma	+
C57SV	C57BL/6	*b*	SV40-transformed embryo fibroblast	+
MC57G	C57BL/6	*b*	Methylcholanthrene-induced sarcoma	+
G26-23	C57BL/6	*b*	Methylcholanthrene-induced glioma	+
P-815-X2	DBA/2	*d*	Methylcholanthrene-induced mastocytoma	−
L-1210	DBA/2	*d*	Methylcholanthrene-induced leukemia	−
A-10	A/He	*a*	Spontaneous mammary adenocarcinoma	−
C-1300NA	A	*a*	Spontaneous neuroblastoma	−
Spleen	DBA/2	*d*	—	−
Spleen	C57BL/6	*b*	—	−

H-2-unrestricted. These effector cells were classified as T cells because they were sensitive to anti-Thy-1.2 serum, passed through nylon wool, were nonadherent, and were resistant to an antiimmunoglobulin-plus-complement treatment that did destroy B cells. This activity was found only in the ascitic mass of the tumor-bearing animal, as though the growing ascites acted as an *in vivo* solid-phase immunoadsorbent and a filter to which all such cells in the body remained immobilized.

A second intriguing observation was made by Biddison and Palmer (1977). On day 10, when the T killer cells were found in the ascitic mass, the P815Y tumor cells obtained from the same Sta-put gradient were sensitive to these killer cells (the tumor size on day 10 varied among animals from 1 to 10×10^7 cells per animal). Those mice that were untouched for 16 days after inoculation of 1000 cells all had much larger ascitic tumors, some as large as $40–50 \times 10^7$ cells per animal. When the 16-day ascitic tumors were separated on the Sta-put gradient, some killer-cell activity was seen in the slowest-sedimenting fraction. However, the P815Y tumor cells obtained from these gradients were completely resistant to the day 10 or day 16 DBA/2-anti-P815Y killer cells. These tumor cells were not resistant to allogeneic C57BL/6 anti-DBA/2 spleen killer cells. Not only were the 16-day tumor cells resistant to direct lysis, but also they would not inhibit DBA/2-anti-P815Y killing in a cold-target inhibition test. It was concluded that the P815Y had undergone antigenic modulation and had lost the TATA by an unknown mechanism. The data suggested that the modulation was reversible, since after the 16-day tumor cells were cultured for several days, they again became sensitive to the ascitic killers. Antibody was not found in the ascitic fluid or on the tumor cells at that time.

We have obtained much greater insight into this phenomenon of antigenic modulation during the last few months. We have been evaluating the number of H-2-antibody-binding sites of both L-5178Y and P815Y tumor cells growing *in vivo* either as an ascites or as a solid tumor (Manson and Fleisher, 1980). The H-2-binding capacity of cells, either grown in tissue culture or *in vivo,* is determined by incubating the cells under saturating conditions with a variety of H-2 antisera, then detecting the bound antibody with an [^{125}I]-rabbit-anti-Fab. The reagent we used in these studies was prepared by Dr. Michael Cancro and is especially efficient at detecting IgM. Since normal immunoglobulin binds nonspecifically to the tumors, we must always compare the binding of normal serum to immune serum to evaluate specific binding. In Tables 2 and 3 are shown the results of two experiments, one with L-5178Y growing as a solid tumor and one with P815Y growing as an ascites tumor in DBA/2 mice. What is notable in both experiments, and these are just two examples of many such experiments, is that with time *in vivo*, the H-2-antibody-binding capacity of the tumor cells disappears. This appears to be due to an increase in the binding capacity of the *in vivo* grown cells with the [^{125}I]-anti-Fab reagent directly (cells incubated in buffer) and no further increase in the capacity of the *in vivo* grown cells to bind additional amounts of H-2 antibody. This increase in background binding is progressive with time, as can be seen by comparing the day 16 cells with the day 10 tumor cells. To date, we know that no significant amounts of antitumor immunoglobulin are detectable in the day 10 or day 16 ascitic fluid or in the serum of the tumor-bearing animals. Control experiments have shown that prior incubation of P815Y cells in undiluted 16-day ascitic fluid or in undiluted DBA/2 serum does not prevent to any significant extent the subsequent binding of specific H-2 antibodies. Other control experiments indicate that the molecules detected by

TABLE 2. H-2-Binding Activity of P815Y Grown in DBA/2 Mice as Ascites[a]

Antiserum	T.C. controls	Day 10	Day 16
Buffer	754	4,742	11,550
Normal	2,593	5,186	10,034
α L-5178Y	14,619 *12,026*	12,902 *7,716*	15,219 *4,001*
D-31	5,578 *2,985*	8,484 *3,278*	13,534 *1,984*
D-13	10,884 *8,291*	10,551 *5,365*	12,690 *1,140*

[a] All antisera were used at a 1:100 dilution. Values are cpm/0.25 × 10⁶ cells. The input [^{125}I]-anti-Fab was 4 × 10⁵ cpm/0.1 ml. The values in italics were obtained by subtracting the radioactivity bound to cells treated with normal serum from that found after immune-serum treatment.

TABLE 3. H-2-Binding Activity of L-5178Y Grown
in Vivo as a Solid Tumor in DBA/2 Mice[a]

Antiserum	T.C. controls		Day 15	
Buffer	803 ± 103		17,735 ± 726	
Normal	8,667 ± 211		16,182 ± 844	
α L-5178Y	32,418 ± 227	*23,751*	34,964 ± 591	*18,783*
D-31	14,313 ± 273	*5,646*	18,315 ± 300	*2,134*
D-4	18,199 ± 997	*9,533*	17,225 ± 377	*1,044*

[a] All antisera were used at a 1:50 dilution. Values are cpm/0.25 ×
10^5 cells. The input [^{125}I]-anti-Fab was 7.0×10^5 cpm/0.1 ml. The
values in italics were obtained by subtracting the radioactivity
bound to cells treated with normal serum from that found after
immune-serum treatment.

radioactive reagents on the *in vivo* grown cells appear to be IgM-like,
and their presence on the cells inhibits these cells from binding additional
amounts of H-2 antibody. To date, we have carried out a few experiments
in which H-2-binding sites were assayed on cells raised *in vivo* that were
also tested for sensitivity to ascitic killer cells. In one such case, the 16-
day cells were resistant, and they appeared saturated with respect to H-
2-antibody-binding. In another case, the tumors were extremely large,
the tumor cells were sensitive to the killer cells, and they did show the
capacity to bind additional H-2 antibody. Many more such experiments
must be carried out before anecdotal data described above can be
considered as even indicating a trend, let alone proving the point.

In an investigation parallel to the *in vivo* studies, we have been
investigating the biochemical properties of the H-2 antigens of the L-
5178Y cells (Manson and Moav, 1979). In DBA/2 spleen cells, we have
found, as have many others, that from Nonidet P-40 lysates of labeled
cells, two major peaks are seen when immunoprecipitates are analyzed
in sodium dodecyl sulfate–polyacrylamide gel electrophoresis (SDS-
PAGE), one a glycoprotein of 45,000 daltons and a protein peak of
11,500, β2-microglobulin. From L-5178Y immunoprecipitates with standard anti-*H-2*^{d} antisera, we see a complex of additional glycoproteins,
behaving in SDS-PAGE as though they were of 8000, 33,000, and 55,000
daltons in size. The data suggest that these additional glycoproteins are
hydrophobically associated with the *H-2K* and *D* gene products in the
membrane.

There is a reasonable explanation that fits all the data cited above.
There may be in these tumor lines *H-2*-associated peptides in the
membrane complex that create additional antigenic determinants that the
immune system of the syngeneic host sees as foreign or interprets to be
"allogeneic." As the tumor grows, a "strong" primary cell-mediated

immune response develops, which we see as nonrestricted T cell killers. In parallel to this cell-mediated response, there also develops a primary IgM humoral response to the same determinants. This tumor antigen may be different from the TATA that we observed in our early studies, because T cell killers to that antigen were not cross-reactive nor were they *H-2*-unrestricted (Manson *et al.*, 1975). To differentiate this antigen from the antigen involved in inducing the primary responses just described, I will call the latter *emergence-associated tumor antigen* (EATA), since it is the responses to this latter antigenic system that permit the tumor to escape immune surveillance. The high degree of cross-reactivity manifested by the killer cells suggests that this antigen can be found on a variety of transplantable tumor lines differing greatly in their origin. This in itself is difficult to accept, let alone the concept that what is being seen with these long-transplantable tumors resembles what is found in the case of the spontaneous, autochthonous tumor emerging in the original host. It is also clear that some tumors do not fall into this class; we have reported one such case just recently (Tax and Manson, 1979), the A-10 tumor in the A/J mouse. In this latter case, no TATA or EATA at all was demonstrable.

The data that we have accumulated suggest that some tumors grow progressively from small inocula even though they can induce "strong" primary immune responses, both humoral and cell-mediated. The mechanism of escape from the T-cell-mediated response may be via the formation of an antibody that binds firmly to the target site on the tumor cell to which the T cell would normally bind. For the response to develop as rapidly as we have seen with L-5178Y or P815Y, the antigen should be considered "strong" rather than "weak." One might expect an "altered H-2-antigen complex" to be such an antigen, since the immune system would then react to this "altered H-2-antigen" as though it were allogeneic to the host's immune system. In the original description of immunological surveillance, it was postulated that tumors are "weakly" antigenic. Very few attempts have been made to evaluate the *in situ* immune responses. As a consequence, a strong immune response that localizes effectors at the tumor site might appear to be weak or nonexistent when effectors are looked for in lymph nodes, spleen, or serum. It is to be hoped that a more careful examination of *in vivo* responses, especially at the tumor site, will provide further support for the concepts proposed in this review.

ACKNOWLEDGMENTS. The author is indebted to the excellent collaboration he has had with his colleagues, Drs. Biddison, Goldstein, Moav, Palmer, Tax, and Thorn and Mr. E.P. Cowan and Mr. L.A. Fleisher.

Much of the technical assistance which made these studies possible was due to the excellent cooperation given to us by Mr. M. Alexander and by Mss. Chang, A. Guarini, S. Mannion, M. McGuigan, and B. Van Dyke. The studies were supported by Research Grants CA-07973 and CA-10815 from the National Cancer Institute and Grant RR-05540 from the Division of Research Resources.

References

Biddison, W.E., and Palmer, J.C., 1977, Development of tumor cell resistance to syngeneic cell-mediated cytotoxicity during growth of ascitic mastocytoma P815Y, *Proc. Natl. Acad. Sci. U.S.A.* **74**:329.

Biddison, W.E., Palmer, J.C., Alexander, M.A., Cowan, E.P., and Manson, L.A., 1977, Characterization and specificity of murine anti-tumor cytotoxic effector cells within an ascitic tumor, *J. Immunol.* **118**:2243.

Goldstein, L.T., 1976, Immunological Studies of the Murine Lymphoma L-51784 in Its Syngeneic Host, Ph.D. thesis, University of Pennsylvania.

Goldstein, L.T., and Manson, L.A., 1975, Specificity of the immune response in an L-5178Y-DBA/2 syngeneic mouse system, *Transplant. Proc.* **1**:513.

Goldstein, L.T., Klinman, N.R., and Manson, L.A., 1973, A microtest radioimmunoassay for noncytotoxic tumor-specific antibody to cell-surface antigens, *J. Natl. Cancer Inst.* **51**:1713.

Manson, L.A., and Fleisher, L.A., 1980, The development of a primary humoral immune response during progressive growth of murine ascites tumors (to be submitted).

Manson, L.A., and Moav, N., 1979, Additional glycoproteins associated with the MHC-gene products in a murine lymphoma L-5178Y, *Fed. Proc. Fed. Am. Soc. Exp. Biol.* **38**:806.

Manson, L.A., Goldstein, L.T., Thorn, R., and Palmer, J.C., 1975, Immune response against apparently host-compatible transplantable tumors, *Transplant. Proc.* **8**:161.

Möller, G., and Möller, E., 1979, Immunologic surveillance revisited, *Transplant. Proc.* **11**:1041.

Tax, A., and Manson, L.A., 1979, An immunologic analysis of A strain mice bearing the A-10 mammary adenocarcinoma, *Cancer Res.* **39**:1735.

Thorn, R.M., Palmer, J.C., and Manson, L.A., 1974, A simplified ^{51}Cr-release assay for killer cells, *J. Immunol. Methods* **4**:301.

7

Self-*HLA-D*-Region Products Restrict Human T-Lymphocyte Activation by Antigen

E. Thorsby, B. Bergholtz, and H. Nousiainen

1. Introduction

Numerous recent studies in rodents have demonstrated that T-cell immune responses to antigen are restricted by products of the major histocompatibility complex (MHC) of the animal under study [for references, see Paul and Benacerraf (1977) and Thorsby (1978), as well as Chapters 1, 3, and 8]. Available data may be summarized as follows:

1. Macrophage-dependent antigen activation of T cells involves corecognition of antigen and products of the MHC immune-response (*I*) region.

2. T-cell help for B-cell antibody production involves recognition of the MHC *I*-region products expressed in the B cells.

3. T-cell cytotoxicity against virus-infected or chemically modified target cells, or target cells expressing minor histocompatibility antigens, involves corecognition of the MHC *D*- or *K*-region products.

These and other observations have led to the concept that T cells can only be activated by foreign antigen, or help B cells produce antibodies to antigens, in the context of self-MHC products, either because: (1) the foreign antigen in complex with self-MHC products produces new antigenic determinants (NADs) that are the immunogenic principle being recognized on macrophages, B cells, or other target cells

E. Thorsby, B. Bergholtz, and H. Nousiainen • Tissue Typing Laboratory, Rikshospitalet (The National Hospital), Oslo, Norway.

("altered self"); or because (2) T cells have two receptors, one of low avidity for self-MHC, the other for foreign antigen (x), and both must combine to trigger a T-cell response ("dual recognition").

The self-MHC restriction appears to be imposed on T cells during their development in the fetal thymus, and is independent of antigen also being recognized. Antigen activation of T cells in the periphery requires that antigen be presented by cells expressing the same MHC-region products as those that T cells met during thymic development (Zinkernagel *et al.*, 1978a,b; Waldmann *et al.*, 1979).

These observations have important implications for the mechanism of gene control of the immune response. It has been known for many years that the MHC includes immune-response (*Ir*) genes that control the ability of T cells to respond to given antigens. One explanation for their function has been that they either code for or influence the specificity of the T-cell receptor (Benacerraf and McDevitt, 1972). Some recent data are difficult to fit in with this concept, for example, the fact that most workers have had great difficulties in detecting *I*-region-encoded cell-membrane products, the immune-associated (Ia) antigens, on resting T cells (Hämmerling, 1976). More important, recent data have shown that T lymphocytes of low-responder MHC type, which operationally lack the corresponding *Ir* gene, can be converted to a high-responder type if permitted to develop in a thymus from high-responder animals (Press and McDevitt, 1977; Zinkernagel *et al.*, 1978c; Billings *et al.*, 1978; von Boehmer *et al.*, 1978). Thus, high or low responsiveness to a given antigen appears to be determined by the MHC alleles expressed in the thymus and peripheral environment, and not by the MHC alleles expressed in the T cells. This would further indicate that the MHC products that restrict the T-cell immune responses (the self-Ia molecules for the T helper cells and the self-D/K molecules for the cytotoxic T cells) may be identical to the *Ir*-gene products. For example, Ia and D/K molecules expressing different allotypic variants may differ in their ability to display antigenic determinants in an immunogenic way to T lymphocytes, because of differences in capacity either to combine with or to be modified by antigen. (For discussion, see also Benacerraf and Germain, 1978; Thorsby, 1978.)

The concept of MHC restriction of T-cell immune responses of course has important implications for clinical immunology and histocompatibility. The human MHC, the *HLA* complex, is structurally and functionally closely related to the rodent MHC, and it was to be expected that human T-cell immune responses are similarly restricted by self-*HLA* products.

In the following, a short review of some of our own recent studies on self-*HLA-D/DR* restriction of human T-cell immune responses will be given. Some clinical and biological implications of these findings will also be discussed.

2. The *HLA-D/DR* and Rodent *I*-Region Cell-Membrane Products are Analogous

It is necessary first to briefly discuss this assumption. The known cell-membrane products of the *HLA-D* region carry alloantigenic determinants that induce T-cell proliferative responses, *D determinants,* and determinants that induce alloantibody production, D-related (*DR*) *determinants.* The former have mainly been detected on macrophages and B lymphocytes (references in Albrechtsen and Lied, 1978), but also appear to be present on some skin cells, endothelial cells, and possibly sperm (for references, see Thorsby *et al.,* 1977). Similarly, the antibody-inducing DR determinants are present on macrophages and B lymphocytes, as well as on the macrophage-like Langerhans cells in the epidermis, endothelial cells, and possibly sperm (references in Thorsby *et al.,* 1977, 1978). In addition, some subpopulations of human T cells appear to express the DR determinants, namely, the T cells initially responding to the mitogen concanavalin A (Con A) (Albrechtsen *et al.,* 1977a), as well as the suppressor T cells that can be generated in mixed-lymphocyte cultures (MLCs) (Hirschberg and Thorsby, 1977). Other functionally different subsets of T cells were not found to express DR determinants in a resting stage (Albrechtsen *et al.,* 1977a), but may express them after blastic transformation (Fu *et al.,* 1978; Evans *et al.,* 1978).

This tissue distribution is very similar to that found for the murine Ia determinants (Hämmerling, 1976; Niederhuber and Frelinger, 1976; Murphy *et al.,* 1976; Ahmann *et al.,* 1978). A summary is given in Table 1.

The HLA-DR molecules are composed of two noncovalently linked glycosylated polypeptides of molecular weight 29,000 and 33,000, and thus also biochemically closely resemble the murine Ia molecules (Barnstable *et al.,* 1978). Furthermore, both the *HLA-D* and the *H-2I* region control the strongest MLC-activating determinants, and anti-DR antibodies (Albrechtsen *et al.,* 1977b) and anti-Ia antibodies (Meo *et al.,* 1975) specifically inhibit the stimulating but not the responding cells in MLCs. In the mouse, different loci in the *H-2I* region appear to control Ia antigens (Shreffler *et al.,* 1977). There is little evidence of more than one locus in the *D* region determining DR antigens (see Bodmer *et al.,* 1978), but some more recent studies have indicated that additional *HLA* loci coding for other "DR-like" specificities may exist (Abelson and

TABLE 1. Distribution of DR and Ia Antigens on
Lymphoid Cells

Cells	DR (man)	Ia (mouse)
Macrophages	+	+
B lymphocytes	+	+
T cells		
Proliferating to antigen	$-^a$	−
Responding in MLC	$-^a$	−
Cytotoxic	$-^a$	−
Suppressor	$+^b$	$+^c$
PHA-sensitive (progenitor)	−	−
Con-A-sensitive (progenitor)	$+^b$	$+^d$

[a] May express DR after activation.
[b] DR antigen may be different from those expressed on macrophages
and B cells.
[c] Determined by the I-J subregion.
[d] May express both I-A- and I-J-coded determinants.

Mann, 1978; Tosi et al., 1978). Taken together, available data support
the assumption that the HLA-D and the murine I regions are analogous.

The exact relationship between the T-cell-activating D determinants
and those inducing antibody production, the DR determinants, is not
known, but most available data suggest that they are present on the same
gene product [for discussion, see Thorsby (1979) and Vol. 1, Chapter
12]. For this reason, the term D/DR is used to designate these cell-
membrane molecules.

3. Self-HLA-D/DR Restriction of T Cells Sensitized in Vivo

3.1. The T-Cell Proliferative Response to PPD in Vitro Is Macrophage-Dependent

To study possible HLA-D restriction of human T-cell immune
responses, we first selected purified protein derivative (PPD) of tuberculin
as antigen, since most individuals in this country are immunized with
BCG as teenagers and react positively to skin-testing with PPD. First,
we demonstrated that an in vitro response to this antigen requires T cells
from sensitized individuals and that antigen be presented by viable
macrophages.

Table 2 presents the results of an experiment in which T cells from
four different sensitized donors were cultured with or without PPD and
with or without autologous adherent macrophages (details in Bergholtz
and Thorsby, 1979a). It can be clearly seen from this table that the PPD
response was macrophage-dependent and that there was no significant

TABLE 2. T-Lymphocyte Stimulation by PPD Macrophages[a]

Cell donor	No macrophages		5 × 10³ Autologous Macrophages (Mφ)		
	PPD (2.5 μg/ml)	Wells "pulsed" with PPD	No PPD	PPD (2.5 μg/ml)	Mφ pulsed with PPD[b]
E.B.	198 ± 61	72 ± 33	140 ± 44	1,274 ± 248	1,766 ± 131
E.T.	214 ± 30	102 ± 26	158 ± 40	4,158 ± 473	3,429 ± 360
A.T.	903 ± 207	349 ± 52	429 ± 131	11,635 ± 323	13,256 ± 885
B.B.	230 ± 81	93 ± 17	307 ± 88	3,531 ± 388	4,166 ± 248

[a] In this experiment, 5 × 10⁴ T lymphocytes [produced by rosetting with S,2-aminoethylisothiouronium (AET)-treated sheep red blood cells (SRBC)] were cultured with or without 2.5 μg PPD and with or without 5 × 10³ adherent cells in RPMI 1640 with antibiotics and 20% normal human serum for 5 days in the wells of flat-bottomed microtiter plates. The adherent cells were prepared by culturing peripheral-blood mononuclear cells for 20 hr in tissue culture flasks removing non-adherent cells. [³H]Thymidine was added 24 hr before harvesting. Values are mean cpm ± S.E.
[b] In these experiments, 5 × 10³ adherent cells were first incubated for 24 hr with 2.5 μg PPD/ml, and then washed, before T cells were added.

difference in stimulating activity whether T cells were cocultured with macrophages and soluble PPD or PPD-pulsed macrophages. Macrophages alone did not respond to PPD (Bergholtz and Thorsby, 1977). In other experiments (Bergholtz and Thorsby, 1979a), we also showed that the macrophages had to be viable to be able to induce a PPD-specific response, and that the macrophages could not be replaced by supernatants from antigen-pulsed macrophages or by 2-mercaptoethanol.

The requirement for T cells from sensitized donors was studied in experiments using T cells and macrophages from newborn babies (Bergholtz and Thorsby, 1979a). Table 3 shows the results of one experiment. It can be seen from this table that in the presence of autologous macrophages, T cells from the adult sensitized donor (A) will respond to

TABLE 3. Requirement of the PPD Response for Sensitized T Cells[a]

T cells	PPD	Macrophages			PHA + Mφ
		−	A	N	
Adult (A)	−	233 ± 51	277 ± 90	299 ± 102	12,195 ± 1351
(5/8)[b]	+	470 ± 104	2192 ± 631	1989 ± 511	
		237	1915	1690	
Neonate (N)	−	136 ± 13	411 ± 38	326 ± 91	9,209 ± 740
(5/8)[b]	+	143 ± 54	421 ± 90	289 ± 50	
		7	10	0	

[a] Values are mean cpm ± S.E. Values beneath the line in the PPD+ rows are the incremental responses (Δcpm).
[b] *HLA-D* phenotype of the donor.

PPD. On the other hand, T cells from the newborn (N) in the presence of autologous macrophages (N) will not respond to PPD, but respond normally to phytohemagglutinin (PHA). Similar results were found using other cell donors, both newborn and nonimmunized youths. Table 3 also reveals another interesting phenomenon. While T cells from the neonatal donor are not able to respond to PPD, his macrophages can induce a PPD response in T cells from sensitized *HLA-D*-identical adults. Thus, macrophages need not stem from sensitized donors.

3.2. The Antigen-Presenting Macrophages Must Share at Least One HLA-D/DR Determinant with the T-Cell Donor

To study whether the PPD response was *HLA-D*-restricted, T cells were stimulated with PPD and macrophages from *HLA-D*-identical, semiidentical, or totally incompatible donors. The results of one of a series of experiments (Bergholtz and Thorsby, 1977, 1978) are given in Table 4. It can be seen that allogeneic macrophages that are of type Dw3/Dw8, and thus share one HLA-D/DR determinant (Dw3) with the T-cell donor (Dw3/Dw3), can induce a PPD response of the T cells of approximately the same magnitude as the PPD response with autologous macrophages (Dw3/Dw3), while totally *HLA-D*-incompatible macrophages (Dw7/−) are not capable of doing this.

Figure 1 gives the combined results of these experiments. The PPD response is expressed as the percentage relative antigen-specific stimulation (RAgS), relating the PPD response obtained with allogeneic macrophages (after subtraction of the allogeneic response without PPD) to that obtained with autologous macrophages and PPD [(= 100%) see footnote *b* in Table 4 for explanation]. It can be clearly seen that an optimal PPD response generally requires that the donors of the T cells

TABLE 4. *HLA-D* Restriction of T Cell–Macrophage Collaboration

5 × 10³ Macrophages	Responses of 5 × 10⁴ Dw3/Dw3 T cells			
HLA-D phenotype	Without PPD[a]	PPD (2.5 μg/ml)[a]	Δcpm	RAgS[b]
—	5 ± 3	231 ± 127	**226**	—
Dw3/Dw3	38 ± 31	4830 ± 331	**4792**	100
Dw3/Dw8	1487 ± 22	5393 ± 234	**3906**	81
Dw7/−	1807 ± 106	2191 ± 193	**348**	3

[a] Values are the mean cpm of triplicate determinations ± S.E.

[b] (RAgS) Relative antigen-specific stimulation = (Δ*cpm* with allogeneic Mφ − Δ*cpm* without Mφ)/(Δ*cpm* with autologous Mφ − Δ*cpm* without Mφ), where Δ*cpm* is the difference in [³H]thymidine uptake between PPD-stimulated cultures and the same cultures without PPD added.

and macrophages share at least one HLA-D determinant. These observations have recently also been confirmed by Hansen Sønderstrup *et al.* (1978). We have also recently found a similar *HLA-D/DR* restriction of the *in vitro* proliferative response of T cells from herpes-simplex-virus (HSV) sensitized individuals to HSV antigen (Berle and Thorsby, 1980).

3.3. Lack of Cooperation between Cells from *HLA-D*-Disparate Donors Is Not Due to Suppression or Cytotoxicity Caused by the Allogeneic Responses

The data summarized above indicate that self-*HLA-D* expressed in macrophages participates in inducing a T-cell response to foreign antigen (PPD). However, in all combinations of macrophages and T cells from *HLA-D*-disparate donors, even without antigen a proliferative response will occur, induced by the foreign *HLA-D*-region product expressed in the macrophages (see Table 4). It could be speculated that the lack of cooperation between cells from *HLA-D*-disparate donors is due to suppressive factors also being generated.

One argument against this is that the allogeneic response seen in the combinations sharing only one HLA-D determinant was usually not much less than when the donors were incompatible for both (Table 4). However, to study this further, experiments were performed in which T cells were stimulated with PPD in the presence of autologous macrophages, *HLA-D*-incompatible macrophages, or a mixture of both. Table 5 shows the results of two different experiments. It can be seen that the PPD-specific response found when the T cells and autologous macrophages were cocultured was only slightly inhibited by the simultaneous

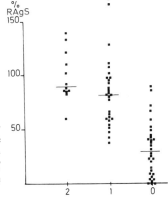

Figure 1. PPD responses of allogeneic T lymphocyte–macrophage combinations expressed as relative antigen-specific stimulation (RAgS), and grouped according to whether they share 2, 1, or no (0) HLA-D/DR determinants. The distributions and medians are plotted.

presence of allogeneic *HLA-D*-disparate macrophages, even though an allogeneic response is clearly seen in the latter three-cell combinations.

It can still be argued that since killed macrophages are not able to induce a PPD response in sensitized T cells, the inability of *HLA-D*-disparate macrophages to induce an antigen-specific response could be due to their being killed through generation of cytotoxic T cells in the allogeneic cell mixture. Experiments were performed to investigate this possibility (Bergholtz and Thorsby, 1979a). Macrophages and *HLA*-incompatible T cells were cocultured for 5 days. The cultures were then irradiated (2000 rads) before the addition of PPD and 5×10^4 freshly prepared T cells from the macrophage cell donor. After another 5 days, the PPD response was assayed. Control cultures were included in which macrophages were precultured alone before the addition of PPD and T cells. The results obtained in these experiments are given in Fig. 2. It can be seen that the preculturing of macrophages with T cells from an *HLA*-incompatible individual did not reduce their ability to cooperate with autologous T cells. In fact, a significant increase in the PPD response was seen after this preculture.

On the basis of these experiments, it can be concluded that the lack of cooperation between macrophages and T cells from *HLA*-disparate donors is not due to generation of cytotoxicity or to suppression generated as a result of the allogeneic response.

TABLE 5. PPD Responses in Autologous T Lymphocyte–Macrophage Combinations: Influence of the Presence of *HLA-D*-Incompatible Macrophages in the Cultures

T-lymphocyte donor[a]	Mφ[b] donor	Without PPD[c]	PPD (2.5 μg/ml)[c]	Δcpm
A 3/–	A	112 ± 26	3723 ± 243	**3611**
A	B	1342 ± 178	2193 ± 416	**851**
A	A + B	1694 ± 424	4543 ± 818	**2849**
B 1/2	B	323 ± 116	2892 ± 333	**2569**
B	A	826 ± 102	1157 ± 200	**331**
B	B + A	1002 ± 183	3247 ± 326	**2245**
C 5/8	C	63 ± 30	1326 ± 221	**1263**
C	D	703 ± 143	950 ± 117	**247**
C	C + D	690 ± 131	1551 ± 297	**961**
D –/–	D	79 ± 14	1066 ± 132	**987**
D	C	541 ± 36	459 ± 14	**0**
D	D + C	563 ± 91	1662 ± 393	**1099**

[a] The donor *HLA-D* phenotypes are given.   [b] (Mφ) Macrophages.
[c] Values are mean cpm ± S.E.

3.4. Anti-DR Antibodies Will Specifically Inhibit the Antigen-Specific Response

If the self-D/DR molecules participate in antigen activation of T cells, antibodies reacting with the appropriate self-D/DR molecules should be able to inhibit the response. To investigate this, we used our anti-DR antisera produced by planned immunization (Albrechtsen *et al.,* 1977c). Different combinations of cells from unrelated donors homozygous or heterozygous at the *HLA-D* locus were stimulated with PPD in the presence or absence of these heat-inactivated anti-DR antisera (Bergholtz and Thorsby, 1978). Table 6 shows the results of a typical experiment. It can be seen that the two anti-DR antisera exerted a pronounced inhibitory effect on the PPD response provided the antiserum recognized the HLA-DR antigens shared by the macrophages and T-cell donor, i.e., those present in the initial sensitizing environment *in vivo.* The inhibition was significantly less when the antigen recognized "irrelevant" DR antigens—i.e., DR antigens expressed only by the macrophages and not by the T-cell donor—and no inhibition was seen if the antiserum recognized DR antigens carried by the T-cell donor but absent from the antigen-presenting macrophages (data not shown).

The combined results of these experiments are given in Fig. 3, expressed as the percentage residual stimulation. Again, it can be seen that significant inhibition was observed only when the antiserum recognized DR antigens shared by the macrophages and T-cell donor, i.e., the restricting HLA-D determinant present during initial sensitization. That this was a specific effect was shown by the much less or no inhibitory action of antisera recognizing the irrelevant DR antigen expressed in the macrophages only. Similar experiments were performed with anti-HLA-

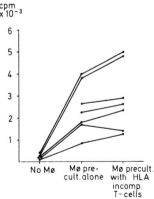

cpm
x 10⁻³

Figure 2. PPD responses of 5 × 10⁴ T cells cultured with PPD and without (No Mφ) or with 5 × 10³ autologous Mφ. Before being added to the T cells and PPD, the Mφ were precultured for 5 days either alone or together with 5 × 10⁴ *HLA*-incompatible T cells.

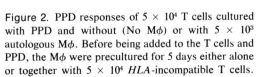

A and -B antisera (Bergholtz and Thorsby, 1978). These behaved differently in that inhibition was seen when the antisera recognized HLA-A and/or -B antigens carried by the T cells, irrespective of whether or not the macrophages also possessed the same antigens. Again, only weak or no inhibition was seen when the antiserum reacted only with the macrophages. Thus, the effects of the antisera cannot be explained by nonspecific distortion of the macrophage cell membrane. Only when the expression of the restricting HLA-DR determinant was disturbed by antibody was strong inhibition seen.

3.5. Clonal Distribution of *HLA-D/DR*-Restricted Antigen-Specific T Cells

The studies summarized above strongly suggest that T lymphocytes from individuals previously sensitized with antigen will respond *in vitro* only when confronted with antigen together with one of the HLA-D/DR molecules present in the initial sensitizing environment. Thus, the response is restricted by self-HLA-D/DR. This would indicate that, for example, in parallel with data from studies in the guinea pig (Rosenthal *et al.,* 1977), in *HLA-D/DR*-heterozygous donors, two separate T-cell clones exist, one recognizing PPD together with the self-HLA-D/DR determinant derived from the one parent, the other recognizing PPD together with the self-HLA-D/DR determinant inherited from the other parent. To test this assumption, we performed studies using our previously reported "hot-pulse suicide technique," eliminating cells that synthesize DNA and proliferate in response to antigen stimulation *in vitro,* by adding "hot-pulse" [³H]thymidine (Hirschberg and Thorsby, 1973). Part of the results of one of our experiments are given in Table 7.

We first showed that the technique could be used to eliminate the PPD-responsive clones of T cells from individuals sensitive to this

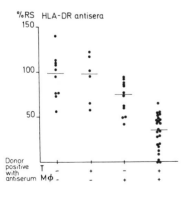

Figure 3. Inhibitory effects of anti-HLA-DR antisera on the PPD responses of allogeneic T lymphocyte–macrophage combinations sharing at least one HLA-D/DR determinant. The data, expressed as percentage residual stimulation (%RS) on the ordinate, are grouped according to the reactivity of the antiserum with the T-lymphocyte and macrophage donors, indicated by + or − along the abscissa.

TABLE 6. Inhibition of the PPD Stimulation of Different Combinations of T Lymphocytes and Macrophages with Anti-DR Antisera

T lymphocytes[a]	Mφ[a]	PPD	NS[b] (cpm ± S.E.)[d]	Anti-DRw2 cpm ± S.E.[d]	% RS[c]	Anti-DRw3 cpm ± S.E.[d]	% RS[c]
A (2/2)	A (2/ 2)	−	131 ± 43	87 ± 30		119 ± 41	
		+	1155 ± 127	564 ± 58		1091 ± 91	
			1024	**447**	44	**972**	95
A (2/2)	C (2/3)	−	1046 ± 97	493 ± 88		334 ± 60	
		+	2818 ± 37	795 ± 53		1228 ± 191	
			1772	**302**	17	**394**	50
B (3/3)	B (3/3)	−	49 ± 7	83 ± 18		141 ± 32	
		+	4993 ± 297	2459 ± 125		1607 ± 46	
			4444	**2376**	53	**1466**	33
B (3/3)	C (2/3)	−	612 ± 129	329 ± 52		354 ± 72	
		+	2685 ± 120	2062 ± 143		1243 ± 93	
			2073	**1743**	84	**889**	43

[a] HLA-DR phenotype indicated in parentheses.
[b] (NS) Normal serum.
[c] (% RS) Percent relative stimulation (i.e., response in antiserum/response in normal serum × 100).
[d] The third value in each group (centered beneath the two cpm ± S.E. values) is the incremental cpm (cpm with antigen − cpm without antigen).

antigen. When T cells from a PPD-sensitive donor (A; D/DRw1/4) were first precultured with autologous or allogeneic (D) macrophages, without PPD but with [³H]thymidine of high specific activity, for 48 hr, they were still able to give a PPD-specific response together with autologous or allogeneic macrophages sharing either one (B; D/DRw 1/1) or the other (C; D/DRw 4/4) D/DR determinant of the T-cell donor (lines 1 and 2 in

TABLE 7. Recognition of PPD in HLA-D/DR-Heterozygous Donors by Two Separate HLA-D/DR-restricted T-Cell Clones

Hot-pulse culture[a]	Not restim- ulated	Restimulated with macrophages from[b]: A (1/4) PPD −	+	Δ	B (1/1) PPD −	+	Δ	C (4/4) PPD −	+	Δ
T_A + Mφ_A	107	108	2116	**2008**	181	1163	**982**	132	3999	**3867**
T_A + Mφ_D	791	1194	5703	**4509**	1816	2922	**1106**	2368	7668	**5300**
T_A + Mφ_A + PPD	314	204	456	**252**	277	386	**109**	295	686	**391**
T_A + Mφ_B + PPD	444	269	1278	**1009**	286	543	**257**	318	2563	**2245**
T_A + Mφ_C + PPD	507	593	1921	**1328**	392	1880	**1488**	609	526	**−83**

[a] [³H]Thymidine of high specific activity was added after 24 and 48 hr. After 72 hr, 5×10^4 T cells were restimulated with 1×10^4 macrophages + PPD as given in the right hand side of the table. Values are the median cpm of triplicate determinations.
[b] Restimulation was with macrophages [e.g., non-T cells ($\approx$ 30% latex-ingesting cells)] in the absence (−) or in the presence (+) of PPD (2.5 μg/ml). (Δ) Incremental response (i.e., response with PPD − response without PPD).

Table 7). However, when the T cells were precultured together with autologous macrophages, PPD, and hot-pulse thymidine, a response against PPD together with the autologous or compatible macrophages (B and C) was no longer seen (line 3). More important, when the T cells from A (1/4) were hot-pulse precultured together with PPD and macrophages from B (1/1), the PPD response together with macrophages from B and not C (4/4) was abolished (line 4). Opposite results were obtained when the T cells were first hot-pulse precultured with macrophages from C and PPD (line 5).

Similar results were obtained in another experiment involving other cell donors (Hirschberg *et al.*, 1979) and demonstrate that in *D/DR*-heterozygous individuals, two separate *HLA-D/DR*-restricted antigen-specific T-cell clones exist.

3.6. B Lymphocytes Expressing Self-HLA-D Are Not Able to Substitute for Macrophages in Antigen Activation

In the experiments hitherto reported, macrophage-enriched cell suspensions were used as antigen-presenting cells. However, B cells also express the HLA-D/DR determinants. The question therefore arises whether B cells in conjunction with antigen might also be able to elicit an *HLA-D/DR*-restricted antigen activation of sensitized T cells.

To study this, we prepared B-cell-enriched, macrophage-depleted cell suspensions by first culturing the T-cell-depleted suspensions overnight in tissue culture flasks, then performing a new *S*, 2-aminoethyli-sothiouronium–sheep red blood cell (AET-SRBC) rosetting, followed by incubation in a glass-bead column. The resulting cell suspensions contained less than 1% latex-ingesting cells and more than 60% cells that carried cell-membrane-bound Ig and expressed DR antigens (Bergholtz and Thorsby, 1979b).

Table 8 shows the results using T cells and different numbers of macrophages and B cells from two different donors. It can be seen that an optimal PPD response occurred at a T/Mϕ ratio of 5 : 1 or 10 : 1, and that B-enriched, macrophage-depleted cells, even at a T/B ratio of 1 : 1, were not able to induce a significant PPD response. In other experiments (Bergholtz and Thorsby, 1980b), we could show that any PPD-specific response induced in the presence of the B-cell fraction was in all probability due to contaminating macrophages.

We also investigated whether autologous B cells might provide the self-*HLA-D/DR* restriction "signal" when antigen is presented by *HLA-D/DR*-incompatible allogeneic Mϕ. In two experiments, T cells from a total of six donors were stimulated with PPD in the presence of autologous Mϕ or *HLA-D/DR*-incompatible allogeneic Mϕ either alone or

TABLE 8. PPD Presentation by Different Non-T Fractions

T-cell donor (5 × 10⁴ cells)	APC[a]	PPD (μg/ml)	Number of autologous APC[b]					
			0	200	1000	5000	10,000	50,000
E.S.	Mφ (91%)	0	66 ± 12	77 ± 25	307 ± 30	355 ± 12	409 ± 18	395 ± 50
		2.5	206 ± 36	1065 ± 36	2990 ± 174	6350 ± 274	4,780 ± 143	1911 ± 59
			140	**988**	**2683**	**5995**	**4371**	**1516**
	B (<1%)	0	—	65 ± 17	97 ± 3	73 ± 13	125 ± 28	237 ± 60
		2.5	—	204 ± 19	200 ± 21	203 ± 11	210 ± 61	534 ± 81
				139	**103**	**130**	**85**	**297**
E.T.	Mφ (95%)	0	129 ± 40	303 ± 96	150 ± 44	179 ± 60	211 ± 57	1292 ± 450
		2.5	568 ± 50	2064 ± 414	4777 ± 334	7707 ± 425	10,936 ± 281	2170 ± 198
			439	**1761**	**4627**	**7528**	**10,725**	**868**
	B (<1%)	0	—	118 ± 29	221 ± 86	95 ± 46	185 ± 34	336 ± 79
		2.5	—	269 ± 115	183 ± 51	247 ± 53	623 ± 128	558 ± 155
				151	**0**	**152**	**438**	**222**

[a] (APC) Antigen-presenting cells (percentage of latex-ingesting cells in parentheses).

[b] The first two values in each case are mean cpm ± S.E. the Third value (centered beneath the first two) is the incremental response.

mixed with autologous B-enriched cells (these B cells were not as "pure" as used in the aforementioned experiments, containing approximately 10% Mφ). All experiments yielded consistent results. Table 9 shows results obtained with two of the donors. An optimal T-cell response was obtained only with autologous Mφ. Addition of an equal number of autologous B-enriched cells did not affect this response. More important, the very poor incremental PPD response obtained with *HLA-D/DR*-incompatible Mφ was also not improved by the presence of 5×10^3 autologous B-enriched cells.

These studies show that although they certainly express the HLD-D/DR determinants, B cells have no ability to induce an *HLA-D/DR*-restricted, antigen-specific response. Since we have shown previously that it is mainly PPD bound to the accessory cells that stimulates T cells (see Section 3.1), the simplest explanation of the inability of B cells to substitute for macrophages is that B cells lack the capacity to nonspecifically bind or process enough antigen. A selective purification of B cells bearing specific Ig receptors for PPD might yield a B-cell fraction capable of binding and presenting PPD to T cells. We have not been able to perform this kind of experiment. However, trinitrophenyl (TNP)-treated "pure" B cells seem to be able to induce an *HLA-D/DR*-restricted, hapten-specific response in T cells primed to TNP-modified autologous non-T cells (see Section 4.4).

The poor T-cell response to PPD in conjunction with *HLA-D/DR*-incompatible allogeneic Mφ was not improved by the addition of autologous (*HLA-D/DR*-bearing) B cells. This indicates that the activation of T cells by PPD requires that both PPD and autologous HLA-D/DR molecules be displayed on the surface of the same cell.

4. Self-*HLA-D/DR* Restriction of T Cells Sensitized *in Vitro*

4.1. *In Vitro* Priming against TNP-Treated Autologous Cells

To investigate whether an *HLA-D/DR* restriction could be seen after primary sensitization *in vitro*, we used the system first described by Shearer (1974) for murine cells, and later by Newman *et al.* (1977) for human cells, demonstrating that T cells can be primed in *vitro* to trinitrophenyl (TNP)-conjugated autologous cells.

In preliminary experiments, we found that an optimal secondary response was observed when T cells were first stimulated with TNP-treated autologous non-T cells (i.e., B cells and macrophages) for 9–10 days *in vitro*, and then restimulated with the same TNP-treated autologous non-T cells for 48–72 hr.

The results of two experiments are given in Table 10 (details in

TABLE 9. T-Cell Response to PPD in the Presence of *HLA-D/DR*-Incompatible Macrophages Mixed with Autologous B Cells[a]

T-cell donor (5 × 10⁴ cells)	PPD (µg/ml)	Accessory cells					
		None	Autol. Mφ[b]	Autol. B[c]	Autol. Mφ[b] + autol. B[c]	Allog. Mφ[d]	Allog. Mφ[d] + autol. B[c]
A.K.	0	252 ± 109[a]	240 ± 44	291 ± 156	239 ± 33	1495 ± 201	1720 ± 327
	2.5	197 ± 39	1273 ± 230	521 ± 240	1221 ± 81	1059 ± 402	1746 ± 302
		0	**1033**	**230**	**982**	**0**	**26**
E.G.K.	0	604 ± 81	680 ± 294	297 ± 71	345 ± 71	2392 ± 231	2202 ± 26
	2.5	1382 ± 194	8447 ± 872	1765 ± 95	7785 ± 405	4277 ± 402	3306 ± 463
		778	**7767**	**1468**	**7440**	**1885**	**1104**

[a] The first two values in each case are mean cpm ± S.E. The third value (centered beneath the first two) is the incremental response.
[b] 5 × 10⁴ macrophages.
[c] 5 × 10³ B-enriched cells (contaminated with < 10% macrophages).
[d] *HLA-D/DR*-incompatible with T-cell donor.

TABLE 10. *In Vitro* Priming against Autologous Cells

Expt. No.	T cells primed to[a]:	—	Restimulated with[b]: Nontr. non-T	TNP non-T	Δ[c]
I	—	197 ± 91	985 ± 123	1,762 ± 358	777
	Nontr. non-T	265 ± 44	4956 ± 201	5,202 ± 435	246
	TNP-non-T	240 ± 76	3077 ± 125	14,262 ± 935	11,185
II	—	168 ± 15	2054 ± 749	2,688 ± 494	634
	Nontr. non-T	153 ± 10	2666 ± 349	3,387 ± 563	721
	TNP-non-T	306 ± 43	3008 ± 294	9,293 ± 481	6,285

[a] Equal amounts of T cells and X-ray-irradiated (2000 rads) autologous non-T cells (prepared by rosetting with AET-treated SRBC) were cultured together in tissue culture tubes and serum-supplemented RPMI 1640 for 9–10 days.

[b] For restimulation, 10^5 of the primed T cells were restimulated with an equal amount of X-ray-irradiated non-T cells for 72 hr in the wells of microtiter plates.

[c] TNP-specific response: mean of cpm in primed cultures restimulated with TNP-treated autologous cells minus restimulation response when confronted with nontreated cells.

Thorsby and Nousiainen, 1979). A clear TNP-specific response can be seen (compare results of TNP-primed cells when restimulated with TNP-treated cells vs. restimulated with nontreated cells). In ten different experiments performed, a TNP-specific response was seen in nine, with a range of incremental responses of 11,420–2255 cpm (mean ± S.E. = 5675 ± 1268). It can also be seen, particularly in Expt. No. 1, that T lymphocytes can apparently be primed to non-treated cells (compare response of primed and nonprimed cells). This effect was, however, more variable than the secondary TNP-specific response.

4.2. *HLA-D/DR* Restriction of the TNP-Specific Response

To study this question, cells were prepared from different unrelated donors sharing HLA-A,B,C and/or -D/DR antigens with the autologous priming cells. The results of one of a series of five different experiments (see Thorsby and Nousiainen, 1979) are depicted in Table 11. It can be seen from the table that TNP-treated allogeneic cells that are *HLA-D/DR*-identical with the autologous priming cells induced a TNP-specific response of the primed cells that varied from 47 to 101% of the TNP-specific response seen when restimulated with autologous cells, In contrast, the *HLA-D/DR*-different cells gave rise to a restimulation response of only 12 and 21%, and the incremental TNP-specific response was not much higher than that of the nonprimed cells. It also appears that the nonprimed cells gave a much higher response to the allogeneic *HLA-D/DR*-different cells than to the identical cells (as expected),

TABLE 11. Priming with Autologous TNP-Treated Cells and Restimulation with Autologous and Allogeneic Cells[a]

| | Autologous cells[b] | | | Allogeneic cells[c] | | | | | | | | | |
| | | | | HLA-D-identical | | | | | HLA-D-different | | | | |
	Nontr.	TNP	Δ	ABC[d]	Nontr.	TNP	Δ	%[e]	ABC[d]	Nontr.	TNP	Δ	%[e]
Non-primed	901	1,447	546	2	2236	3,288	**1,052**	—	1	9554	12,305	**2751**	—
				4	3107	3,452	**345**	—	0	9027	11,171	**2144**	—
				0	3542	4,252	**710**	—					
Primed	3139	14,559	11,420	2	7749	14,765	**7,016**	61	1	7211	9,617	**2406**	21
				4	5482	17,038	**11,556**	101	0	6153	7,466	**1313**	12
				0	2196	7,516	**5,320**	47		—	—	—	—
Mean (5 expts.)			100%					71.5 ± 8.2 (N = 13)					30.8 ± 6.1 (N = 8)
								$p < 0.005$					

[a] The experimental conditions were as given in Table 10. Values are median cpm of triplicate determinations.

[b] HLA: A1, 9; B8, 15; Cw3; Dw3,4.

[c] HLA: A2,28; B27,15; Cw2,3; Dw3,4

A1,2; B8,15; Cw3; Dw3,4 } HLA-D-identical with priming cells.

A2; B12; Dw3,4

A2,11; B5,40; Cw3; Dw2, –

A3,28; B18,27; Cw2; Dw –, – } HLA-D-different from priming cells.

[d] Number of HLA-A,B,C antigens shared between priming and restimulating cells.

[e] TNP-specific response when restimulated with allogeneic cells as a percentage of TNP-specific response when restimulated with autologous cells (= 100%).

whereas after autologous priming, this difference was less pronounced or no longer seen.

The mean relative TNP-specific restimulation responses of all 5 experiments involving different responding cells and a total of 13 *HLA-D/DR*-identical and 8 *HLA-D/DR*-different cells (sharing no HLA-D/DR antigens with the autologous priming cells) are given at the bottom of Table 11. The difference between the two groups is highly significant ($p < 0.005$) as estimated by Wilcoxon's rank sum test. Thus, after priming *in vitro* with hapten-conjugated autologous cells, the secondary hapten-specific response is restricted by self-*HLA-D/DR*. Very similar results were obtained by Seldin and Rich (1978) and Charmot and Mawas (1979), by using nonfractionated peripheral-blood mononuclear cells as responding and stimulating cells.

4.3. Is the TNP-Specific Response Also Restricted by *HLA-A,B,C*?

The results of the experiment presented in Table 11 indicate that the effects of sharing of HLA-A,B,C antigens between autologous priming and allogeneic restimulating cells are less than sharing of HLA-D. However, due to the high degree of nonrandom associations between certain HLA-B and -D determinants, it was difficult to select enough informative allogeneic cells. For this reason, and since most T cells do not express the HLA-D determinants, T lymphocytes that had been primed with autologous TNP-treated non-T cells were also restimulated with a similar number of TNP-treated autologous T cells, in some experiments together with autologous nontreated macrophages (80,000 T + 20,000 Mϕ). The results of two of a series of eight experiments are

TABLE 12. Priming against Autologous Non-T Cells and Restimulation with Autologous Cells[a]

Expt. No.	T cells primed to	Non-T —	nontr.	TNP	Δ	T cells Nontr.	TNP	Δ	ΔMφ[b]
	—	96	495	591	96	59	35	—	—
I	Nontr.	157	2,879	2,115	—	392	164	—	—
	TNP-non-T	111	1,393	3,648	2255	234	278	44	—
	—	127	1,505	2,962	1457	250	155	—	186
II	Nontr.	598	13,587	11,502	—	516	530	14	591
	TNP-non-T	332	4,413	6,765	2352	427	643	216	879

[a] The experimental conditions were as given in Table 10. Values are mean cpm of triplicate determinations.
[b] TNP-specific response in the presence of nontreated macrophages.

given in Table 12. T lymphocytes primed against HLA-A,B,C- and -D-expressing TNP-treated autologous cells gave only weak responses when restimulated with nontreated or TNP-treated T cells, and no response or only a weak TNP-specific response was seen. The TNP-specific response was slightly increased after addition of nontreated autologous macrophages ($\Delta_{M\phi}$ in Table 12), but in all experiments much less than when restimulation was performed with TNP-treated non-T cells. Thus, to obtain a secondary hapten-specific proliferative response, sharing of HLA-A,B,C between priming and restimulating cells was not sufficient.

We also found that it was possible to prime T cells against nontreated autologous non-T cells *in vitro*, and that this autosensitization appeared to be restricted by self-*HLA-D/DR* and not -*A,B,C* (Thorsby and Nousiainen, 1979). The nature of the autoantigenic complex being recognized by T cells in this case is not known. Possibly, during *in vitro* culture, tissue-culture constituents or cell metabolites may modify the cell membranes to a certain extent, making them immunogenic.

4.4. Can B Cells Substitute for Macrophages in the Secondary TNP-Specific Response?

The nature of the TNP-modified autologous cell-membrane components that are recognized by the T lymphocytes *in vitro* is not known. Since self-*HLA-D* products of the modified cells apparently are involved in the activation, one might suggest that TNP directly modifies self-*HLA-D* molecules, which are then recognized as foreign. However, Thomas *et al.* (1978) could not detect any TNP-modified Ia antigens in similar experiments in the guinea pig. We have also found that when T lymphocytes are primed to either untreated or TNP-treated allogeneic cells, restimulation with the same allogeneic cells, whether TNP-treated or not, gives rise to the same early increased response, indicating that many of the *HLA-D*-activating determinants have not been altered (Thorsby and Nousiainen, unpublished).

In Section 3.6, we presented data showing that B cells expressing self-*HLA-D/DR* could not replace macrophages in inducing an *HLA-D/DR*-restricted antigen-specific response to PPD. We proposed that this, at least in part, might be due to too few B cells binding PPD. Since TNP apparently binds to most cell membranes, it might be that with this hapten, B cells might be able to replace macrophages in secondary stimulation.

To study this, T cells were primed with TNP-treated autologous non-T cells (B cells + macrophages) and then restimulated with TNP-treated non-T cells (B cells + macrophages), TNP-treated B cells (prepared as described in Section 3.6), or TNP-treated macrophages. Table 13 shows the results of two out of six experiments involving different donors, all giving essentially the same results. Using 50,000 primed T cells, a clear TNP-specific response was always seen using 10,000 or more TNP-treated B cells for restimulation. Also, the same number of TNP-treated B cells usually caused a stronger restimulation than the same number of TNP-treated macrophages.

These results indicate that while B-cell-enriched suspensions prepared by similar methods were not able, together with antigen, to induce a PPD-specific response of sensitized T cells, these cell suspensions, when treated with TNP, would often induce a strong *HLA-D/DR* restricted TNP-specific response of TNP-sensitized T cells. Our B-cell suspensions contained less than 1% latex-ingesting cells, and this possible contamination of macrophages (500–1000 cells) was not able to induce a secondary TNP-specific response alone. These results are in contrast to the results reported by Thomas *et al.* (1978), who used a similar approach with T cells from guinea pigs sensitized *in vivo* with picryl chloride and restimulated with TNP-treated Ia-rich EN-L_2C B-cell-like leukemic cells. They found that these TNP-treated leukemic cells, in contrast to similarly treated macrophages, were unable to induce a TNP-specific response. The authors state that different results might have been obtained using normal (instead of malignant) B cells.

5. Comments

Taken together, these studies demonstrate that antigen-sensitized human T cells will respond by proliferation *in vitro* only when confronted with antigen together with *HLA-D/DR* determinants present in the initial sensitizing environment *in vivo* or *in vitro,* i.e., they are restricted by self-*HLA-D/DR* molecules. Macrophages which express self-*HLA-D/DR* appear to be the most important antigen-presenting cells, although under particular circumstances other self-*HLA-D/DR*-expressing cells may also possibly substitute for macrophages. Different nonoverlapping T-cell clones apparently exist with specificity for the same antigen but are restricted by different *HLA-D/DR* determinants. Thus, in *HLA-D/DR* heterozygous donors, at least two different populations of T cells with specificity for the same antigen seem to exist.

By analogy with the data on MHC restriction of T cells from studies of rodents, the human T cells which are *HLA-D/DR* restricted include, in all probability, the T helper cells. Thus, one may assume that T-helper-cell activation by antigen requires that antigen be displayed on

TABLE 13. T Cells Primed with TNP-Treated Autologous Non-T Cells and Restimulation with Various Numbers of B Cells or Macrophages

Expt. No.	T cells[a] primed with	Cells used for restimulation	Non-T[b] 50,000 cells	B cells[c] 40,000 cells	20,000 cells	10,000 cells	5,000 cells	Mφ[d] 10,000 cells	5,000 cells	2,500 cells	1,250 cells
I	—	TNP-treated	2437[e]	3817	1751	462	113	126	120	95	71
		Nontreated	959	1828	843	412	109	112	89	88	67
		Δ[f]	1478	1989	908	50	4	14	31	7	4
	TNP-non-T	TNP-treated	8250	9686	5839	2807	360	799	558	228	304
		Nontreated	2084	2546	850	416	195	148	191	145	95
		Δ	6166	7140	4989	2391	165	651	367	83	209
II	—	TNP-treated	1409	2057	1596	—	471	97	110	108	184
		Nontreated	1712	1037	540	—	154	119	205	126	101
		Δ	—	1021	1056	—	317	—	—	—	83
	TNP-non-T	TNP-treated	2726	5794	3824	—	1476	467	348	168	145
		Nontreated	1480	1140	396	—	123	97	94	162	147
		Δ	1246	4654	3428	—	1353	370	354	6	—

[a] Fifty thousand T cells primed with an equal amount of non-T cells.
[b] B cells + macrophages.
[c] < 1% latex ingesting cells; > 60% Ig and HLA-DR positive cells.
[d] (Mφ) Macrophages; > 95% latex ingesting cells.
[e] Median cpm of triplicates.
[f] TNP-specific response.

macrophages expressing the *D/DR* molecules of the T-helper-cell donor, and that T-cell help in antibody production requires that the T helper cells can recognize antigens bound by the B-cell Ig receptor, together with the same D/DR molecules in the B-cell membrane. Similar restrictions, but to the HLA-A,B,C molecules, have been found for cytotoxic T cells from individuals sensitized to minor histocompatibility antigens (Goulmy *et al.,* 1977), influenza virus (McMichael *et al.,* 1977), and dinitrofluorobenzene (Dickmeiss *et al.,* 1977). Most probably, again by analogy with data from studies in rodents, the self-*HLA* restriction is not imposed on the T cells when activated by antigen, but by confrontation with self-HLA molecules during fetal thymic development (Zinkernagel *et al.,* 1978a,b).

The studies in man, in addition to confirming that human T cells are also restricted by self-MHC products, also add one important piece of information that most studies of mainly inbred animals have not provided. All the studies reported here, and most of the studies reported by other groups working with human systems, have used cells from completely *unrelated* donors. They have been selected to share or not share HLA-A,B,C or D/DR molecules on the basis of the reactivity of their cells with cellular or serological reagents. Thus, in the human studies, the restricting elements appear to be the HLA-A,B,C or D/DR molecules as such, and not products of closely linked genes. If products of closely linked genes were to be involved, they would have to be nonrandomly associated to the *A,B,C* or *D/DR* genes of a degree even stronger than that known for the *A,B,C,D* genes themselves. Furthermore, following the results of the antibody-inhibition studies, one also had to postulate close association in the macrophage cell membrane. Of course, our studies cannot add evidence in favor of either the one or the other of the two prevailing theories on how *HLA* restriction functions at the T-cell level.

6. Implications

There are several clinical implications of the concept that T cells are self-*HLA*-restricted in their ability to be activated by antigen. For adoptive immunotherapy with immunocompetent T cells to be effective, it would be a requirement that the recipient and the donor at least share some of the HLA-A,B,C and D/DR determinants.

It is also possible that the same is true for the use of putative antigen-specific products of T cells. The little success with which the clinical trials with ''transfer factor'' have thus far been met has created severe doubt as to whether an antigen-specific "transfer factor" exists at all. Perhaps some of the experiments should be repeated preparing the factor from donors *HLA*-compatible with the recipients.

As pointed out by Zinkernagel *et al.* (1978a), the MHC restriction of T cells has great relevance for attempts at restoring T-cell immune competence with thymic transplants. The data suggest that for this to be successful, the thymic donors should be as *HLA-A,B,C*- and *D/DR*-compatible with their recipients as possible. This is to ensure that the thymus-induced *HLA* restriction of T cells is matched by the *HLA* profile of the interacting lymphoid and antigen-presenting cells. It should be kept in mind, however, that *HLA* restriction of human T cells does not seem to be an all-or-none phenomenon. Some allogeneic foreign HLA molecules may show a sufficient degree of cross-reactivity to be able to substitute for self-HLA.

One could also wonder whether confrontation with minor histocompatibility antigens on cells that are allogeneic, but *HLA*-identical with the recipient, might result in a stronger immune response toward the minor histocompatibility antigens than when they are presented on *HLA*-disparate cells. The reason is that the *HLA*-identical cells, expressing the minor histocompatibility antigens, also provide the HLA-restricting elements. Some preliminary data from experiments in the mouse involving minor histocompatibility antigens add some evidence in favor of this being so (P. Matzinger, personal communication). If confirmed, this would indicate that blood transfusions from *HLA*-matched donors should probably, if possible, be avoided before the use of transplants from *HLA*-identical (or haploidentical) donors. This might be particularly important in bone marrow transplantation.

After it was found that certain HLA antigens occurred with a much increased frequency among patients with particular diseases [e.g., HLA-B27 and ankylosing spondylitis, HLA-D/DRw3 in several different autoimmune diseases and others (see Dausset and Svejgaard, 1977)], HLA typing has become an important diagnostic tool. Several hypotheses have been presented to explain *HLA* and disease associations, the one receiving the greatest support being nonrandom associations between *Ir* genes and certain HLA antigens. However, for some associations (e.g., HLA-B27 and ankylosing spondylitis, Dw3/DRw3 and coeliac disease), this explanation would require that the same nonrandom association exist in different populations and races to a degree previously unknown for the *HLA* system. The recent data that indicate that the MHC products that restrict the T-cell immune responses (i.e., Ia and D/K in mice) may be identical to the *Ir*-gene products (see Section 1) provide a more direct explanation. Thus, the HLA molecules themselves may be directly involved, by differing in their ability to display antigenic determinants in an immunogenic way for T cells. There is already some indirect evidence of this. McMichael (1978) found that sharing of HLA-A and/or -B antigens between influenza-virus-infected target cells and the donor of the cytotoxic T cells was necessary to obtain cytolysis. However, not all HLA-A and -B antigens were equally effective in this respect; for example, HLA-A2 was not very effective.

Following this, many of the *HLA* and disease associations may be explained by the self-HLA molecules themselves influencing the immunological repertoire of the T cells, thus determining resistance to particular infectious agents, and so on (see also Zinkernagel and Doherty, 1977). In man, further proof of this can be obtained only when antigens involved in or present on the agents causing some of these diseases can be purified and used in appropriate *in vitro* tests. Needless to say, *HLA* is of course not the only factor determining disease susceptibility.

This concept would also provide a simple explanation for the extreme degree of polymorphism that exists for MHC antigens. As has also been outlined by others elsewhere (see Zinkernagel and Doherty, 1977), heterozygosity at *HLA* and a high degree of polymorphism will be an advantage for the species. The more allotypic variants to choose from, the higher the chance that some members will have the appropriate display of A,B,C,D molecules to mount an efficient immune response against a given infectious agent. Depending on the environment, different selection pressures would exist in different populations. What is lacking is a clear demonstration of *HLA* associations to an infectious disease that particularly affects young individuals before or during puberty. However, the polymorphism we observe today is of course more a reflection of strong selection pressures in the past.

Perhaps one of the most puzzling facts about the MHC is the high number of T cells with the ability to recognize MHC antigens that also exist in nonsensitized individuals. As many as 2–4% or more of the T cells of a given individual will initially respond when confronted with the MHC products of another member of the same species (Simonsen, 1967; Wilson *et al.*, 1968). At the same time, there seems to be no need for joint recognition of self-MHC products for activation against allo-MHC products to occur.

The MHC restriction of T-cell responses again provides a possible explanation for the high number of histocompatibility-antigen-reactive cells (HARC). Following the altered-self hypothesis, one could postulate that self-MHC molecules modified by given antigens might bear certain similarities to particular allogeneic MHC variants. Alternatively, following the dual-recognition hypothesis, either the one receptor of low avidity for self-MHC products may fortuitously have high avidity for products of the MHC of another member of the species (Janeway *et al.,* 1976), or allogeneic MHC products might combine with both receptors, a "core" part through cross-reactivity with the one T-cell receptor for self-MHC, and the allotypic part with the second receptor for non-MHC antigens (see also Matzinger and Bevan, 1977).

Recent studies have provided some experimental evidence in support of this hypothesis. It was first shown that cytotoxic murine T cells induced against allogeneic MHC may also lyse chemically modified syngeneic cells (Lemonnier *et al.,* 1977; Billings *et al.,* 1977) and that cytotoxic T cells induced against foreign "minor" non-H-2 antigens (together with self-H-2) are also able to lyse allogeneic targets differing solely at *H-2* (Bevan, 1977). More important, Finberg *et al.* (1978) were recently able to demonstrate that apparently the same effector cells that after sensitization to virus-infected autologous cells were able to lyse these cells were also able to lyse certain noninfected allogeneic target cells. Thus, the great number of HARC and the strength of allogeneic products of MHC as transplantation antigens may be considered a by-product of the restricted ability of T cells to combine with antigen-modified self-MHC products or antigen in complex with self-MHC products.

7. Conclusion

The studies reported herein and those of others have demonstrated that T-cell immune responses are restricted by cell-membrane products of the *HLA* complex. Thus, self-*HLA* cell-membrane molecules appear to be directly involved in activating a T-lymphocyte immune response to most foreign antigens. Their involvement in antigen activation of T cells may also lead to an influence on the immunogenicity of foreign antigens. Thus, the self-*HLA* cell-membrane products may have an immune-response-regulating ability.

It follows that the biological function of *HLA* may be to participate in signaling changes in cell-membrane self, and the strong antigenicity of HLA antigens in allogeneic combinations may be a reflection of this function of self-*HLA* in T-cell activation to foreign antigens.

The study of HLA antigens and their role in cell interactions, which was initiated due to the need for better histocompatibility matching in clinical transplantation, has become of major importance for general and clinical immunology.

ACKNOWLEDGMENTS. Our studies have received support from The Norwegian Council for Science and the Humanities, The Norwegian Cancer Society, The Norwegian Society for Fighting Cancer, and Mr. Anders Jahre's Fund for the Promotion of Science. The secretarial help of E. Garmann and K. Goyer is gratefully acknowledged.

References

Abelson, L.D., and Mann, D.L., 1978, Genetic control of B-cell alloantigens: Evidence for gene(s) linked to the HLA-A locus, *Tissue Antigens* 11:101.

Ahmann, G.B., Sachs, D.H., and Hodes, R.J., 1978, Genetic analysis of Ia determinants expressed on Con A-reactive cells, *J. Immunol.* 121:159.

Albrechtsen, D., and Lied, M., 1978, Stimulating capacity of human lymphoid cell subpopulations in mixed lymphocyte cultures, *Scand. J. Immunol.* 7:427.

Albrechtsen, D., Solheim, B.G., and Thorsby, E., 1977a, The presence of Ia-like determinants on a subpopulation of human T lymphocytes, *Immunogenetics* 5:149.

Albrechtsen, D., Solheim, B.G., and Thorsby, E., 1977b, Antiserum inhibition of the mixed lymphocyte culture (MLC) interaction: Inhibitory effect of antibodies reactive with HLA-D-associated determinants, *Cell Immunol.* 28:258.

Albrechtsen, D., Solheim, B.G., and Thorsby, E., 1977c, Serological identification of five HLA-D associated (Ia-like) determinants, *Tissue Antigens* 9:153.

Barnstable, C.J., Jones, E.A., and Crumpton, M.J., 1978, Isolation, structure and genetics of HLA-A, -B, -C and -DRw (Ia) antigens, *Br. Med. Bull.* 34:1978.

Benacerraf, B., and Germain, R.N., 1978, The immune response genes of the major histocompatibility complex, *Immunol. Rev.* 38:70.

Benacerraf, B., and McDevitt, H.O., 1972, Histocompatibility linked immune response genes, *Science* 175:273.

Bergholtz, B., and Thorsby, E., 1977, Macrophage-dependent response of immune human T lymphocytes to PPD *in vitro:* Influence of HLA-D compatibility, *Scand. J. Immunol.* 6:679.

Bergholtz, B., and Thorsby, E., 1978, HLA-D restriction of the macrophage-dependent response of human T lymphocytes to PPD *in vitro:* Inhibition by anti-HLA-DR antisera, *Scand. J. Immunol.* 8:63.

Bergholtz, B., and Thorsby, E., 1979a, Macrophage/T lymphocyte interaction in the immune response to PPD in humans, *Scand. J. Immunol.* 9:511.

Bergholtz, B., and Thorsby, E., 1979b, HLA-D restricted antigen activation of sensitized T lymphocytes: Studies on the ability of HLA-D/DR expressing B cells to substitute for macrophages in antigen activation, *Scand. J. Immunol.* 10:267.

Berle, E., and Thorsby, E., 1980, The proliferative T cell response to herpes simplex virus (HSV) is restricted by self HLA-D, *Clin. Exp.Immunol.* 39:668.

Bevan, M.J., 1977, Killer cells reactive to altered-self antigens can also be alloreactive, *Proc. Natl. Acad. Sci. U.S.A.* 5:2094.

Billings, P., Burakoff, S., Dorf, M.E., and Benacerraf, B., 1977, Cytotoxic T lymphocytes induced against allogeneic I-region determinants react with Ia molecules on trinitro-phenyl-conjugated syngeneic target cells, *J. Exp. Med.* 146:623.

Billings, P., Burakoff, S.J., Dorf, M.E., and Benacerraf, B., 1978, Genetic control of cytolytic T-lymphocyte responses. II. The role of the host genotype in parental → F_1

radiation chimeras in the control of the specificity of cytolytic T-lymphocyte responses to trinitrophenyl-modified syngenic cells, *J. Exp. Med.* **148**:352.

Bodmer, W.F., Batchelor, J.R., Bodmer, J.G., Festenstein, H., and Morris P.J. (eds.), 1978, *Histocompatibility Testing 1977,* Munksgaard, Copenhagen.

Charmot, D., and Mawas, C., 1979, The *in vitro* cellular response of human lymphocytes to trinitrophenylated autologous cells: HLA-D restriction of proliferation but apparent absence of HLA restriction of cytolysis, *Eur. J. Immunol.* **9**:723.

Dausset, J., and Svejgaard, A. (eds), 1977, *HLA and Disease,* Munksgaard, Copenhagen.

Dickmeiss, E., Soeberg, B., and Svejgaard, A., 1977, Human cell-mediated cytotoxicity against modified target cells is restricted by HLA, *Nature (London)* **270**:526.

Evans, R.L., Faldetta, T.J., Humphreys, R.E., Pratt, D.M., Yunis, E.J., and Schlossman, S.F., 1978, Peripheral human T cells sensitized in mixed leucocyte culture synthesize and express Ia-like antigens, *J. Exp. Med.* **148**:1440.

Finberg, R., Burakoff, S.J., Cantor, H., and Benacerraf, B., 1978, Biological significance of alloreactivity: T cells stimulated by Sendai virus-coated syngeneic cells specifically lyse allogeneic target cells, *Proc. Natl. Acad. Sci. U.S.A.* **75**:5145.

Fu, S.M., Chiorazzi, N., Wang, C.Y., Montazeri, G., Kunkel, H.G., Ko, H.S., and Gottlieb, A.B., 1978, Ia-bearing T lymphocytes in man: Their identification and role in the generation of allogeneic helper activity, *J. Exp. Med.* **148**:1423.

Goulmy, E., Termijtelen, A., Bradley, B.A., and van Rood, J.J., 1977, Y-antigen killing by T cells of women is restricted by HLA, *Nature (London)* **226**:544.

Hämmerling, G.J., 1976, Tissue distribution of Ia antigens and their expression on lymphocyte subpopulations, *Transplant. Rev.* **30**:64.

Hansen, G., Rubin, B., Sørensen, S.F., and Svejgaard, A., 1978, Importance of HLA-D antigens for cooperation between human monocytes and T lymphocytes, *Eur. J. Immunol.* **8**:520.

Hirschberg, H., and Thorsby, E., 1973, Specific *in vitro* elimination of histocompatibility antigen reactive cells (HARC), *J. Immunol. Methods* **3**:251.

Hirschberg, H., and Thorsby, E., 1977, Activation of human suppressor cells in mixed lymphocyte cultures, *Scand. J. Immunol.* **6**:809.

Hirschberg, H., Bergh, O.J., and Thorsby, E., 1979, Clonal distribution of HLA restricted antigen-reactive T cells in man, *J. Exp. Med.* **150**:1271.

Janeway, C.A., Jr., Wigzell, H., and Binz, H., 1976, Two different V_H gene products make up the T-cell receptors, *Scand. J. Immunol.* **5**:993.

Lemonnier, F., Burakoff, S.J., Germain, R.N., and Benacerraf, B., 1977, Cytolytic thymus-derived lymphocytes specific for allogeneic stimulator cells crossreact with chemically modified syngeneic cells, *Proc. Natl. Acad. Sci. U.S.A.* **3**:1229.

Matzinger, P., and Bevan, M.J., 1977, Why do so many lymphocytes respond to major histocompatibility antigen?, *Cell Immunol.* **29**:1.

McMichael, A., 1978, HLA restriction of human cytotoxic lymphocytes specific for influenza virus: Poor recognition of virus associated with HLA-A2, *J. Exp. Med.* **148**:1458.

McMichael, A.J., Ting, A., Zweerink, H.J., and Askonas, B.A., 1977, HLA restriction of cell-mediated lysis of influenza virus-infected human cells, *Nature (London)* **270**:524.

Meo, T., David, C.S., Rinjbeek, A.M., Nabholtz, M., Miggiano, V.C., and Shreffler, D.C., 1975, Inhibition of mouse MLR by anti-Ia sera, *Transplant. Proc.* **7**:(Suppl. 1):127.

Murphy, D.B., Herzenberg, L.A., Okumura, K., Herzenberg, L.S., and McDevitt, H., 1976, A new I subregion (I-J) marked by a locus (Ia-4) controlling surface determinants of suppressor T lymphocytes, *J. Exp. Med.* **144**:699.

Newman, W., Stoner, G.L., and Bloom, B.R., 1977, Primary *in vitro* sensitization of human T cells, *Nature (London)* **269**:151.

Niederhuber, J.E., and Frelinger, A.F., 1976, Expression of Ia antigens on T and B cells and their relationship to immune-response functions, *Transplant. Rev.* **30**:101.

Paul, W.E., and Benacerraf, B., 1977, Functional specificity of thymus-dependent lymphocytes: A relationship between the specificity of T lymphocytes and their functions is proposed, *Science* **195**:1293.

Press, J.L., and McDevitt, H., 1977, Allotype-specific analysis of anti-(Tyr, Glu)-Ala-Lys antibodies produced by Ir-1A high and low responder chimeric mice, *J. Exp. Med.* **146**:1815.

Rosenthal, A.S., Barcinski, M.A., and Blake, J.T., 1977, Determinant selection is a macrophage dependent immune response gene function, *Nature (London)* **267**:156.

Seldin, M.F., and Rich, R.R., 1978, Human immune responses to hapten-conjugated cells. I. Primary and secondary proliferative responses *in vitro*, *J. Exp. Med.* **147**:1671.

Shearer, G.M., 1974, Cell-mediated cytotoxicity to trinitrophenyl-modified syngeneic lymphocytes. *Eur. J. Immunol.* **4**:527.

Shreffler, D.C., David, C.S., Cullen, S.E., Frelinger, J.A., and Niederhuber, J.E., 1977, Serological and functional evidence for further subdivision of the I regions of the H-2 complex, *Cold Spring Harbor Symp. Quant. Biol.* **41**:477.

Simonsen, M., 1967, The clonal selection hypothesis evaluated by grafted cells reacting against their hosts, *Cold Spring Harbor Symp. Quant. Biol.* **32**:517.

Thomas, D.W., Clement, L., and Shevach, E.M., 1978, T lymphocyte stimulation by hapten-conjugated macrophages: A model system for the study of immunocompetent cell interactions, *Immunol. Rev.* **40**:181.

Thorsby, E., 1978, Biological function of HLA, *Tissue Antigens* **11**:321.

Thorsby, E., 1979, The human major histocompatibility complex HLA: Some recent developments, *Transplant. Proc.* **11**:616.

Thorsby, E., and Nousiainen, H., 1979, *In vitro* sensitization of human T lymphocytes to hapten (*TNP*)-conjugated and nontreated autologous cells is restricted by self-HLA-D, *Scand. J. Immunol.* **9**:183.

Thorsby, E., Albrechtsen, D., Hirschberg, H., Kaakinen, A., and Solheim, B.G., 1977, MLC-activating HLA-D determinants: Identification, tissue distribution and significance, *Transplant. Proc.* **9**:393.

Thorsby, E., Albrechtsen, D., Bergholtz, B.O., Hirschberg, H., and Solheim, B.G., 1978, Identification and significance of products of the HLA-D region, *Transplant. Proc.* **10**:313.

Tosi, R., Tanigaki, N., Centis, D., Ferrara, G.B., and Pressman, D., 1978, Immunological dissection of human Ia molecules, *J. Exp. Med.* **148**:1592.

von Boehmer, H., Haas, W., and Jerne, N., 1978, Major histocompatibility complex-linked immune responsiveness is acquired by lymphocytes of low responder mice differentiating in thymus of high responder mice, *Proc. Natl. Acad. Sci. U.S.A.* **75**:2439.

Waldmann, H., Pope, H., Bettles, C., and Davies, A.J.S., 1979, The influence of thymus on the development of MHC restrictions exhibited by T-helper cells, *Nature (London)* **277**:137.

Wilson, D.B., Blyth, J.L., and Nowell, P.C., 1968, Quantitative studies on the mixed lymphocyte interaction in rats. III. Kinetics of the response, *J. Exp. Med.* **128**:1157.

Zinkernagel, R.M., and Doherty, P.C., 1977, Possible mechanisms of disease-susceptibility association with major transplantation antigens, in: *HLA and Disease* (J. Dausset and A. Svejgaard, eds.), pp. 256–268, Munksgaard, Copenhagen.

Zinkernagel, R.M., Callahan, G.N., Althage, A., Cooper, S., Klein, P.A., and Klein, J.,

1978a, On the thymus in the differentiation of "H-2 self-recognition" by T cells: Evidence for dual recognition?, *J. Exp. Med.* **147**:882.

Zinkernagel, R.M., Callahan, G.N., Altage, A., Cooper S., Streilein, J.W., and Klein, J., 1978b, The lymphoreticular system in triggering virus plus self-specific cytotoxic T cells: Evidence for T help, *J. Exp. Med.* **147**:897.

Zinkernagel, R.M., Althage, A., Cooper, S., Callahan, G., and Klein, J., 1978c, In irradiation chimeras, K or D regions of the chimeric host, not of the donor lymphocytes, determine immune responsiveness of antiviral cytotoxic T cells, *J. Exp. Med.* **148**:805.

8

How Strict Is the MHC Restriction of T Cells?

Rolf M. Zinkernagel

1. Introduction

Thymus-derived lymphocytes (T cells) are generally specific for a self determinant (self-H) expressed on the target-cell surface and coded by the major histocompatibility gene complex (MHC) (reviewed in Paul and Benacerraf, 1977; Katz, 1977; Zinkernagel and Doherty, 1979). T cells that mediate nonlytic functions, such as T helper cells, proliferating T cells, and T cells involved in delayed-type hypersensitivity against contact allergens or intracellular bacteria, are specific for H-2I determinants, whereas lytic T cells are specific for H-2K or D structures. Specificities both for self-H and for any foreign antigen (X) are clonally expressed and highly specific. It is still unclear whether this dual specificity reflects T-cell expression of a single receptor for a neoantigenic determinant combining self-H complexed with X or T-cell expression of two independent receptor sites for self-H and for X.

How T cells acquire specificity for self-H during ontogeny has been the focus of several experiments with chimeras formed either by lethally irradiating mice and then reconstituting them with lymphohemopoietic stem (bone marrow) cells from various sources (reviewed in Bevan and Fink, 1978; Zinkernagel, 1978) or by using mice that lack thymuses and T cells and reconstituting them with grafted thymuses. These experiments have revealed the following: (1) Precursor T cells select the receptor specificity for self-H independent of antigens in the thymus; radioresistant

Rolf M. Zinkernagel • Department of Immunopathology, Scripps Clinic and Research Foundation, La Jolla, California 92037. Present address: Department of Pathology, Universitatsspital, 8091 Zürich, Switzerland.

thymic cells seem to be responsible for this selection (Zinkernagel *et al.*, 1978a; Fink and Bevan, 1978; Miller *et al.*, 1979; Waldmann *et al.*, 1979). (2) Apparently, thymic selection of the restriction specificity alone is not sufficient for T cells to mature to immunocompetence. For example, H-2^k mice lacking a thymus on being reconstituted with transplanted F_1 (H-2^k × H-2^d) thymuses do not express H-2^d restriction specificity (Zinkernagel, 1978). However, if the thymus graft is eliminated and lymphohemopoietic cells of H-2^d type are transfused, such animals may eventually express H-2^d-restricted T cells. Therefore, T-cell maturation seems to occur in at least two steps: thymic and posthymic. Whether the second step involves some *I*-region-dependent amplification of T cells that are relatively rare and "committed" or whether this step influences and/or promotes diversification of the T-cell repertoire for X is unknown. (3) Thymic selection of the restriction specificity simultaneously includes selection of the immune-response *(Ir)* phenotype expressed by T cells (von Boehmer *et al.*, 1978; Zinkernagel *et al.*, 1978b; Kappler and Marrack, 1978; Mullbacher and Blanden, 1979). Thus, selection of a restriction specificity for a strain's *K, D,* or *I-A* allele that regulates the responsiveness of that strain's cytotoxic or nonlytic T cells, respectively, automatically fixes the strain's responder phenotype. Apparently, then, *Ir*-gene products and *K, D,* or *I-A* products involved in T-cell restriction are identical. Therefore, *Ir* phenomena may simply be a direct consequence of T cells' being restricted. That is, *Ir* phenomena arise because a T cell's function is determined by that cell's restriction specificity and because the selection of a particular receptor for self-H that mediates the T cell's effector function (lysis via *K, D,* or further differentiation via *I-A*) influences the receptor repertoire available to recognize X (Langman, 1978; Cohn and Epstein, 1978; von Boehmer *et al.*, 1978; Zinkernagel, 1978).

Thus, MHC restriction reflects T cells' performance of a particular effector function according to what kind of self-H they recognize along with X. For example, T cells kill in response to K and D, which are receptors for lytic signals; alternatively, they trigger-cell differentiation in response to I determinants, which are receptors for cell differentiation signals. *In vivo,* MHC-restricted cytotoxic T cells are crucially involved in early antiviral recovery, whereas nonlytic T cells act antivirally or antibacterially via *I*-mediated macrophage activation (reviewed in Zinkernagel, 1978). MHC products define the effector function and also influence the receptor repertoire that can be expressed by T cells.

All immunological specificity is relative, and there is no doubt that the same is true for T-cell specificity for self-major transplantation antigens. Nevertheless, T-cell restriction specificity seems rather exquisite. This restriction seems to fit two possible models for T-cell receptors: (1) T cells express a single receptor site for a neoantigenic determinant resulting when self-H forms a complex with X on the cell surface or (2) T cells express two receptor sites, one for self-H, the other for X (reviewed in Zinkernagel and Doherty, 1979). These models make quite distinct predictions in terms of T-cell receptor repertoires. The single-receptor model predicts no *a priori* restriction of the repertoire; the two-receptor-site model does. If the specificity for self-H is great, detection of great differences in precursor frequencies among T cells specific for self-H vs. non-self-H should be easy. If specificity is weak, then it may be difficult to differentiate a two-receptor model from a single-receptor model. It has been reported recently that specificities of restriction expressed by T cells may in fact be much less stringent than thought so far (Bennink and Doherty, 1978; Doherty and Bennink, 1979; Matzinger and Mirkwood, 1978).

The purpose of this chapter is to quantitate restriction specificity as expressed by virus-specific cytotoxic T cells, regardless whether such specificity is mediated by suppression. We conclude that the T cells have a high degree of specificity for self-H.

2. Materials and Methods

2.1. Mice

C3H $(H-2^k)$, C57BL $(H-2^b)$, B10.D2 $(H-2^d)$, BALB/c $(H-2^d)$, C3H.OH $(H-2^{oz1})$, A.TL $(H-2^{t1})$, B10.BR $(H-2^k)$, CBA $(H-2^k)$, B10.A (5R) $(H-2^{i5})$, F_1 hybrids, and genetically thymus-deficient nude mice were obtained either from the Strong Foundation, San Diego, California; from the Jackson Laboratory, Bar Harbor, Maine; or from the breeding colony at Scripps Clinic.

2.2. Virus and Immunization

Vaccinia virus WR was a gift from Dr. W. Joklik, Duke University, Durham, North Carolina, and was grown in L cells as described elsewhere (Zinkernagel *et al.*, 1978). Lymphocytic choriomeningitis virus (LCMV) came from Dr. M.B.A. Oldstone, Scripps Clinic. LCMV was titrated on BHK 21/13S cells in agarose suspension as described by Pulkkinen and Pfau (1970).

2.3. Chimeras

Chimeras were produced by using the general protocol of Sprent *et al.* (1975). The mice were irradiated with a supralethal dose of 900–950 rads from a cesium source and on the same day were reconstituted with $1.5–2.5 \times 10^7$ anti-Θ plus complement (C)-treated bone marrow cells or fetal (14–16 day) liver cells injected intravenously (i.v.). Chimeras were analyzed individually 10–80 weeks later.

To form thymus chimeras, thymuses were taken from 15- to 17-day-old fetal mice and transplanted under the kidney capsules of 6- to 8-week-old nude mice (Kindred, 1979; Miller and Osoba, 1967). The only successful method for producing nude F_1 mice with functional grafts from both parents was to transplant 15- to 17-day-old fetal thymus lobes from donors of one parental strain under the recipient's left kidney capsule and from the other parental strain under the recipient's right kidney capsule on the same day (Zinkernagel et al., 1979). In all cases, the functional test and the restriction specificity of mature T cells correlated with the engrafted and histologically normal thymus.

2.4. Cell Preparations and H-2 Typing

All cells were prepared and used in minimal essential medium (MEM) supplemented with nonessential amino acids, pyruvate, bicarbonate, antibiotics, and 10% heat-inactivated fetal calf serum. All these ingredients were from Flow Laboratories, Inc. (Inglewood, California). Spleen cells from the virus-infected mice were processed and typed for H-2 as described previously (Zinkernagel et al., 1978a,b, 1979). In each typing assay, positive and negative control cells were included to confirm the specificity of the antisera treatment and the activity of C.

2.5. Cytotoxicity Assay

The assay and target cells used have been described (Zinkernagel et al., 1978a,b, 1979). L929 (H-2K) cells originate from C3H mice, MC57G (H-2^b) cells come from C57BL/6 mice, and D2 (H-2^d) are a methylcholanthrene-induced line of B10.D2 origin. The D2 line spontaneously released the most ^{51}Cr (20–30% for 6 hr, 30–45% for 16 hr), whereas MC57G released 8–12% during a 6-hr test and 12–25% over 16 hr, and L929 released 15–25% and 20–40%, respectively. The percentage of ^{51}Cr release was calculated as the percentage of water release (100%) and was corrected for medium release. Water usually released about 80–85% of the ^{51}Cr.

2.6. Antiviral Protection Assay in Vivo

Well-established techniques were used (Mims and Blanden, 1972; Blanden et al., 1975; Zinkernagel and Welsh, 1976). Donor mice were injected i.v. with 5×10^2 plaque-forming units (PFU) of LCMV, and their immune spleen cells were harvested 7–8 days later. Single spleen cell suspensions were made as described in Section 2.4. Recipient mice were injected i.v. with about 3×10^3 PFU 15–24 hr before transfer of usually 1×10^8 immune spleen cells. Recipients were sacrificed 24–30 hr later. Control spleens were from infected recipient mice that had received no cells or only normal cells. Individual spleens were homogenized with Teflon-coated pestles in glass grinder tubes in 2 ml MEM.

2.7. Statistical Methods

Means and S.E.M. of triplicates were determined and compared by Student's t test. The S.E.M. was usually less than 3%, and always less than 5%.

3. Results

3.1. Quantitation of the Restriction Specificity Expressed *in Vivo* and *in Vitro* by Virus-Specific Cytotoxic T Cells from Unmanipulated Mice

The comparison of the cytotoxic activity of C3H $(H\text{-}2^k)$ vaccinia-immune spleen cells on infected $H\text{-}2^k$ vs. infected $H\text{-}2^b$ targets revealed that histocompatible targets are lysed at least 30–100 times more efficiently than incompatible targets. Vice versa, $H\text{-}2^b$ immune T cells lysed infected $H\text{-}2^b$ targets at least 30–100 times better than infected $H\text{-}2^k$ targets. Similar differences exist for other haplotype combinations as shown in Fig. 1. The limitations of this titration are technical; for geometrical reasons, killer target-cell ratios greater than 40 cannot be used, and the assay time cannot be extended beyond 16 hr because of increase in spontaneous ^{51}Cr release and other factors. Therefore, the foregoing estimates must be minimal rather than exaggerated.

These limitations in quantitations of the cytotoxic activities *in vitro* were much less pronounced when the antiviral activity of K- or D-restricted T cells was measured *in vivo*. In this experiment, 5×10^7 immune spleen cells from mice infected for 7 days with LCMV were transferred to normal recipient mice that had been challenged with about 10^3 PFU of LCMV some 12–18 hr prior to cell transfer. At 24 hr after cell transfer, the number of PFU was assessed in recipients of immune and normal cells. Usually, spleens of recipients of immune cells contained $2\text{–}5 \log_{10}$ less PFU than controls. When the protective potential of $H\text{-}2$- or $H\text{-}2I$-incompatible LCMV-immune spleen cells was compared with the efficiency of D-compatible immune spleen cells, the difference was about $4 \log_{10}$ (Fig. 2). Thus, in this test system, which measured virtually

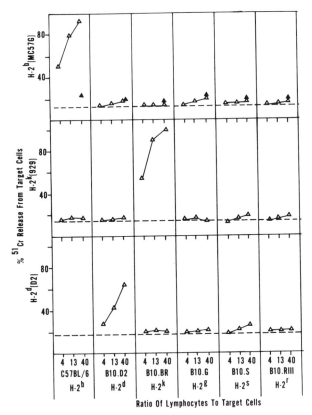

Figure 1. Cytotoxic activity of vaccinia-virus-immune spleen cells tested on infected ($\triangle$) or uninfected ($\blacktriangle$) target cells of various H-2 haplotypes for 6 hr. (---) Spontaneous ^{51}Cr release. The values are not corrected for spontaneous ^{51}Cr release.

exclusively T-cell activities, the specificity of restriction between H-2^k- and H-2^d-restricted T cells was a factor of at least 10,000.

3.2. Comparison of the Restriction Specificities Expressed by Virus-Specific Cytotoxic T Cells from Chimeric Mice

Chimeras were used to study differentiation of T cells and of their restriction specificities, because as summarized in Section 1, the restriction specificity is generally selected by the MHC of the chimeric host or thymus, rather than by the genotype of the T cell itself.

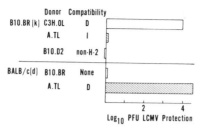

Figure 2. Adoptive transfer of anti-LCMV protection. Antiviral protection conferred by adoptive transfers of 1×10^8 LCMV-immune spleen cells in normal recipient mice that had been challenged with about 2×10^3 PFU of LCMV 14 hr prior to cell transfer. Recipients were sacrificed 30 hr after cell transfer. Protection is measured as the difference in PFU formed per spleen in control mice that had received normal cells or no cells and recipients of immune spleen cells. From Zinkernagel and Welsh (1976).

3.2.1. Irradiation Chimeras

Chimeras of the general type $(A \times B) \rightarrow (A \times C)$ were formed by reconstituting lethally irradiated (950 rads) $(BALB/c \times C3H)F_1$ mice with T-cell-depleted $(C3H \times C57BL)F_1$ bone marrow cells. The chimeras were infected with vaccinia virus 15 months after reconstitution (Table 1). The chimeric lymphocytes lysed only infected $H-2^k$ target cells that were histocompatible with both chimeric recipient and donor. Neither infected $H-2^d$ nor $H-2^b$ targets were lysed to any substantial level. Thus, the restriction specificity expressed by such chimeric T cells seems to be comparable to that expressed by T cells from nonchimeric mice.

3.2.2. Thymic Reconstitution of Nude Mice

$(C57BL \times BALB/c)F_1$ hybrid mice carrying the nude mutant gene were negative when tested for T-cell immunocompetence. However, when transplanted with thymuses from one or the other parent, these F_1 nude mice subsequently formed T cells with restriction specificities corresponding to the thymus graft. Therefore, a $(C57BL \times BALB/c)F_1$ nude mouse reconstituted with a C57BL $(H-2^b)$ thymus graft generated vaccinia-virus-specific cytotoxic T cells active against infected $H-2^b$ but not $H-2^d$ targets. The extent of restriction demonstrated by these chimeric T cells was again comparable to that expressed by T cells from nonchimeric mice (Fig. 3). F_1 nude mice transplanted with thymus grafts from fetal donors of both parental $H-2$ types formed T cells that were restricted to one or the other parental $H-2$ type. This result is interesting because theoretically F_1 nude mice reconstituted with thymus grafts of both parental types should show complete suppression of any immunocom-

TABLE 1. Restriction Specificities of T Cells from Irradiation Bone Marrow Chimeras

Bone marrow donor	Irradiated recipient	H-2^k(L929) Vacc.	Nor.	H-2^d(D2) Vacc.	Nor.	H-2^b(MC57G) Vacc.	Nor.
(C3H × C57BL)F$_1$ →	(BALB/c × C3H)F$_1$^{a}	61	0	5	2	5	3
(k × b) →	(d × k)	37	1	0	0	0	1
		14	1	0	0	0	0
Controls							
C57BL (b)		2	2	N.T.	N.T.	57	2
		0	0	—	—	30	1
		0	0	—	—	11	0
CBA (k)		49	1	6		1	0
		32	0	3		6	3
		12	0	5		3	3
B10.D2 (d)		1	1	43		0	0
		0	0	19		0	0
		0	0	4		0	0

^{a} Chimera was infected 15 months after reconstitution.

petence (or suppression of one restriction specificity by the "dominant" second one) if thymus-dependent suppression directed against the second host haplotype is responsible for the thymic influence on restriction specificities. Thus, suppression of one thymic maturational pathway does not seem to suppress the other and therefore cannot readily explain the results obtained with one parental thymus graft in F$_1$ nude mice.

3.2.3. H-2D-Compatible, H-2K,I-Incompatible Chimeras

Chimeras that are made with stem cells after lethal irradiation and are histoincompatible for all of *H-2* or for *H-2I* are only marginally immunocompetent when tested for their capacity to respond to virus. If selected restriction specificities overlap to a certain degree between various haplotypes, such chimeras should express at least some immunocompetence. The question is not whether there are any restricted T cells, but rather how the frequency of precursors generated in such incompatible chimeras compares with that found in *H-2*-compatible chimeras or in nonchimeric control mice.

Since we have no *in vitro* assay for determining absolute or relative precursor frequencies, we tested the delayed-type hypersensitivity response to LCMV in histocompatible chimeras and compared the capacity of these chimeras to eliminate the virus with the capacity of the control groups.

As shown in Table 2, F$_1$ → parental type chimeras and nonchimeric

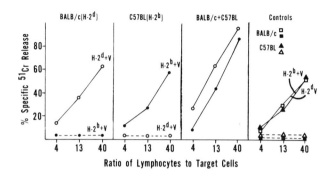

Figure 3. (C57BL × BALB/c)F₁ nu/nu mice reconstituted with fetal thymus grafts. (C57BL × BALB/c)F₁ nude mice reconstituted with one parental or simultaneously with both parental thymus grafts were tested for their capacity to generate virus-specific cytotoxic T cells. F₁ nude mice with a BALB/c thymus graft lysed infected *H-2ᵈ*, those with a C57BL graft lysed infected *H-2ᵇ*, and those with both parental grafts lysed both infected *H-2ᵈ* and infected *H-2ᵇ* targets. Virus-immune spleen cells from control mice were tested on both target cells [right most panel; BALB/c on infected *H-2ᵈ* (□) and on infected *H-2ᵇ* (■); C57BL on infected *H-2ᵇ* (▲) and on infected *H-2ᵈ* (△)]. Modified from Zinkernagel *et al.* (1979).

mice swell sizably at the site of the virus injection by day 9 and by day 15 have cleared all virus. In contrast, chimeras (5R → D2) given stem cells from a donor that is histocompatible for the *D* region but not for the *K* or *I-A* regions do not make a significant delayed-type hypersensitivity response and do not eliminate virus. Thus, if T-cell restriction specificities do overlap, the frequency is undetectable and of no practical consequence for the capacity of *H-2*-incompatible chimeras to deal with intracellular parasites.

4. Discussion

Discussing how specific T-cell restriction functions has the practical possibility of providing a sensible rationale for reconstituting immunodeficient patients and the theoretical potential of offering some insight into the nature of T-cell recognition, at least until we have direct biochemical evidence of it. The fact that T cells from unmanipulated mice are restricted with a great degree of specificity is undisputed, particularly for virus-specific T cells (see Figs. 1 and 2). However, the degree of restriction specificity expressed by T cells from chimeras is debatable. Some researchers believe that the specificity of restriction in chimeras is comparable to that of nonchimeric mice (Zinkernagel, 1978;

TABLE 2. Delayed-Type Hypersensitivity to Virus and Elimination of Virus in Chimeras[a]

Stem-cell donor		Irradiated recipient	Specific footpad swelling (%)	Log_{10} PFU of LCMV per 10 μl blood
5R $(K^b I^{b/d} D^d)$	→	D2[1] $(K^d I^d D^d)$	0	2.7
(C3H × BALB/c) $(k \times d)$	→	(C3H)[1] (k)	95	< 1
Control 5R			100	< 1

[a] Chimeras were tested 4 months after reconstitution. 10^6 PFU in 30 μl LCMV were injected into the left, control medium into the right footpads. Footpad swelling was assessed at day 9, viremia on day 15.

Bevan and Fink, 1978); others find that specificity is comparatively less strict (Blanden and Andrew, 1979; Matzinger and Mirkwood, 1978), but still "preferential" for one vs. the other haplotype. Still other investigators cannot document restriction specificity in chimeras (D.H. Katz, personal communication). As is usually the case, there are several technical details in the experiments that may explain the differences. The contamination of stem cells with immunocompetent T cells and the survival of T cells in so-called "lethally irradiated" mice are possibly the most important variables. Since serological typing of cells is usually not sensitive enough to detect this contamination, these variables cannot be stabilized for the time being. Therefore, we tend to take the experiments with chimeras that demonstrate most extensive restriction as the most meaningful; however, this somewhat arbitrary selection may be wrong if suppression should be responsible for the host influence on selection of restriction specificities.

The findings that incompatible or D-compatible chimeras do not generate measurable primary antiviral T-cell responses and do not eliminate virus efficiently strongly suggest that the immunocompetence of such chimeras is very low compared to histocompatible chimeras or nonchimeric mice. Therefore, the overlap of restriction specificities is not great enough so the cellular immune system can differentiate sufficiently to deal with virus infection. Still, any of the chimeras could conceivably have T cells with a restriction specificity that cross-reacts with H-2 antigens expressed by the thymus and by lymphohemopoietic cells. A procedure that selectively restimulates such rare T-cell precursors (or possibly contaminating immunocompetent cells that have not undergone differentiation in the chimeras) to sizable (measurable) numbers may give a different picture. Whether these explanations for the results of negative selection experiments or from repeated restimulation of chimeric lymphocytes are correct is speculative (Bennink and Doherty, 1978; Doherty and Bennink, 1979; Matzinger and Mirkwood, 1978).

If we accept a relatively high degree of restriction specificity, as the experiments summarized here document, how can it be explained? We favor the two-receptor site model for T-cell recognition as an explanation; nevertheless, until the receptor sites are characterized biochemically, single-receptor models will not be excluded unequivocally. Alternative explanations, such as suppression, may explain the findings with chimeras. For example, in (A × B) → A chimeras, perhaps restriction specificities that recognize self-B are suppressed. Despite intensive search, evidence for such suppression is still lacking (Bevan and Fink, 1978; Zinkernagel and Althage, 1979). Since acquisition of restriction specificities by T cells in allophenic mice (zygote aggregation chimeras) seems comparable to that in irradiation bone marrow chimeras, the implication is that either suppression is not responsible for the selection of restriction specificities or, alternatively, suppression is responsible for the very existence of restriction even in unmanipulated mice.

ACKNOWLEDGMENTS. Work reported in this chapter has been supported by USPHS grants No. AI-13779 and No. AI-00248. The excellent technical assistance of Ms. Alana Althage, Mrs. Elizabeth Waterfield, and Mr. Pierre Pincetl, and the secretarial and editorial help by Ms. Annette Parson, Phyllis Minick, and Andrea Rothman, are gratefully acknowledged. This paper is Publication No. 1814 and was submitted in May 1979.

References

Bennink, J.R., and Doherty, P.C., 1978, Different rules govern help for cytotoxic T cells and B cells, *Nature (London)* **276**:829–831.

Bevan, M.J., and Fink, P.J., 1978, The influence of thymus H-2 antigens on the specificity of maturing killer and helper cells, *Immunol. Rev.* **42**:4–19.

Blanden, R.V., and Andrew, M.E., 1979, Primary anti-viral cytotoxic T cell responses in semiallogeneic chimeras are not absolutely restricted to host H-2 type, *J. Exp. Med.* **149**:535–538.

Blanden, R.V., Bowern, N.A., Pang, T.E., Gardner, I.D., and Parish, C.R., 1975, Effects of thymus-independent (B) cells and the H-2 gene complex on antiviral function of immune thymus derived (T) cells, *Aust. J. Exp. Med. Sci.* **53**:187.

Cohn, M., and Epstein, R., 1978, T-cell inhibition of humoral responsiveness. II. Theory on the role of restrictive recognition in immune regulation, *Cell. Immunol.* **39**:125–153.

Doherty, P.C., and Bennink, J.R., 1979, Vaccinia-specific cytotoxic T-cell responses in the context of H-2 antigens not encountered in thymus may reflect aberrant recognition of a virus-H-2 complex, *J. Exp. Med.* **149**:150–157.

Fink, P.J., and Bevan, M.J., 1978, H-2 antigens of the thymus determine lymphocyte specificity, *J. Exp. Med.* **148**:766–775.

Kappler, J.W., and Marrack, P., 1978, The role of H-2 linked genes in helper T cell function. IV. Importance of T cell genotype and host environment in I-region and *Ir* gene expression, *J. Exp. Med.* **148**:1510–1522.

Katz, D.H., 1977, *Lymphocyte Differentiation, Recognition and Regulation*, Academic Press, New York.

Kindred, B., 1979, Nude mice in immunology, *Prog. Allergy* **26**:137–238.

Langman, R.E., 1978, The role of the major histocompatibility complex in immunity: A new concept in the functioning of a cell-mediated immune system, *Rev. Physiol. Biochem. Pharmacol.* **81**:1.

Matzinger, P., and Mirkwood, G., 1978, In a fully H-2 incompatible chimera, T cells of donor origin can respond to minor histocompatibility antigens in association with either donor or host H-2 type, *J. Exp. Med.* **148**:84–92.

Miller, J.F.A.P., and Osoba, D., 1967, Current concepts in the immunological function of the thymus, *Physiol. Rev.* **47**:437–520.

Miller, J.F.A.P., Gamble, J., Mottram, P., and Smith, F.I., 1979, Influence of thymus genotype on acquisition of responsiveness in delayed-type hypersensitivity, *Scand. J. Immunol.* **9**:29–38.

Mims, C.A., and Blanden, R.V., 1972, Antiviral action of immune lymphocytes in mice infected with lymphocytic choriomeningitis virus, *Infect. Immunol.* **6**:695.

Mullbacher, A., and Blanden, R.V., 1979, H-2 linked control of cytotoxic T cell responsiveness to alphavirus infection: Presence of $H-2D^k$ during differentiation and stimulation converts stem cells of low responder genotype to T cells of responder phenotype, *J. Exp. Med.* **149**:786–790.

Paul, W.E., and Benacerraf, B., 1977, Functional specificity of thymus-dependent lymphocytes, *Science* **195**:1293.

Pulkkinen, A.J., and Pfau, C.J., 1970, Plaque size heterogeneity: A genetic trait of lymphocytic choriomeningitis virus, *Appl. Microbiol.* **20**:123.

Sprent, J., von Boehmer, H., and Nabholz, M., 1975, Association of immunity and tolerance to host H-2 determinants in irradiated F_1 hybrid mice reconstituted with bone marrow cells from one parental strain, *J. Exp. Med.* **142**:321.

von Boehmer, H., Haas, W., and Jerne, N.K., 1978, Major histocompatibility complex-linked immune-responsiveness is acquired by lymphocytes of low-responder mice differentiating in thymus of high-responder mice, *Proc. Natl. Acad. Sci. U.S.A.* **75**:2439–2442.

Waldman, H., Pope, H., Bettles, C., and Davies, A.J.S., 1979, The influence of thymus on the development of MHC restrictions exhibited by T-helper cells, *Nature (London)* **277**:137–138.

Zinkernagel, R.M., 1978, Thymus and lymphohemopoietic cells: Their role in T cell maturation, in selection of T cells' H-2-restriction-specificity and in H-2 linked *Ir* gene control, *Immunol. Rev.* **42**:224–270.

Zinkernagel, R.M., and Althage, A., 1979, Search for suppression of T cells specific for the second nonhost H-2 haplotype in $F_1 \rightarrow P$ irradiation bone marrow chimeras, *J. Immunol.* **122**:1742–1749.

Zinkernagel, R.M., and Doherty, P.C., 1979, MHC-restricted cytotoxic T cells: Studies on the biological role of polymorphic major transplantation antigens determining T cell restriction-specificity function and responsiveness, *Adv. Immunol.* **27**:52–142.

Zinkernagel, R.M., and Welsh, R.M., 1976, H-2 compatibility requirement for virus-specific T cell-mediated effector functions *in vivo*. I. Specificity of T cells conferring antiviral protection against lymphocytic choriomeningitis virus is associated with H-2K and H-2D, *J. Immunol.* **117:**1495–1502.

Zinkernagel, R.M., Callahan, G.N., Althage, A., Cooper, S., Klein, P.A., and Klein, J., 1978a, On the thymus in the differentiation of "H-2 self-recognition" by T cells: Evidence for dual recognition?, *J. Exp. Med.* **147:**882.

Zinkernagel, R.M., Althage, A., Cooper, S., Callahan, G., and Klein, J., 1978b, In irradiation chimeras, K or D regions of the chimeric host, not of the donor lymphocytes, determine immune responsiveness of antiviral cytotoxic T cells, *J. Exp. Med.* **148:**805.

Zinkernagel, R.M., Althage, A., and Callahan, G., 1979, Thymic reconstitution of nude F_1 mice with one or both parental thymus grafts, *J. Exp. Med.* **150:**693–697.

II

Clinical Aspects of Transplantation: Association with Disease

9

The Role of Histocompatibilty Antigens in Clinical Transplantation

Kent C. Cochrum and Deanne M. Hanes

1. Introduction

Controversy surrounding the influence of *HLA-A* and *-B* matching in clinical kidney transplantation has not abated since its inception. Clearly, the excellent graft survival of *HLA*-identical siblings seemed to underline the efficacy of histocompatibility testing. However, *HLA-A* and *-B* matching in unrelated donor–recipient pairs, particularly in heterogeneous populations, has not been as successful as anticipated. *HLA-D* matching, as evidenced by mixed-lymphocyte culture (MLC), has proven to be an excellent indication of graft survival especially in living–related situations. Recent developments, i.e., *DRw* typing and the beneficial effects of blood transfusions, appear to offer evidence of even better graft survival. In this chapter, we will relate our experience with donor–recipient matching in renal transplants and attempt to place our results in some perspective with evidence from other centers.

2. *HLA-A* and *-B* Matching

Large European kidney-exchange programs such as Eurotransplant, Scandiatransplant, and France Transplant were organized specifically to offer the best *HLA-A* and *-B*-matched kidneys to their existing patient

Kent C. Cochrum and Deanne M. Hanes • Department of Surgery, University of California, San Francisco, California 94143.

populations. The arguments concerning the efficacy of *HLA-A* and *-B* matching and graft survival continue, although the consensus, in both Europe and the United States, appears to be in favor of *HLA* matching for improving graft survival (Festenstein *et al.*, 1976; Persijn *et al.*, 1978). The agreement is not enthusiastic, for even at best, *HLA* matching improves graft survival only 10–20% when the best- and the worst-matched grafts are compared (van Rood *et al.*, 1979). Our results (Vincenti *et al.*, 1978) with 510 unrelated pairs showed virtually no advantage in matching for serological determinants alone in cadaver transplants (Fig. 1). However, since the number of three- and four-antigen matches is so low in our population (number of four-antigen matches = 2), it is difficult to compare our data with data from other centers where three- and four-antigen matches are more frequent.

The differences apparent in European and American data probably stem from the racial characteristics of the two populations. Since, in relatively homogeneous populations, linkage dysequilibrium exists between the *HLA-A* and *-B* loci and the *HLA-D* locus (van Hooff *et al.*, 1974), it is probable that serological matching also matches for *HLA-D* locus. Thus, the improvement in graft survival with closely matched pairs evident from the European statistics probably reflects this beneficial linkage dysequilibrium. Transplant centers in the United States select from a relatively small, hetergeneous recipient pool; consequently, close

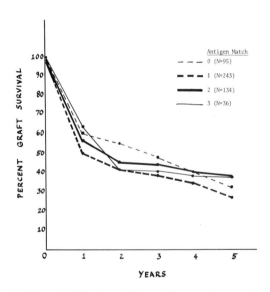

Figure 1. Effect of *HLA-A* and *-B* matching on cadaver-graft survival.

matches are infrequent and linkage dysequilibrium tends to disappear. Because of these factors, the benefits of *HLA* matching have been less discernible in the United States.

At present, it has not been shown conclusively that products of the *HLA-D* locus can be determined serologically, and since MLC testing cannot be used for cadaver transplants, *HLA-A* and *-B* matching supported by careful crossmatching remains the best method for improving graft survival in unrelated pairs.

Interestingly, the lack of relative population homogeneity and linkage dysequilibrium was instrumental in the recognition of two important factors in allograft survival: HLA-D compatibility and pretransplant blood transfusions.

3. *HLA-D* Matching

Our initial report in 1973 (Cochrum *et al.*, 1973) suggested that minimal *HLA-D* disparity, as measured by MLC testing, was crucial in living–related kidney transplantation. For almost nine years, we have been preselecting our intrafamilial transplant pairs using the MLC. The results obtained support our initial findings that renal-allograft survival is inversely correlated with the magnitude of the MLC response between recipient and donor. Figure 2 demonstrates this inverse correlation in 175 related pairs. All *HLA-A* and *-B*-identical siblings (N = 59) were also *HLA-D*-identical, with MLC stimulation indices [SIs of 2 or less (SIs = (R + D/RR + DD)/2, where R is recipient lymphocytes, D is donor lymphocytes, RR is recipient lymphocytes control culture, and DD is donor lymphocyte control)]. Graft survival in this group is excellent. One-haplotype pairs with MLC SIs between 2 and 8 also had excellent graft survival (91%) and had graft survivals not significantly different from the *HLA*-identical pairs. But the one-haplotype pairs with significant *HLA-D* disparity (MLC SI > 8) had only 52% graft survival at 1 year, which is significantly lower than the pairs with minimal or moderate *HLA-D* disparity. Comparison of the two groups with high and low MLC SIs illustrates the advantage of MLC testing in living–related transplantation.

Our results emphasize the observation that graft survival is highest among *HLA-A*-, -B-, -C-, and -D-locus identical siblings. In these siblings, the MLC is important in confirming *D*-locus identity and excluding a possible *HLA-B/D* recombination. Although we have not transplanted a "two-haplotype"-identical (*HLA-A*, *-B*, *-C*) sibling pair with high MLC reactivity (*HLA-B/D* recombination), poor graft survival has been reported in this situation (Garovoy *et al.*, 1978). Instead, we

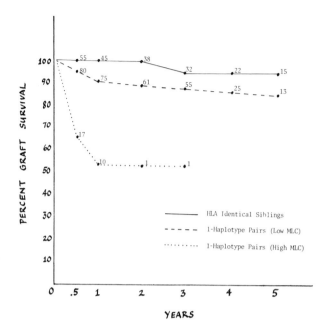

Figure 2. Correlation between MLC reactivity (*HLA-D* disparity) and living–related allograft survival. Stimulation Index (S.I.) = (R + D / RR + DD)/2. The numbers on the curves indicate the number of patients studied for each time interval (see text for explanation).

have chosen to select one-haplotype donors with minimal *HLA-D* disparity and have had excellent graft survival with these pairs.

In one-haplotype-matched pairs, our data clearly show that MLC reactivity affects transplant outcome. Other investigators have confirmed our results and have shown that the MLC assay is extremely beneficial in choosing the one-haplotype donor with the best prognosis for a successful graft (Ringden and Berg, 1977; Cerilli *et al.*, 1978). In our study on the correlation of MLC reactivity and graft survival, the results reveal that the survival of one-haplotype-matched transplants is related not only to the degree of *HLA-D* disparity, but also to the magnitude of the response existing between donor and recipient in the MLC assay. Since the one-haplotype-matched transplant recipient shares only one *HLA-D*-locus antigen with the donor, the recipient's response to the D-locus difference becomes an important factor in graft survival. Thus, the number of D-locus antigens shared between recipient and donor may not by itself be adequate in predicting graft status.

We have found that complete family studies involving *HLA-A* and -*B* serotyping and MLC testing eliminates several problems routinely encountered in selecting donor–recipient pairs: the assignment of haplotypes in individuals with unidentified HLA-A, -B, and C antigens; the assignment of haplotypes in families who share or have homozygous HLA antigens; and the assignment of haplotypes in individuals with crossovers among the various *HLA* loci. Problems with donor selection can arise even if four HLA-A and -B antigens are identified in donor–recipient pairs.

In a large retrospective study (Cochrum *et al.*, 1975), we confirmed the relevance of *HLA-D* matching in cadaveric transplants (N = 219). Figure 3 shows the graft survival in high- and low-MLC pairs. Clearly, the findings in unrelated transplants are as striking as in intrafamilial transplantation. In these patients, there was no correlation between the number of HLA antigens shared and the degree of *HLA-D* disparity as measured by MLC. However, a comparison shows that the low-MLC group in unrelated transplants (Fig. 3) has a lower graft survival than the low-MLC group does in related transplants (Fig. 2). This emphasizes the importance of factors other than *HLA-D* matching in transplantation and stresses the importance of other minor histocompatibility loci.

Recently, several other centers have confirmed our initial findings of

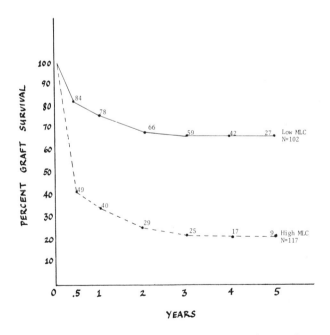

Figure 3. MLC reactivity and unrelated graft survival. The numbers on the curves indicate the number of patients studied for each time interval (see text for explanation).

the importance of *HLA-D* matching in unrelated-graft survival. Walker *et al.* (1978), in a study involving cadaveric pairs (N = 240), showed that those pairs with low MLCs demonstrated greater graft survival than those with high MLCs. The development of serological detection of *D*-locus-related antigens (*DR* typing) should facilitate identification of these important antigens in cadaveric transplantation. Nevertheless, MLC testing with its ability to measure the immunological response generated by various degrees of *D*-locus incompatibility offers a necessary and important supplement in the evaluation of histocompatibility.

In our experience, the most important variables affecting MLC results are bacterial and viral infections, recent blood transfusions, and various drugs (e.g., aspirin, steroids). These must be carefully controlled so that MLC testing will give meaningful data. Also, histocompatibility laboratories should not attempt to apply the SI values determined elsewhere. Rather, a sensitive and standardized MLC technique should be developed that will correlate with graft outcome at any transplant center. To accomplish this, further communication among MLC laboratories regarding standardization seems essential. Although there seems to be no question of the efficacy of *HLA-D* in renal transplant, it is also obvious that there are other important factors governing allograft survival. One of the most important of these factors is the effect of blood transfusions.

4. Blood Transfusions

The intentional administration of pretransplant blood transfusions to allograft recipients is one of the most controversial and exciting issues in clinical transplantation. Previously, transfusions were thought to have a deleterious effect on kidney-graft survival. But in 1973, Opelz *et al.* (1973) reported a positive effect of blood transfusions and showed a direct correlation between the number of transfusions given prior to transplantation and graft outcome. Since their initial report, most transplant centers in the United States and Europe have confirmed that pretransplant transfusions improve kidney-allograft prognosis in cadaver transplantation. Also, their work has been substantiated by additional clinical studies (Festenstein *et al.*, 1976; Fuller *et al.*, 1977) and by experimental work in the dog (Abouna *et al.*, 1977). The positive correlation between pretransplant transfusions and unrelated graft survival at the University of California at San Francisco (Vincenti *et al.*, 1978; Feduska *et al.*, 1979) agrees with most published data (Fig. 4).

In contrast, the beneficial effects of transfusions in related transplants are still controversial. Solheim *et al.* (1977) could not demonstrate

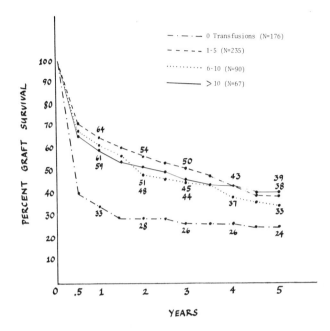

Figure 4. Effect of blood transfusions on graft survival in 568 cadaver transplants. The numbers on the curves indicate the number of patients studied for each time interval (see text for explanation).

a transfusion effect in related donors, but reported a strongly positive effect on cadaver kidney-graft survival. However, Brynger et al. (1977) found an impressively beneficial effect of transfusions in related- as well as unrelated-allograft survival. When we analyzed the effect of transfusions in our related-transplant population, there was a significant improvement in graft survival in the transfused patients when the patients were grouped according to the degree of HLA-D disparity. Those related one-haplotype pairs with considerable HLA-D disparity (high MLC reactivity) demonstrated the beneficial effect of pretransplant transfusions (Fig. 5), while those patients with minimal HLA-D disparity did not show as significant an improvement in graft survival with transfusions (Fig. 6). This well-matched, low-MLC group had a 91% 1-year graft survival, and therefore the additional favorable effect of blood transfusions would not be as apparent in this group as it is in the high-MLC group.

Next, we evaluated the effect of HLA-D disparity and pretransplant transfusions in the cadaveric-transplant situation (Fig. 7). Graft survival was improved substantially by transfusion in both high- and low-MLC groups. These results support the reports (Persijn et al., 1978; van Rood

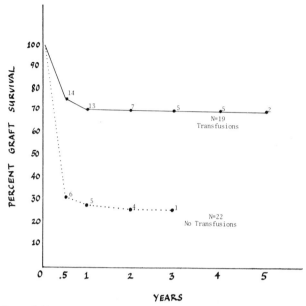

Figure 5. Effect of blood transfusions on graft survival in high-MLC, one-haplotype-related pairs. The numbers on the curves indicate the number of patients studied for each time interval (see text for explanation).

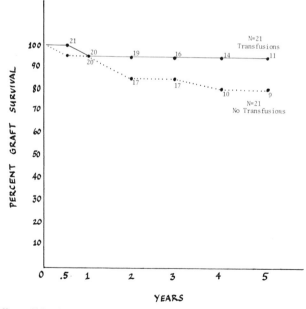

Figure 6. Effect of blood transfusions on graft survival in low-MLC, one-haplotype-related pairs. The numbers on the curves indicate the number of patients studied for each time interval (see text for explanation).

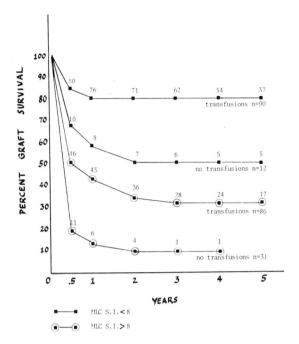

Figure 7. Effect of blood transfusions on unrelated graft survival (high and low MLC.) The numbers on the curves indicate the number of patients studied for each time interval.

et al., 1979) that *HLA-DR* matching and transfusions will lead to significant improvements in related and unrelated transplants. Serologically detected HLA-DR antigens, on B lymphocytes, are closely linked to HLA-D determinants that stimulate in the MLC test. Donor–recipient pairs that are *HLA-DR*-identical are frequently *HLA-D*-identical, although not all *DR*-identical pairs have negative or low MLC tests.

The improvement in graft survival by matching for two DR determinants was expected, since low or negative MLCs between related and unrelated donor–recipient pairs have excellent graft survival (Figs. 2, 3, 6, and 7). But the improved graft survival in pairs who share only one HLA-DR determinant was not expected, since these pairs frequently have high MLCs. Our demonstration (Fig. 5) that blood transfusions are enhancing in sibling and parent–child pairs despite high MLC reactivity is informative. These results illustrate the syngeneic effect of *HLA-D* matching on the nonspecific beneficial effect of transfusions. In addition, these results suggest that matching for one HLA-DR determinant in related and perhaps unrelated donor–recipient pairs improves graft survival if the recipient has been transfused before transplantation.

No consensus exists concerning the type of blood used or the number or timing of transfusions that should be given to maximize the beneficial effects observed. At present, there is also controversy about the sensitizing effects of blood transfusions. At some centers, no deleterious sensitization was observed, although many centers have reported an increased incidence of sensitization following transfusions and have recommended reducing the number of transfusions to avoid sensitization that may preclude transplantation.

We have reported an increased incidence of patient sensitization due to unrelated transfusion. This effect was particularly evident in patients receiving more than ten transfusions (Feduska et al., 1979). But the development of lymphocytotoxins against a random panel does not always prevent the patient from receiving a successful transplant in the future. In an earlier report (Salvatierra et al., 1977), we demonstrated a graft survival in highly sensitized patients that was comparable to the graft survival in less-sensitized recipients. In addition, a distinction should be made between sensitization against the donor's HLA-A and -B antigens and against his HLA-DR (B-cell) antigens. Antibodies directed against the donor's HLA-A and -B antigens have a detrimental effect on allograft survival whether present before transplantation or developing posttransplant. In contrast, antibodies directed against B-cell antigens may be harmless (Ettenger et al., 1976a) or possibly advantageous if present pretransplant (Morris et al., 1977). However, the appearance of B-cell antibodies posttransplant is related to graft rejection (Ettenger et al., 1976b; Cochrum et al., 1979). Although the consensus indicates that pretransplant transfusions result in better graft survival, recipient sensitization due to random transfusions is still a great problem. An undetermined number of patients become so broadly sensitized by transfusions that transplantation becomes difficult if not impossible. Therefore, we felt that it was important to formulate a transfusion protocol that would improve transplant survival without incurring sensitization to the specific renal donor.

Experimental animal work has shown that transfusion of donor-specific blood effectively induces specific suppression of allograft rejection (Marquet et al., 1971; Fabre and Morris, 1972 a,b; van Es et al., 1977). In rats, prolonged graft survival by pretreatment with whole blood has been described (Jenkins and Woodruff, 1971), and in dogs, donor blood pretransplant also had specific immunosuppressive activity (Halasz et al., 1964). Obertop et al. (1975) treated beagle littermates with a single intravenous transfusion of specific blood 14 days before transplantation. They found that in a few dogs, transfusions led to sensitization and slightly accelerated rejection, but in the majority of the dogs receiving donor-specific transfusions, no antibody production occurred and there was prolonged graft survival.

In the past, attempts to induce passive or active enhancement in humans have been limited. Batchelor et al. (1970) were able to produce passive enhancement in a child to his mother's kidney, and in another report, donor-lymphocyte injections given with prednisone and azathioprine were used to enhance a patient before kidney transplantation (Newton and Anderson, 1973). Allograft enhancement has also been suggested in skin grafts on human volunteers immunized with donor lymphocytes (Rapaport et al., 1968).

We have recently reported our preliminary results (Cochrum et al., 1979) utilizing donor-specific pretransplant transfusions to attain specific and nonspecific benefits from transfusions. Donor-specific transfusions were performed with well-defined HLA-D-disparate pairs who shared a single haplotype. Ferrara et al. (1978) have shown that the degree of HLA disparity between blood donor and recipient correlated directly with the frequency with which the recipient developed antibodies against the donor. In one-haplotype pairs, the number of incompatible antigens is decreased and the probability that sensitization will occur in the donor–recipient relationship is considerably lessened. In addition, donor-specific transfusions were performed with HLA-D-disparate parent–child pairs to facilitate detection of humoral and cellular sensitization to the mismatched haplotype.

Two or three donor-specific-blood transfusions, each consisting of 200–500 ml fresh, whole, citrated blood or packed cells, were administered intravenously to recipients at 2-week intervals before kidney transplantation. All recipients were tested extensively over the transfusion period for humoral and cellular sensitization. Of the donor-specific-transfused patients, 30% became sensitized and were not transplanted. Patients who had negative T- and B-cell cross-matches following the transfusions were transplanted and have normally functioning allografts 2 months to 1.5 years posttransplant. Table 1 shows recipient and donor HLA genotypes, pretransfusion MLC, cell-mediated (CML), lymphocytotoxicity and random-panel cross-match values, and the number of pretransplant unrelated-blood transfusions in six of these patients. Both MLC and in vitro CML values in these patients were not changed significantly by the donor-specific-blood transfusions.

It has been suggested that the capacity of a recipient to respond immunologically to blood transfusions may influence his graft survival (Opelz and Terasaki, 1978). In addition, a distinction has been made between high and low responders on the basis of the "broadness" of the cytotoxic reactivity pattern of the recipient's sera against a random panel of lymphocytes. High responders were shown to have a poorer graft survival than low responders. Table 2 shows representative cross-match data from two patients transfused with donor-specific blood. Patient No.

TABLE 1. Immunological Parameters of Donor-Specific-Transfused Patients

Patient No.	HLA genotype	MLC SI[a]		CML[b]	Lymphocytotoxins against random panel[c]	Unrelated-blood transfusion (units)	Time graft at risk (months)
		2-Way	1-Way				
1	Aw29 B12/A11 B18 (R) Aw29 B12/A1 Bw35 (D)	8	8	N.D.	0%	0	13
2	A2 B40/A1 Y (R) A2 B40/X B7 (D)	28	18	26%	38%	7	8
3	Aw24 B18/A1 B8 (R) Aw24 B18/A2 B7 (D)	36	50	16%	12%	6	7
4	A2 B17/X Bw49 (R) A2 B17/A1 Bw39 (D)	8	14	14%	75%	0	5
5	A1 B8/X B14 (R) A1 B8/A2 B40 (D)	22	21	22%	0%	2	4
6	A11 B35/A29 Y (R) A11 B35/A29 Bw49 (D)	12	26	50%	0%	8	3

[a] SI: 1-way = RDx/RRx; 2-way = (R + D/RR + DD)/2.
[b] Chromium-51 release.
[c] Before donor-specific transfusion.

2 is obviously immunologically competent, since he responded to the unrelated-blood transfusions by developing lymphocytotoxins, and would certainly be classified as a high responder, since he developed antibodies against 100% of the random panel. But this patient graphically demonstrated a selective ability to respond to the unrelated transfusions while remaining unresponsive to three transfusions from his mother. This patient has never experienced a rejection crisis and is 1 year posttransplant.

Two of our patients had weak preexisting lymphocytotoxins to their donor at 4 and 23°C, but not at 37°C. These patients did not show an ammestic response to the donor transfusions, but in fact their antibody titers disappeared during the donor-transfusion course. These patients were transplanted and have had excellent graft survival. The disappearance of the antibodies is indicative of a suppressive effect, although the mechanism of suppression in these patients is unclear. Blocking factors in the serum seem unlikely, since the MLC responses in all the transfused patients remained high after transfusion and were not inhibited by the recipient's plasma. This suggests that blocking antibodies against the donor's mismatched HLA-D locus were not significant.

Iwaki et al. (1978) recently reported that antibodies directed against B cells may play a role in the transfusion phenomenon. These antigens appear to be governed by loci outside HLA and are most readily recognized in the cold (4°C).

We attempted to evaluate the possible existence of a link among blood transfusions, cold B-cell antibodies, and graft protection in our donor-specific-transfused patients, but were unable to consistently detect B-cell antibodies that reacted primarily at 4°C. In addition, we did not find warm B-cell antibodies (37°C) in these patients' sera. Although some investigators have found that the presence of preformed warm B-cell antibodies was followed by poor transplant outcome (Iwaki et al., 1978), others have not observed this (d'Apice and Tait, 1979; Ting and Morris, 1978).

Our results using related one-haplotype blood donors to accomplish the benefits of random transfusions are encouraging. The immunological monitoring of these transfused patients is much easier because the immunizing haplotype is known. In addition, the risk of a related donor's transmitting hepatitis or another viral disease is obviously less than with an unrelated blood donor. But most important, the use of blood donors who share one haplotype greatly reduces the risk of sensitization because of fewer antigenic differences. Indeed, following our transfusion protocol, only 30% of the patients became sensitized to their specific donor's cells and were not transplanted. This should be compared with Fig. 2, which

TABLE 2. Selected Cross-Match Data for Two Donor-Specific-Transfused Patients

	Blood transfusions[a]	Lymphocytotoxins against random panel	Cross-match vs. donor					
			T cells			B cells		
			4°C	23°C	37°C	4°C	23°C	37°C
Patient 2								
Pretransplant	5 units (Unr)	38%	–	–	–	–	–	–
Posttransplant								
0 Weeks	200 cc (DSp)	38%	–	–	–	–	–	–
2 Weeks	200 cc (DSp)	17%	–	–	–	–	–	–
4 Weeks	200 cc (DSp)	38%	–	–	–	–	–	–
6 Weeks	—	—	–	–	–	±	–	–
8 Weeks	2 units (Unr)	100%	–	–	–	–	–	–
Transplant	—	100%	–	–	–	–	–	–
Patient 6								
Pretransplant	3 units (Unr)	0%	±	±	–	±	±	–
Posttransplant								
0 Weeks	250 cc (DSp)	0%	±	±	–	–	±	–
2 Weeks	200 cc (DSp)	0%	–	±	–	–	+	–
4 Weeks	200 cc (DSp)	0%	–	–	–	±	±	–
6 Weeks	5 units (Unr)	0%	–	–	–	–	–	–
Transplant	—	0%	–	–	–	±	–	–

[a] (Unr) Unrelated; (DSp) donor-specific.

shows a 50% allograft rejection rate at 1 year in *HLA-D* disparate related pairs, where virtually all recipients also developed antibodies.

Donor-specific transfusions not only seem to restrict sensitization, but also appear to select out potentially poor grafts before transplantation. In addition, if the recipient becomes sensitized, it is sensitization against only the one disparate donor haplotype instead of broad sensitization. Therefore, these recipients would be much less restricted in relation to future unrelated allografts. The transfusion of potential cadaver recipients with *HLA*-typed blood from relatives could confer the benefits of transfusion with low sensitization of the recipient. Although *HLA-A* and -*B* typing and particularly cross-matching are important to good graft survival, *HLA-D* matching appears to be most important to graft acceptance and may be key in the initiation of suppressor mechanisms and enhancing antibodies following blood transfusions. And since *HLA-D* typing correlates closely with *HLA-DR* matching, which can be performed serologically, the most practical means of improving graft survival, at present, appears to be a combination of DR typing, blood transfusions, and immunosuppression. Because of the apparent restrictive polymorphism of the *DR* locus, a much-reduced recipient pool will be necessary to find well-matched donor–recipient pairs in cadaver transplantation.

ADDENDUM. To date, we have transfused 32 one-haplotype HLA-D disparate living related pairs with donor-specific blood. Nine patients (28%) were sensitized by the donor-specific transfusions. Twenty-three patients with negative T- and B-cell crossmatches have been transplanted; 22 patients have functioning grafts at 2 months to 2 years. One graft was rejected at 3 months posttransplant after the patient discontinued her immunosuppressive drugs.

ACKNOWLEDGMENTS. We wish to gratefully thank Victor Lim, Frances Sturtevant, Marianne Gumbert, and Margaret Rheinschmidt for their valuable assistance and Janet Mulhern for her careful preparation of this manuscript.

References

Abouna, G.M., Barabas, A.Z., Pazderka, V., Boyd, N., Vetters, J.M. Kinniburgh, D.W., Lao, V.S., Shlaut, J., Kovithavongs, T., and Dossetor, J.B., 1977, Effect of pretreatment with multiple blood transfusions and with skin grafts on the survival of renal allografts in mongrel dogs, *Transplant. Proc.* **9**:265.

Batchelor, J.R., French, M.E., Camerons, J.S., Ellis, F., Bewick, M., and Ogg, C.S., 1970, Immunological enhancement of human kidney grafts, *Lancet* **2**:1007.

Brynger, H., Frisk, B., Ahlmen, J., Blohme, I., and Sandberg, L., 1977, Blood transfusion and primary graft survival in male recipients, *Scand. J. Urol. Nephrol. (Suppl.)* **42**:76.

Cerilli, J., Newhouse, Y., and Williams, M.A., 1978, The correlation of tissue typing, mixed lymphocyte culture and related donor renal allograft survival, *Transplant. Proc.* **10**:953.

Cochrum, K.C., Perkins, H.A., Payne, R.O., Kountz, S., and Belzer, F.O., 1973, The correlation of MLC with graft survival, *Transplant. Proc.* **5**:391.

Cochrum, K.C., Salvatierra, O., Perkins, H.A., and Belzer, F.O., 1975, MLC testing in renal transplantation, *Transplant. Proc.* **3**:659.

Cochrum, K.C., Hanes, D., Potter, D., Vincenti, F., Amend, W., Feduska, N., Perkins, H., and Salvatierra, O., 1979, Donor-specific blood transfusions in HLA-D disparate 1-haplotype related allografts, *Transplant. Proc.* **11**:1903.

d'Apice, A.J.F., and Tait, B.D., 1979, The positive B cell cross match: A marker of active enhancement?, *Transplant. Proc.* **11**:954.

Ettenger, R.B., Terasaki, P.I., and Opelz, G., 1976a, Successful renal allografts across a positive cross-match for donor B lymphocyte alloantigens, *Lancet* **2**:56.

Ettenger, R.B., Teraski, P.I., and Ting, A., 1976b, Anti-B lymphocytotoxins in the renal allograft rejection. *N. Engl. J. Med.* **295**:305.

Fabre, J.W., and Morris, P.J., 1972a, The effect of donor strain blood pretreatment on renal allograft rejection in rats, *Transplantation* **14**:608.

Fabre, J.W., and Morris, P.J., 1972b, The mechanism of specific immunosuppression of renal allograft rejection by donor strain blood, *Transplantation* **14**:638.

Feduska, N.J., Vincenti, F., Amend, W., Duca, R., Cochrum K., and Salvatierra, O., 1979, Do blood transfusions enhance the possibility of a compatible transplant?, *Transplantation* **27**:35.

Ferrara, G.B., Tusi, R., Longo, A., Castellanii, A., Viviani, C., and Carminati, G., 1978, A safe blood transfusion procedure for immunization against major histocompatibility complex determinants in man, *Transplantation* **26**:150.

Festenstein, H., Sachs, J.A., Paris, A.M.I., Pegrum, G.D., and Moorhead, J.F., 1976, Influence of HLA matching and blood-transfusion on outcome of 502 London Transplant Group renal-graft recipients, *Lancet* **1**:157.

Fuller, T.C., Delmonico, F.L., Cosimi, A.B., Huggins, C.E., King, M., and Russell, P.S., 1977, Effects of various types of RBC transfusions on HLA alloimmunization and renal allograft survival, *Transplant. Proc.* **9**:117.

Garovoy, M.R., Person, A., and Carpenter, C.B., 1978, Correlation of mixed lymphocyte culture (MLC) reactivity and graft survival in 1-haplotype matched recipients, *Proc. Dialysis Transplant. Forum* **8**:74.

Halasz, N.A., Orloff, M.J., and Hirose, E., 1964, Increased survival of renal homografts in dogs after injection of graft donor blood, *Transplantation* **2**:453.

Iwaki, Y., Terasaki, P.I., and Park, M.S., 1978, Enhancement of human kidney allografts by cold B-lymphocyte cytotoxins, *Lancet* **1**:1228.

Jenkins, A.L., and Woodruff, M.F.A., 1971, Specific immunosuppression of cardiac allograft rejection in rats, *Transplantation* **12**:57.

Marquet, R.L., Heystek, G.R., and Timbergen, W.J.,, 1971, Specific inhibition of organ allograft rejection by donor blood, *Transplant. Proc.* **3**:708.

Morris, P.J., Ting, A., Oliver, D.I., Bishop, M., Williams, K., and Dunhill, M.S., 1977, Renal transplantation and a positive serological crossmatch, *Lancet* **2**:1288.

Newton, W.T., and Anderson, C.B., 1973, Planned preimmunization of renal allograft recipients, *Surgery* **74**:430.

Obertop, H., Jeckel, J., Vriesendorp, H.M., MacDicken, I., and Westbrock, D.L., 1975, The effect of donor blood on renal allograft survival in DL-A typed beagle littermates, *Transplantation* **20**:49.

Opelz, G., and Teraski, P.I., 1978, Absence of immunization effect in human kidney retransplantation, *N. Engl. J. Med.* **299**:369.

Opelz, G., Sengar, D.P.S., Mickey, M.R., and Terasaki, P.I., 1973, Effect of blood transfusions on subsequent kidney transplants, *Transplant. Proc.* **5**:253.

Persijn, G.G., Gabb, B.W., van Leeuwen, A., Nagtegaal, A., Hoogeboom, J., and van Rood, J.J., 1978, Matching for HLA antigens of A, B, and DR loci in renal transplantation by Eurotransplant, *Lancet* **1**:1278.

Rapaport, F.T., Dausset, J., Lawrence, H.S., and Converse, J.M., 1968, Enhancement of skin allograft survival in man, *Surgery* **64**:25.

Ringden, O., and Berg, B., 1977, Correlation between magnitude of MLC and kidney graft survival in intrafamilial transplantation, *Tissue Antigens* **10**:364.

Salvatierra, O., Perkins, H.A., Amend, W., Feduska, N., Duca, R.M., Potter, D.E., and Cochrum, K.C., 1977, The influence of presensitization on graft survival, *Surgery* **81**:146.

Solheim, B.G., Flatmark, A., Jervell, J., and Arnesen, E., 1977, Influence of blood transfusions on kidney transplant and uremic patient survival, *Scand. J. Urol. Nephrol. (Suppl.)* **42**:65.

Ting, A., and Morris, P.J., 1978, Cold and warm B cell antibodies in renal transplantation, *Lancet* **2**:478.

van Es., A.A., Marquet, R.L., van Rood, J.J., Kalff, M.W., and Balner, H., 1977, Blood transfusions induce prolonged kidney allograft survival in rhesus monkeys, *Lancet* **1**:506.

van Hooff, J.P., Hendriks, G.F., Schippers, H.M.A., and van Rood, J.J., 1974, Influence of possible HLA haploidentity on renal-graft survival in Eurotransplant, *Lancet* **2**:1130.

van Rood, J.J., Persijn, G.G., van Leeuwen, A., Goulmy, E., and Gabb, B.W., 1979, A new strategy to improve kidney graft survival: The induction of CML non-responsiveness, *Transplant. Proc.* **11**:736.

Vincenti, F., Duca, R.M., Amend, W., Perkins, H.A., Cochrum, K.C., Feduska, N.J., and Salvatierra, O., 1978, Immunologic factors determining survival of cadaver kidney transplants, *N. Engl. J. Med.* **299**:793.

Walker, J., Opelz, G., and Terasaki, P.I., 1978, Correlation of MLC response with graft survival in cadaver and related donor kidney transplants, *Transplant. Proc.* **10**:949.

10

HLA-Linked Regulation of Immune Responsiveness in Man

Role of *I*-Region-Gene Products

Leonard J. Greenberg

1. Introduction

During the past decade, there has been an ever-increasing interest in the interaction between the immune system and the major histocompatibility complex (MHC) of the species. The impetus for this intense scientific focus derives for the most part from the discovery that immune responsiveness is genetically controlled by genes mapping in the *H-2* complex of the mouse, i.e., the observation of linkage between the *Ir-1* locus and *H-2* (McDevitt and Chinitz, 1969). Since that time, many associations between immune-response (*Ir*) genes and the MHC have been detected in inbred strains of mice (Martin *et al.*, 1971; Vaz and Levine, 1970; McDevitt *et al.*, 1969) and guinea pigs (Green and Benacerraf, 1971; Ellman *et al.*, 1970; Green *et al.*, 1970). This subject has been extensively reviewed in several books (McDevitt, 1978; Sercarz *et al.*, 1977; Snell *et al.*, 1976; Klein, 1975) and will not be dealt with in any detail in this chapter.

Although many genes, located within the MHC region of the chromosome, have been shown to be involved in immune functions, their precise mode of action is still unclear. These studies have nevertheless led to the presumption that the observed associations are meaningful for survival and therefore have been preserved in evolution. As a conse-

Leonard J. Greenberg ● Department of Laboratory Medicine and Pathology, University of Minnesota Medical School, Minneapolis, Minnesota 55455.

quence, many investigators have searched for and described human counterparts. These studies have primarily involved association between human histocompatibility antigens (*HLA*) and susceptibility to specific diseases, a subject that has been extensively reviewed (Dausett and Hors, 1975; van Rood *et al.*, 1975; Svejgaard *et al.*, 1975). Although a number of diseases show a definite association with an *HLA-B* allele, some show an even stronger association with *HLA-D*. These more recent observations have led to the notion that disease associations are due to the effect of genes in the *HLA-D* region or to genes in strong linkage dysequilibrium with *HLA-D* genes. Although very little is known about the number and function of genes in this region, since *D*-region genes code for membrane determinants that elicit mixed-lymphocyte culture (MLC) reactivity, it has been assumed that the *D* region is the human analogue of the *I* region in the mouse. Aside from a definite role in the initiation of MLC reactivity, *I*-region genes code for immune-associated (Ia) antigens and regulate immune responsiveness (*Ir* genes) (Shreffler and David, 1975) and immune suppression (Debre *et al.*, 1975). At present, it is not known whether or not Ia and *Ir* are separate genetic entities; however, it appears that Ia antigens form an integral part of antigen-specific T-cell-receptor molecules (Tada and Taniguchi, 1976; Taussig *et al.*, 1976). Thus, if indeed *HLA-D*-region genes and *I*-region genes are analogous, then at least some disease associations could very well be due to aberrant regulation, by *Ir* or *Is* genes, of immune responses to specific antigens. Although neither of these genes has been conclusively demonstrated in man nor is there hard evidence linking them to disease susceptibility, some recent studies indicate that such a genetic mechanism could be operative.

In the sections to follow, I will try to provide the reader with some feeling for the state of the art of this area of human immunogenetics. It should be kept in mind, however, that the type of studies and the rate of progress are influenced to a considerable extent by the outbred nature of man and by restrictions in human experimentation. The latter consideration becomes abundantly manifest when one examines the way in which *Ir* genes were discovered. The immune system was challenged with antigens of restricted heterogeneity and specificity. The types of antigens employed were: (1) synthetic polypeptides with a limited number of different L-amino acids and their hapten conjugates; (2) weak native antigens differing slightly from host protein; and (3) strong native antigens injected in limiting doses, i.e., a dose range that is immunogenic for only some individuals within a strain or certain strains within a species. One major consideration is the fact that these immune responses can also be determined *in vitro* by measuring the proliferative response { rate of incorporation of [^{3}H]thymidine ([^{3}H]-TdR) into DNA} of lymphoid cells cultured together with antigen (Tyan, 1972; Tyan and Ness, 1971). Leukocytes from high-responder mice synthesize 10–100 times more DNA at a lower antigen concentration than do leukocytes from low-responder mice.

2. Association between *HLA* and Immune Response

In view of the aforementioned limitations in human experimentation, efforts to define *Ir* genes in man have relied for the most part on the assessment of immune reactivity subsequent to immunization with ethical antigens, skin-testing, and following natural infection. In the sections that follow, representative studies involving these approaches will be described.

2.1. Response to Ethical Antigens

During the past few years, several studies have been described in which efforts were made to uncover an association between immune responsiveness to vaccination with different commonly used viruses and *HLA*. Haverkorn *et al.* (1975) studied the antibody response to poliomyelitis virus, rubella, measles, diphtheria toxoid, and influenza in 143 twin pairs of the same sex, living in the same household, and attending the same elementary school. The study included 71 monozygotic and 72 dizygotic twin pairs. In the latter group, there were 18 pairs sharing no *HLA* haplotypes, 31 pairs sharing one haplotype, and 23 sharing haplotypes. The degree of similarity of antibody response within a twin pair was estimated as the ratio of antibody titers. Thus, if linkage between *HLA* and immune responsiveness exists, it would lower the ratios of *HLA*-identical twin pairs as compared to those of *HLA*-nonidentical twin pairs. Evidence of possible linkage to *HLA* was observed only in the case of response to measles.

Spencer *et al.* (1976) studied the antibody response subsequent to intranasal administration of a live, attenuated influenza A vaccine to 99 volunteers, a placebo solution to 50 volunteers, and a single intramuscular injection of a standard bivalent inactivated influenza vaccine to 50 additional volunteers. Subjects with *HL-A* type W16 had, as a group, a mean convalescent-phase hemagglutination-inhibition antibody titer of 14, which was significantly lower ($P < 0.001$) than the mean titer of 36 in subjects without W16. No association with *HLA* was observed in those subjects who were immunized by intramuscular injection with an inactivated influenza vaccine; examination of both acute-phase and convalescent-phase titers revealed no significant difference among subjects with different *HLA* types. The authors interpreted these data to mean that the lowered antibody response observed in the W16 subjects is due to increased resistance to infection, rather than to a suppressed immune response, since other individuals with W16 had normal responses to killed influenza vaccine. Although a limited amount of data was presented and no mention was made of the level of significance, the geometric mean titers of acute-phase and of convalescent-phase sera from these W16-positive subjects were both lower than the titers of sera from non-W16 subjects.

In a subsequent study, Spencer *et al.* (1977) measured antibody responses following immunization with live, attenuated RA 27/3 rubella vaccine and analyzed the data in terms of sex, age, *HLA,* and ABO types. Children in the youngest age group (1–5 yr) had the highest convalescent-phase, geometric mean, antibody titer. Girls in the 1- to 5- and 6- to 12-year age categories had higher mean titers than boys of the same age groups. Subjects with type AB blood had significantly higher convalescent-phase titers ($p = 0.05$) than non-AB subjects. With respect to *HLA,* subjects with BW17, B18, and AW23 had the lowest convalescent-phase titers, whereas vaccinees with B14 and BW22 had the same high titer (152). Nine children, from 3 to 14 years of age, had titers of 512 or higher. Four of these children were HLA-A28, whereas only 8% of the total study population had this antigen ($\chi^2 = 12.06; p = 0.0005 \times 26 = 0.01$). Although 28% of the test population had clinical symptoms, no correlation could be found with any *HLA* type. The results of this study differ markedly from those of the previous study by Spencer *et al.* (1976), which employed attenuated influenza A vaccine. The authors suggest that the different routes of administration of virus, influenza A intranasally and RA 27/3 rubella vaccine subcutaneously, may be responsible for the differences in immune responsiveness to the two vaccines. It was suggested that subcutaneous administration might bypass some cutaneous defense mechanisms. One final note on this study that intrigued the authors was the fact that the RA 27/3 rubella vaccine was prepared by growing virus in human WI 38 tissue culture cells, on which the only known HLA antigen is HLA-A2. Their notion was that the vaccine may have contained determinants derived from the culture that could facilitate a tolerant infection without a humoral antibody response in those individuals sharing the same histocompatibility determinants as the WI 38 cells. Four of six nonresponders expressed HLA-A2, and three of six nonresponders expressed B12 and BW17. This interpretation, of course, will have to await the elucidation of the complete HLA phenotype of WI 38 cells.

Whereas the studies just described have dealt only with possible association between antibody response to vaccination and *HLA,* deVries *et al.* (1977) examined the relationship between immune response both *in vitro* and *in vivo* and HLA phenotype in 79 individuals subsequent to a primary immunization with vaccinia virus. A low *in vitro* response was observed when lymphocytes from vaccinated individuals were cultured together with heat-inactivated virus. Low response was associated with HLA-Cw3. Antibody titers were higher in subjects tested after 5–11 weeks than in those tested 3–4 weeks postimmunization. In neither case, however, was there a correlation between the degree of lymphocyte reactivity *in vitro* and antibody titer, nor was the frequency distribution of the titers bimodal. Only in the subjects tested after 5–11 weeks was there a significantly increased titer in Cw3-positive subjects as compared to Cw3-negative ones. Although no mechanism of interaction between HLA-Cw3 and the response to vaccinia is immediately apparent, the authors advanced the following possibilities: (1) Low *in vitro* response may involve immune-suppression (*Is*) genes that are in linkage dysequilibrium with HLA-Cw3; (2) Cw3-positive subjects might have a higher intracellular virus load that could interfere with DNA synthesis in the *in vitro* test; and (3) *Ir* genes in linkage dysequilibrium with Cw3 might facilitate a faster response and elimination of virus.

Another aspect of the immune response to vaccinia virus, which may have some bearing on this latter consideration, was studied by Perrin *et al.* (1977). In this study, 12 normal, healthy adults, who had been vaccinated with vaccinia virus during childhood and revaccinated 2 or more years prior to the study, were given vaccinia virus vaccine. Peripheral-blood lymphocytes (PBL) harvested at different days after vaccination showed peak activity to lyse virus-infected target cells on day 7. The cytotoxicity, however, was not related to *HLA* markers, inasmuch as autologous, homologous, and heterologous target cells were all lysed with the same efficiency. Cytotoxicity involved Fc-receptor bearing cells that did not rosette with sheep erythrocytes. Cytotoxic activity could be almost completely abrogated by rabbit Fab'$_2$ anti-human IgG. Nonimmune PBL, on the other hand, lysed vaccinia-infected target cells in the presence of specific antibody against vaccinia virus. The authors concluded that although vaccination produces specific antiviral antibodies and cytotoxic K cells, antibody-dependent cellular cytotoxicity may be of major importance in the way in which humans successfully handle virus infections.

The final studies in this area of response to ethical antigens deal with non-infectious protein antigens, diphtheria and tetanus toxoids (DT and TT), both of which have been shown to give variable responses in humans (Haverkorn *et al.*, 1975). McMichael *et al.* (1977) studied the response to DT in ten families that were tissue-typed for *HLA-A,B* and *D*. All subjects were given 0.5 ml (1.5 Lf) of alum-precipitated diphtheria by intramuscular injection, and venous blood was taken at intervals thereafter for assay. All members of the study were bled between 3 and 6 weeks after immunization, a time period that kinetic studies had shown to be optimal and in which immunological reactivity had reached a plateau. Both antibody-binding capacity (ABC) and the blastogenic activity of lymphocytes from test subjects, subsequent to culture *in vitro* with DT, were assessed. On the basis of an analysis for heritability and linkage to *HLA*, neither of which was described in the text or referenced, the authors offer two alternatives to explain the data. The first is that responsiveness to DT is controlled by a single dominant gene. With the exception of two families, 1 and 9, in which low-responder parents had high-responder children, the authors claim that this interpretation is compatible with the data. The second possible explanation invokes the presence of two linked genes controlling responsiveness to DT such that two low-responder parental haplotypes could complement each other and produce high-responder children. The possibility that response is an autosomal recessive trait was ruled out by data from a family in which high-responder parents had low-responder children. With respect to antibody responses in test subjects, there did not appear to be any correlation between ABC and blastogenic reactivity. The authors point to the fact that the lower mean titer in parents (ABC = 1.5 μg/ml) as compared to that in children (ABC = 9.3 μg/ml) may be a reflection of inadequate immunization in the parents. Since the standard boosting dose of DT is 1/30th of the normal three-injection priming dose given to children, the long interval in the parental generation since previous immunization might mean that even high responders would fail to respond to a single low dose of antigen. The authors contend that lymphocyte blastogenesis induced by DT is probably partially controlled by a dominant gene that is not closely linked to *HLA*. However, in view of the complexity of the antigens employed and ambiguities about the histories of previous immunizations, it is difficult to arrive at any conclusion about possible genetic control of response to DT.

Recently, Sasazuki *et al.* (1978) examined the response to TT in Japanese and found that while there was no association between *HLA* and high response to TT by immune lymphocytes *in vitro,* significant association between HLA-B5 and low responsiveness was manifest. An even stronger association was observed with HLA-DHO, a D specificity in linkage dysequilibrium with B5. This association between low responsiveness to TT and *HLA* is similar to the findings of deVries *et al.* (1977), who described an association between HLA-Cw3 and low response to vaccinia vaccine. Sasazuki *et al.* (1978) feel that if low responsiveness is under genetic control, it might be determined by dominant *Is* genes (Debre *et al.,* 1975). This was also one of the possibilities suggested by deVries *et al.* (1977). However, Sasazuki *et al.* (1978) have ruled out control by *Ir* genes on the basis that if response to TT was under *Ir*-gene control, then low responsiveness could occur only in the absence of the specific *Ir* gene. Low responders would have to be homozygous at that locus. MLC reactivity with *HLA-DHO* homozygous typing cells and lymphocytes from low responders revealed that most individuals were heterozygous for that particular D antigen.

2.2. Response to Skin-Test Antigens

2.2.1. Immediate Cutaneous Reactions

The elucidation of immunogenetic mechanisms underlying allergic reactions in experimental animals has proceeded along rather conventional lines. Vaz and Levine (1970) have demonstrated that histocompatibility-linked genes control specific IgE as well as IgG antibody responses. Histocompatibility-linked *Ir* genes controlling IgE antibody responses to pollen allergens (Chang and Marsh, 1974) and *Ascaris* allergens (Patrucco and Marsh, 1974) have also been demonstrated. Efforts to identify allergen-specific *Ir* genes in man have relied for the most part on a search for association between *HLA* and immediate-type skin reactions to various natural allergens. These studies have involved both the random population and families and have employed allergens of varying degrees of purity, a complication that might account for the lack of strong associations and agreement among studies with the same class of allergen.

Employing a highly purified ryegrass preparation, Marsh (1976) observed significant association between immediate skin reactivity and HLA-B8 ($p = 0.005$), with a p value of 0.007 for the presumptive *A1-B8* haplotype. Another study implicating the *A1-B8* haplotype involved the response to mite antigen (Dasgupta *et al.*, 1976); however, the level of significance was much lower ($p = 0.05$). The most convincing data in this area derive from family studies in which high-titer anti-ragweed IgE antibodies (Levine *et al.*, 1972) and immediate skin reactions to ragweed antigen (Blumenthal *et al.*, 1974) were found to segregate with HLA. In both studies, the authors suggested that the response to allergen is controlled by an *HLA*-linked *Ir* gene.

These interpretations, however, have been challenged by Bias and Marsh (1975) from a number of points of view. A major criticism derived from the fact that in neither study were the data appropriately analyzed for linkage. In the study by Levine *et al.* (1972), several spouses of subjects were not studied, and consequently it would be impossible to assume that a common trait such as an *Ir* gene for antigen E might not be present in these people. In these cases, sensitivity to antigen E in their progeny could have been inherited from a parent who was not studied, whether or not specific allergy was expressed. Bias and Marsh (1975) also raised one additional criticism of this study, namely, that the probable high frequency of *Ir* AgE genes and the differential expressivity in IgE-mediated reactions in different family members present a difficult problem to analyze without the positive identification of the mating types, which is impossible when only one parent is studied. The study by Blumenthal *et al.* (1974) suggesting linkage between *IrE* and *HLA* is dependent on a grandfather and his son being transmitters in that they have seasonal allergy and thus have genes required for the expression of allergy. They possess the postulated *IrE*-linked haplotype, but have negative skin tests to antigen E and a crude ragweed preparation. Blumenthal *et al.* (1974) also postulated a rather high incidence of recombinants between *IrE* and *HLA* (20%), which would place an *IrE* locus well outside the MHC.

Subsequent to the critique by Bias and Marsh (1975), Blumenthal and his collaborators performed genetic analysis on the distribution of immune responses in two ragweed-sensitive families. This analysis revealed that a positive skin test to antigen E or personal history of seasonal allergy, or both, were inherited in an autosomal dominant fashion. Furthermore, they demonstrated by linkage analysis that this locus was linked to *HLA-B* with an estimated recombination frequency of 0.1 in males and 0.5 in females and a log of the odds (lod) score of 2.47. More recently, Black *et al.* (1976), employing four different highly purified pollen antigens (ragweed antigens E, Ra3, and Ra5 and ryegrass Group I), studied IgE-mediated skin sensitivity, serum IgG antibody, and antigen-induced lymphocyte proliferation *in vitro* in 76 members of 13 large families. No evidence for association between specific *HLA* haplotype and immune responses by any of the indices tested was found. In some instances, individuals exhibited lymphocyte responsiveness to antigens, but had no detectable specific IgE or IgG antibody. Conversely, a few individuals with marked IgE or IgG responses, or both, to a given antigen showed no measurable lymphocyte response to that antigen, but did respond to other nonimmunologically cross-reacting antigens.

It is not immediately apparent from the studies just described whether or not *HLA*-linked *Ir* genes control immune responsiveness to allergens. If linkage does indeed exist, the effect may be masked by a number of factors both genetic and nongenetic in nature. Although much more work has to be done to elucidate any underlying genetic mechanisms, the current feeling is still positive and focused in the general direction of two possible genetic controls, one that is linked to *HLA* that controls specific immune responses to allergens and another controlling the level of IgE that is not linked to *HLA*.

2.2.2. Delayed Cutaneous Reactions

The delayed-type hypersensitivity reaction has been studied rather extensively for many years and is commonly used for the assessment of cell-mediated immunity. The delayed reactivity that is seen following intradermal injections of antigens of bacterial, fungal, or viral origin is predicated on prior immunological experience with the antigens under study. However, in the light of our current understanding of the inter-action between the MHC and the immune system, the capacity of an individual to respond in a delayed-type reaction may also depend on genetic background. Although there are many studies demonstrating the delayed-type reaction in man, there are very few examples dealing with the influence of the MHC on the response, and in most instances the studies described involve an *in vitro* counterpart of the delayed skin reaction, i.e., antigen-induced lymphocyte blastogenesis that results when sensitized lymphocytes are cultured together with specific antigen.

Buckley *et al.* (1973) studied both the delayed and immediate skin responses to a large panel of test antigens in three families. Families were selected on the basis of probands with tuberculosarcoidosis, chronic cutaneous moniliasis, and rheumatoid arthritis. Positive associations between *HLA* haplotypes and immediate cutaneous hypersensitivity responses to 5, 8, and 11 of 23 test antigens were identified in the three respective families. However, an increased incidence of delayed cuta-neous unresponsiveness that was not related to *HLA* was observed in each family.

Persson *et al.* (1975) also examined the relationship between HLA, sarcoidosis, and the response to purified protein derivative (PPD) RT23 in an effort to clarify conflicting observations (Hedfors and Moller, 1973; Keuppers *et al.,* 1974) as to whether or not HL-A7 was associated with the disease. These investigators found no increase in HL-A7 in a group of 80 patients. However, in the group of patients not responding to PPD when tested for the first time after diagnosis of sarcoidosis, there was a significant increase in the prevalence of HL-A7 ($P = 0.003$) from 26.8% in controls to 46.8% in patients. In contrast, HL-A7 was completely absent in 28 patients maintaining or developing a positive reaction to PPD after diagnosis ($P = 0.0002$). The difference between these two groups of patients is highly significant ($P = 3 \times 10^{-6}$). The fraction of patients with positive reactions prior to diagnosis was the same in both groups. The authors concluded from these data that the *HLA* system probably did not influence susceptibility to sarcoidosis; however, once the condition developed, individuals expressing HL-A7 would be more likely to lose cellular immunity to PPD and to reveal symptoms.

The next few studies all deal with the *in vitro* response of lymphocytes to streptococcal antigens. Response to these ubiquitous antigens is predicated on the fact that most individuals have had prior immunological experience. However, the precise extent of this type of natural immunization is difficult to assess. Interest in possible MHC control of immune responsiveness to streptococcal constituents derives in part from the involvement of the immune system in the development of streptococcal disease and in part from the observation that heat-killed Group A streptococci have the ability to induce a state of altered reactivity to skin homografts in guinea pigs (Rapaport and Chase, 1965). In this context, Pellegrino *et al.* (1972) studied the relationship between response *in vitro* to streptococcal type M1 protein and *HLA*. These authors observed that lymphocytes from normal, healthy adults underwent a dose-dependent increase in DNA synthesis when cultured with M1 protein. However, the degree of lymphocyte stimulation was not related to either the HLA phenotype or the anti-M1 serum titer of the lymphocyte donor. Inhibition of M1-induced lymphocyte blastogenesis could be achieved with both allo- and heteroantisera directed against *HLA*. This serum inhibitory effect could be abrogated by specific absorption of HLA alloantisera with cultured human lymphoid cells. It was suggested that the serum inhibition by anti-HLA antibodies was brought about by a masking of the M1 protein's mitogenic site that prevented interactions with specific lymphocyte receptors required for induction of the proliferative process. When viewed in the light of our present understanding of human MHC functions, the serum inhibitory effects just described may have been brought about by antibodies directed against *I*-region determinants. This subject will be discussed in more detail in a separate section.

We have also studied the cell-mediated immune response to streptococcal antigens both *in vivo* by measuring the delayed-type skin response and *in vitro* by measuring the degree of antigen-induced blastogenesis. Lymphocytes from a large test panel of normal, healthy adults were cocultured with varying concentrations of SK/SD (Streptokinase-Streptodornase, Lederle), incubated for 120 hr at 37° in CO_2 environment, pulsed with [^{3}H]-TdR, and assayed for radioactivity. Three types of responses were observed: (1) response over the entire range of antigen concentrations; (2) low response to only the highest antigen concentrations; and (3) no response at all. Statistical analysis of the HLA-antigen frequency distribution in each of the population segments revealed that low responders and nonresponders have similar HLA-antigen frequency distributions, whereas the prevalence of HLA-B5 was significantly increased in the responder population (corrected $P = 0.0001$) (Greenberg *et al.*, 1975). Although a limited number of individuals were skin-tested, in general, much greater reactivity was observed with those expressing B5 than in the absence of B5.

Section 3 will deal with our efforts to elucidate possible genetic mechanisms governing the response to streptococcal antigens. However, before describing these studies, I would like to call the reader's attention to a recent report by Kawa *et al.* (1978) on the response of Japanese to SK/SD. In this study, 90 healthy Japanese were tested for their *in vitro* response to 5000 ng SK/SD. Response was distributed in three groups as follows: (1) 52 individuals with a stimulation index (SI) of less than 1.3 (nonresponders); (2) 22 individuals with an SI of between 1.3 and 1.5; and (3) 16 people with an SI of greater than 1.5. No association was found between *HLA* and the degree of SK/SD-induced blastoid transformation. The authors point to a racial difference between their study and that of Greenberg *et al.* (1975) as a possible explanation for the lack of any association between *HLA* and response to SK/SD. It is rather difficult to assess the study of Kawa *et al.* (1978), since no information is given about dose–response conditions, and the data are expressed as SIs. At a dose of 5000 ng/ml, which produced maximal responses (30,000 cpm) in the study by Greenberg *et al.* (1975), Kawa *et al.* (1978) reported only 10 individuals out of 90 with an SI greater than 2.0, of whom 7 are under 2.5. It is not clear from the data presented in this study whether response to SK/SD is bimodally distributed, and therefore attempts at *HLA* association would not be meaningful.

2.3. Conclusion

Studies described in Section 2 have been directed toward the elucidation of the relationship between the *HLA* system and the control of immune responsiveness in man. The antigens employed fell into two categories, infectious agents and noninfectious material. With the possible exception of some studies dealing with immediate cutaneous reaction, in which different doses of purified antigens were used, all immunizations were carried out according to strict human-use protocols, the result being that very heterogenous antigen preparations were employed at a fixed dose. Since the identification of specific murine and guinea pig *Ir* genes depended on the use of antigens of restricted heterogeneity and specificity and the ability to limit antigen dose, it is not surprising that no human counterparts were clearly delineated in these studies. Other major differences between the human studies and the animal model include the route and frequency of administration of antigen and the tissue sources from which samples were obtained for the assessment of immune function. In mice and guinea pigs, spleen, lymph node, or peritoneal cells were employed, but not PBL, whereas in man, PBL were used exclusively.

Although these studies in man did not succeed in identifying any specific human *Ir* gene, except for the postulated *IrE* gene, which is still a controversial matter, one observation that was common to several studies was that of immunological unresponsiveness that was associated with *HLA*. This relationship was observed in the case of low response to vaccinia virus and HLA-Cw3, low response to tetanus toxoid and HLA-DHO, and low response to PPD in patients with sarcoidosis and HLA-B7. In the first two examples, the authors suggested that if low responsiveness is under genetic control, it might be determined by dominant immune-suppression (*Is*) genes. Even if such a mechanism is operative, one is still faced with the problem of developing a test system that is capable of identifying human *Ir* genes, if indeed they do exist.

3. Immunogenetics of Response to Streptococcal Antigens

In Section 2, representative studies were described that were directed toward the identification of MHC-linked genes controlling immune responsiveness in man. For the most part, these studies involved rather complex antigen preparations that were used at one prescribed dose, in a randomly selected test population. Data were analyzed in terms of the relationship between response and HLA-antigen frequency distribution. Although *HLA*-association studies have provided a great deal of useful information about a variety of diseases, this type of statistical approach cannot be employed to elucidate underlying genetic mechanisms. This type of information requires an estimation of linkage, which is determined by the proximity of gene loci on a particular chromosome. Studies to determine linkage must examine families to see whether certain traits are transmitted together from generation to generation.

In this context, the observation that response to streptococcal antigens *in vitro* is associated with HLA-B5 (Greenberg *et al.,* 1975) suggested that an analysis of the response pattern in families to purified streptococcal antigens might provide a means of identifying MHC-linked genes that regulate immune responsiveness. Work that will be described in this section was designed to explore this possibility and was carried out in the author's laboratory in collaboration with Drs. Ricki-Lahn Chopyk, Chuck Eng, and Ernest D. Gray, and Peter W. Bradley, Harriet J. Noreen, Sam Quek, Linda R. Hanson, and Margie Frederickson.

3.1. Purification and Characterization

3.1.1. Group C Antigens (SK/SD)

SK/SD (Streptokinase-Streptodornase, Lederle) is a mixture of extracellular proteins isolated from Group C streptococci, strain H-46A; therefore, it was surprising to find both a striking association between response *in vitro* and HLA-B5 and a relatively large number of nonresponders (Greenberg *et al.*, 1975). This situation might be expected from a purified antigen of restricted heterogeneity and specificity rather than a crude mixture such as SK/SD. However, it can be seen in Fig. 1A, which is a polyacrylamide gel electrophoresis (PAGE) scan of SK/SD, that although SK/SD contains many different proteins, there is only one rather symmetrical peak of blastogenic activity (Fig. 1B). The material under the blastogenic peak was further purified by diethylaminoethyl (DEAE) and carboxymethyl (CM) cellulose chromatography and electrophoresis through 12% acrylamide gel, which resulted in the isolation of a protein that was homogeneous on sodium dodecyl sulfate (SDS)–PAGE with a molecular weight of 38,000. This material, designated PSA-C, is resistant to heat, 70°C for 30 min; has a blocked N-terminus; and induces blastogenesis in responder lymphocytes in a dose-dependent manner (Chopyk *et al.*, 1976).

3.1.2. Group A Antigens

The extracellular constituents of strain C203S were chromatographed on DEAE cellulose and the fractions delineating the peak of blastogenic activity pooled and rechromatographed on CM cellulose. When electrophoresed on acrylamide gel under conditions similar to those for the antigens from Group C, a single peak of blastogenesis occurred (Fig. 2) that was designated PSA-A and was discrete from PSA-C depicted in Fig. 1B. This material was homogeneous on SDS-PAGE with a molecular weight of 17,500. PSA-A is resistant to heat, 100°C for 30 min, and to treatment with RNAase and DNAase, but is inactivated by pronase and trypsin (Gray *et al.*, 1978). PSA-A also induces blastogenesis in responder lymphocytes in a dose-dependent manner.

3.2. PSA-C Response in Families

The response to PSA-C was studied in 15 informative families that were tissue-typed for *HLA-A,-B* and -*C* and in selected instances for *HLA-D*. Peripheral-blood lymphocytes (PBL), purified by floatation on

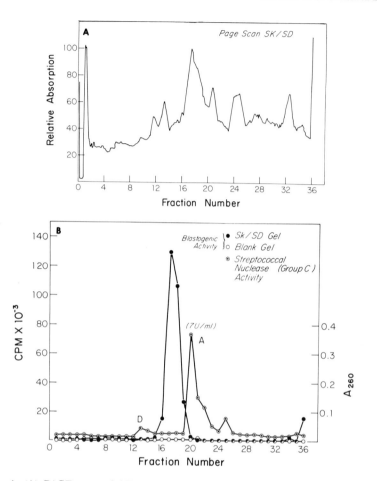

Figure 1. (A) PAGE scan of SK/SD. (B) Analysis of PAGE fractions of SK/SD. (●) Blastogenic activity of SK/SD gel fractions; (○) blastogenic activity of blank gel; (◉) nuclease A activity of SK/SD gel fractions.

Ficoll–Isopaque, were cultured together with varying concentrations of PSA-C. The response pattern was subjected to both segregation and linkage analysis. The mode of inheritance was determined by fitting probability models to the data employing a computer program developed by Morton and MacLean (1974). The best fit was achieved by using a dominant-inheritance model and assuming 100% penetrance. Linkage analysis was performed by using LIPED, a computer program developed by Ott (1974), which generates a set of lod or Z scores. Family data analyzed by LIPED yielded a cumulative lod score of 5.36, which is indicative of highly significant linkage between response to PSA-C and

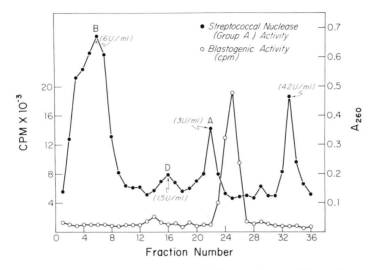

Figure 2. Analysis of PAGE fractions of extracellular constituents of Group A streptococci (strain C203S). (○) Blastogenic activity; (●) nuclease A, B, C, and D activities.

HLA haplotypes. A plot of the antilog of the lod score vs. θ, the recombination fraction, indicates that the probable map distance for the gene controlling response to PSA-C is 8 centimorgans outside *HLA* (Greenberg, 1977). Although work is only in the preliminary stages, response to PSA-A also appears to be controlled by a gene that is linked to *HLA*.

3.3. Mechanisms of Response to Streptococcal Antigens

During the course of analysis of response to PSA-C, an interesting pedigree was identified (Fig. 3) in which response was found to be associated with the maternal *C* haplotype. Sib 1 (*BC*), a nonresponder, expresses only HLA-A3 of the *C* haplotype but is *HLA-C-* and *D-* identical to sib 10, a responder. Sib 2 (*BC/D*), a nonresponder, is an *HLA-A/B* recombinant expressing HLA-B18 of the maternal *D* haplotype. Sib 5 (*AC*), a nonresponder, is *HLA*-identical to sibs 4 and 6, who are both responders. Sibs 4, 5, and 6 are mutually nonstimulatory in mixed-lymphocyte culture (MLC). These findings raise the possibility that recombination has occurred between *HLA-D* and the gene controlling response to PSA-C. In an effort to check this possibility, all family members were analyzed for glyoxalase and PGM3, enzyme markers mapping on chromosome 6 in proximity to *HLA*. This analysis, however, proved uninformative, since the mother was homozygous for GLO-1 and

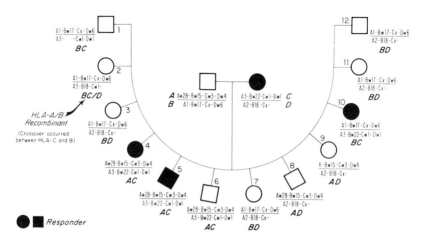

Figure 3. Pedigree of Family 41N. (**AB, CD**) Paternal and maternal haplotypes, respectively. (□) Male and (○) female nonresponders.

the father was homozygous for GLO-2. Both parents were homozygous for the same *PGM3* allele. Alternative explanations for the lack of response exhibited by sibs 1 and 5 might involve the presence of a population of suppressor T lymphocytes or a defect in the way in which these two sibs present antigen.

3.3.1. Cellular Interactions

a. Mixing and Transfer Studies.   In an effort to investigate the possible involvement of suppressor T cells or a defect in antigen presentation in the lack of response to PSA-C by sib 5, mixing and transfer studies were conducted between sibs 5 and 6. The inhibitory action of suppressor cells on the response to PSA-C was ruled out, since the addition of increasing increments of T cells from the nonresponder sib 5 to a culture containing lymphocytes from the responder sib 6 and PSA-C failed to produce inhibition of blastogenesis (Chopyk and Greenberg, 1977). The possibility of a defect in antigen presentation was studied in a cell-transfer system. Cells from sib 5 and sib 6 were incubated separately in replicate glass culture vessels for 2 hr and the supernatant, nonadherent cell suspensions removed and saved. After washing of the adherent cell populations, which were predominantly macrophages, supernatant suspensions from sib 5 were added back to adherent cells from sib 6 and also to cells from sib 5 as a control. In the case of sib 6, the reverse procedure was followed; i.e., supernatant suspensions from sib

6 were added to adherent cells from sib 5 and to cells from sib 6 as a control. All cultures were stimulated with a standard dose of PSA-C and assayed for their blastogenic response as previously described. Response was found to be associated with the nonadherent cells of the responder, sib 6, indicating that nonresponder macrophages are perfectly capable of supporting PSA-C-induced blastogenesis in responder lymphocytes (Chopyk and Greenberg, 1977).

   b. Fractionation and Reconstitution Studies. Although the transfer experiments just described strongly implicate T cells in the response to PSA-C, fractionation and reconstitution studies were initiated in an attempt to better define the nature of the cellular interactions. Ficoll–Isopaque-purified PBL were fractionated by passage over nylon wool (Handwerger and Schwartz, 1974) or by rosetting with neuraminadase-treated sheep red blood cells (E) (Terasaki et al., 1975) to obtain enriched populations of T cells. Nylon-wool-enriched T cells showed no response to PSA-C, whereas E-rosetted cells responded to some extent, possibly due to the presence of contaminant macrophages. Addition of macrophages to both preparations restored the blastogenic response to PSA-C to levels seen with stimulated, unfractionated PBL. Response to phytohemagglutinin (PHA), on the other hand, was in the same order of magnitude as observed in unfractionated PBL, and the reactivity appeared to be independent of the macrophage concentration (Chopyk and Greenberg, 1977).

3.3.2. Serological Inhibition of Response to PSA-C

   Several gene products of the I region in animal systems have already been serologically defined (Hauptfeld et al., 1974; Dickler and Sachs, 1974; Plate and McKenzie, 1973) and have been implicated in the cellular interactions of immune responses (Hauptfeld et al., 1974; Meo et al., 1976; van Leeuwen et al., 1973). Although anti-Ia sera can inhibit a number of in vitro lymphocyte functions, the precise role that Ia antigens play in the mediation of immune function and cooperative cellular interactions is not known. Studies from several laboratories have provided evidence for human analogues of these gene products (Greenberg et al., 1973, 1977; Kunkel et al., 1976; Reinsmoen et al., 1978, 1979).

   The availability of specific antisera prepared by planned immunization between unrelated donors and recipients, identical or compatible at HLA-A and -B (Ferrara et al., 1975), which appeared to contain antibodies against I-region determinants, allowed the study of the effects of these sera on the in vitro response to PSA-C (Greenberg et al., 1978). Three antisera, Fe11/17, FeLD3/3, and Fe81/10 were studied for their effects on the response to both PHA and PSA-C. While all three sera can lyse a panel of leukemic cells, only FeLD3/3 and Fe81/10 can block stimulation in MLC; Fe81/10 can also block response in MLC. At a culture concentration of 2%, both FeLD3/3 and Fe81/10 significantly blocked (p < 0.0005) the blastogenic response of lymphocytes from a panel of responders to PSA-C, but had no inhibitory effect on the response to PHA. When tested for their complement-dependent cytotoxicity on enriched populations of T and B cells, none of the sera manifested cytotoxicity against T cells, nor did inhibition correlate with the capacity to lyse B cells. To put these serological findings to some perspective, I have summarized all the pertinent data as follows: (1) Response to PSA-C appears to be linked to *HLA* and involves an nonadherent cell, presumably a T lymphocyte. (2) Response to PSA-C requires the presence of macrophages. (3) Immunological unresponsiveness to PSA-C does not appear to be a reflection of a defect in the capacity of macrophages to present antigen. (4) Immunological unresponsiveness does not appear to be mediated by the action of suppressor T cells. (5) Serum inhibition is manifest only in culture systems that require cooperativity with macrophages, i.e., MLC reactivity and response to antigen, but not the response to PHA. Since the response to PSA-C requires cooperation between macrophages and T cells and none of the sera under study manifests complement-dependent cytotoxicity for T cells from panel members, one is left with two alternatives to explain the observed serum inhibitory effects. The first possibility involves the action of a blocking antibody for a T-cell determinant that does not bind complement. The second possibility is that inhibition is mediated by antibody directed against a determinant expressed on macrophages, presumably an *I*-region determinant. Whether or not the same presumptive *I*-region determinants are expressed on both B cells and macrophages is not clear at this time. However, the lack of correlation between serum-mediated lysis of panel-member B cells and inhibition of blastogenesis suggests either that different antibodies are involved or that inhibition is brought about by blocking determinants that are expressed exclusively on macrophages.

Of particular relevance are studies demonstrating the ability of anti-Ia antisera to inhibit the proliferation induced in primed T cells by antigen-bearing macrophages in the mouse (Schwartz *et al.*, 1976). It was observed that anti-Ia sera blocked T-cell proliferation with all antigens tested. However, an important exception was manifest in the case of two antigens, (T,G)-A-L and GLT, known to be under the control of *Ir-1* loci mapping a different segments of the *I* region, *I-A* and *I-C*, respectively, Inhibition of T-cell responses was achieved with antisera directed against Ia determinants of the specific subregions; i.e., anti-I-A serum blocked the (T,G)-A-L response and anti-I-C serum blocked the GLT response. Subsequently, Thomas *et al.* (1977), working with strain 2 and 13 guinea pigs, were able to show that T-cell proliferation could be inhibited by antiserum directed against Ia antigens of only stimulator macrophages. The treatment of T cells with anti-Ia serum and complement either before or after priming or both had no effect on their ability to be primed and restimulated with the stimulator macrophages. These authors concluded from this work that T cells primed *in vitro* recognize antigen in association with Ia antigens presented by macrophages and that T-cell Ia antigens may not be involved in the process. They do point out, however, that T cells still exhibit histocompatibility restrictions for the macrophage type used for initial sensitization.

These studies raise the possibility that *Ir* loci and *Ia* loci are one and the same. These gene products, expressed on macrophages, interact with antigen in such a way as to produce an immunogenic stimulus capable of activating specific T-cell clones. Whether or not the antigen–macrophage Ia interaction takes the form of an "altered-self" configuration, retains two completely discrete structures, or forms some intermediate type of complex is not known at this time. Whatever the case maybe, however, sufficient Ia structural identity must be preserved to be recognized by anti-Ia serum and thus permit the observed inhibition of antigen-induced T-cell proliferation.

3.4. Conclusion

Studies presented in Section 3 have dealt primarily with the elucidation of genetic mechanisms that control the response to purified streptococcal antigens. The data presented clearly indicate that *in vitro* blastogenic reactivity to these antigens involves an interaction between macrophages and sensitized T cells. In the case of PSA-C and most likely PSA-A, response is linked to *HLA* haplotypes (lod score 5.36 for PSA-C). A further indication of the involvement of the major histocompatibility system derives from the fact that response to PSA-C can be inhibited by antisera directed against human *I*-region determinants. Since the model under study does not include direct immunization with streptococci or their products, other than by natural infection, an analysis of specific antibody has not as yet been achieved. As a consequence, it is not known whether the observed *HLA*-linked blastogenic response to PSA-C is determined by *Ir* or *Is* genes.

In this context, it is of interest to mention that it has been our experience that patients with rheumatic fever or rheumatic carditis, who have had high serum titers to a number of streptococcal antigens, did not respond to PSA-C or PSA-A stimulation *in vitro*. It is not clear at this point what the significance of this finding is in terms of either regulation of antibody synthesis or relevance to streptococcal disease. However, should neither of these streptococcal constituents be capable of eliciting specific antibody, then their capacity to induce *HLA*-linked *in vitro* blastogenesis may be a reflection of dominantly inherited *Is* gene control. Although it may be premature to speculate about disease, the autoimmune nature of rheumatic fever and the concomitant depression of cell-mediated immune function suggest that susceptibility to this disease may derive from defective *HLA*-linked regulation of immune responsiveness. If susceptibility is associated with immunological unresponsiveness, then the observed *HLA*-linked blastogenic response in normal family members could very well be a marker of resistance to the disease. Work is now in progress to clarify this area.

References

Bias, W.B., and Marsh, D.G., 1975, HL-A linked antigen E immune response genes: An unproved hypothesis, *Science* **188**:375.

Black, P.L., Marsh, D.G., Jarrett, E., Delespesse, D.J., and Bias, W.B., 1976, Family studies of association between HLA and specific immune responses to highly purified pollen allergens, *Immunogenetics* **3**:349.

Blumenthal, M.N., Amos, D.B., Noreen, H., Mendell, N.R., and Yunis, E.J., 1974, Genetic mapping of Ir locus in man: Linkage to second locus of HL-A, *Science* **184**:1301.

Buckley, C.E., III, Dorsey, F.C., Corley, R.B., Ralph, W.B., Woodbury, M.A., and Amos, D.B., 1973, HL-A-linked human immune response genes, *Proc. Natl. Acad. Sci. U.S.A.* **70**:2157.

Chang, E.B., and Marsh, D.G., 1974, Immune responsiveness of inbred mice to pollen allergens, *J. Allergy Clin. Immunol.* **53**:65.

Chopyk, R.-L., and Greenberg, L.J., 1977, Genetic control of immune responsiveness to a purified streptococcal antigen: Definition of cellular mechanisms, *Fed. Proc. Fed. Am. Soc. Exp. Biol.* **36**:4904.

Chopyk, R.-L., Slechta, T., Gray, E.D., and Greenberg, L.J., 1976, Characterization of blastogenic factors isolated from streptococci for use as genetic probes, *Fed. Proc. Fed. Am. Soc. Exp. Biol.* **35**:980.

Dasgupta, A., Misri, N., and Bala, S., 1976, Population and family studies to demonstrate Ir genes: HLA haplotype in atopic allergy, in: *HLA and Allergy* (A.L. de Weck and M.N. Blumenthal, eds.), Monogr. 11, pp. 75–79, Munksgaard, Copenhagen.

Dausset, J., and Hors, J., 1975, Some contributions of the HL-A complex to the genetics of human disease, *Transplant. Rev.* **22**:45.

Debre, P., Kapp, J.A., Dorf, M.E., and Benacerraf, B., 1975, Genetic control of specific immune suppression. II. H-2 linked dominant control of immune suppression by random copolymer L-glutamic acid L-tyrosine (GT), *J. Exp. Med.* **142**:1447.

deVries, R.R.P., Kreeftenberg, H.G., Loggen, H.G., and van Rood, J.J., 1977, *In vitro* immune responsiveness to vaccinia virus and HLA, *N. Engl. J. Med.* **297**:692.

Dickler, H.B., and Sachs, D.H., 1974, Evidence for identity or close association of the Fc receptor of B lymphocytes and alloantigens determined by the Ir region of the H-2 complex, *J. Exp. Med.* **140**:779.

Ellman, L., Green, I., Martin, W.J., and Benacerraf, B., 1970, Linkage between the poly-L-lysine gene and the locus controlling the major histocompatibility antigens in strain 2 guinea pigs, *Proc. Natl. Acad. Sci. U.S.A.* **66**:322.

Ferrara, G.-B, Tosi, R.M., Antonelli, P., and Longo, A., 1975, Serological reagents against "new" lymphocyte surface determinants, in: *Histocompatibility Testing* (F. Kissmeyer-Nielsen, ed.), pp. 608–619, Munksgaard, Copenhagen.

Gray, E.D., Greenberg, L.J., and Wannamaker, L.W., 1978, An extracellular blastogen produced by group A streptococci: Purification and characterization, VIIth International Symposium on Streptococci and Streptococcal Diseases (September 1978) p. 22.

Green, I., and Benacerraf, B., 1971, Genetic control of immune responses to limiting doses of proteins and hapten protein conjugates in guinea pigs, *J. Immunol.* **107**:374.

Green, I., Inman, J., and Benacerraf, B., 1970, Genetic control of the immune response in guinea pigs to limiting doses of bovine serum albumin, *Proc. Natl. Acad. Sci. U.S.A.* **66**:1267.

Greenberg, L.J., 1977, Immunogenetics of response to streptococcal antigens, in: *Histocompatibility Testing* (W. Bodmer, J.R. Batchelor, J.G. Bodmer, H. Festenstein, and P.J. Morris, eds.), p. 339, Munksgaard, Copenhagen.

Greenberg, L.J., Reinsmoen, N., and Yunis, E.J., 1973, Dissociation of stimulation (MLR-S) and response (MLR-R) in mixed lymphocyte culture by serum blocking factors, *Transplantation* **16**:520.

Greenberg, L.J., Gray, E.D., and Yunis, E.J., 1975, Association of HL-A5 and immune responsiveness *in vitro* to streptococcal antigens, *J. Exp. Med.* **141**:935.

Greenberg, L.J., Reinsmoen, N.L., Noreen, H., Chess, L., Schlossman, S.F., and Yunis, E.J., 1977, Serological analysis of MLC determinants, *Transplant. Proc.* **9**:865.

Greenberg, L.J., Chopyk, R.-L., Noreen, H., Gray, E.D., Yunis, E.J., and Ferrara, G.-B., 1978, Serological inhibition of blast transformation to purified streptococcal antigens by planned immunization in HLA (A,B) compatible unrelated individuals, *Vox Sang.* **34**:136.

Handwerger, B.S., and Schwartz, R.H., 1974, Separation of murine lymphoid cells using nylon wool columns, *Transplantation* **18**:544.

Hauptfeld, V., Hauptfeld, M., and Klein, J., 1974, Tissue distribution of I region-associated antigens in the mouse, *J. Immunol.* **113**:181.

Haverkorn, M.J., Hofman, B., Masurel, N., and van Rood, J.J., 1975, HL-A linked genetic control of immune response in man, *Transplant. Rev.* **22**:120.

Hedfors, E., and Moller, E., 1973, HL-A antigens in sarcoidosis, *Tissue Antigens* **3**:95.

Kawa, A., Matsuyama, T., Fujii, H., Nakamura, S., Ogaki, S., Ooe, H., Koreeda, N., Nomoto, K., Arima, N., and Kanehisa, T., 1978, Relations between the HLA-antigens and immune responsiveness to SK/SD in healthy Japanese subjects, *Tissue Antigens* **12**:236.

Keuppers, F., Meuller-Eckhard, C., Heinrich, D., Schwab, B., and Brackertz, D., 1974, HL-A of patients with sarcoidosis, *Tissue Antigens* **4**:56.

Klein, J., 1975, *Biology of the Mouse Histocompatibility Complex*, Springer-Verlag, New York.

Kunkel, H.G., Winchester, R.J., Fu, S.M., and Dupont, B., 1976, Recent studies of Ia like antigens and complement components relating to the human histocompatibility system, in: *The Role of Products of the Histocompatibility Gene Complex in Immune Responses* (D.H. Katz and B. Benacerraf, eds.), pp. 71–75, Academic Press, New York.

Levine, B.B., Stember, R.H., and Fotino, M., 1972, Ragweed hayfever: Genetic control and linkage to HL-A haplotypes, *Science* **178**:1201.

Marsh, D.G., 1976, Allergy: A model for studying the genetics of human response, in: *Nobel Symposium No. 33: Molecular and Biological Aspects of Acute Allergic*

Reactions (S.G.O. Johansson, J. Strandberg, and B. Urnais, eds.), pp. 23–57, Plenum Press, New York.

Martin, W.J., Maurer, P.H. and Benacerraf, B., 1971, Genetic control of immune responsiveness to glutamic acid, alanine, tyrosine copolymer in mice. I. Linkage of responsiveness to H-2 genotype, *J. Immunol.* **107**:715.

McDevitt, H.O., 1978, *Ir Genes and Ia Antigens,* Academic Press, New York.

McDevitt, H.O., and Chinitz, A., 1969, Genetic control of antibody response: Relationship between immune response and histocompatibility (H-2) type, *Science* **163**:1207.

McDevitt, H.O., Shreffler, D.C., and Stimpfling, J.H., 1969, A single chromosome region in the mouse controlling the major histocompatibility antigens and the ability to produce antibody to synthetic polypeptides, *J. Clin. Invest.* **48**:57.

McMichael, A.J., Sasazuki, T., and McDevitt, H.O., 1977, The immune response to diphtheria toxoid in humans, in: *Clinical Histocompatibility Testing* (C.B. Carpenter and W.V. Miller, eds.), pp. 191–194, Grune and Stratton, New York.

Meo, T., David, C.S., and Shreffler, D.C., 1976, H-2 associated MLR determinants: Immunogenetics of the loci and their products, in: *The Role of Products of the Histocompatibility Gene Complex in Immune Responses* (D.H. Katz and B. Benacerraf, eds.), pp. 167–178, Academic Press, New York.

Morton, N.E., and MacLean, C., 1974, Analysis of family resemblance. III. Complex segregation of quantitative traits, *Am. J. Hum. Genet.* **26**:249.

Ott, J., 1974, Estimation of recombination fraction in human pedigrees: Efficient computation of the likelihood for human linkage studies, *Am. J. Hum. Genet.* **26**:588.

Patrucco, R., and Marsh, D.G., 1974, Immune response to ascaris antigen in inbred mice, *J. Allergy Clin. Immunol.* **53**:65.

Pellegrino, M.A., Ferrone, S., Safford, J.W., Hirata, A.A., Terasaki, P.I., and Reisfeld, R.A., 1972, Stimulation of lymphocyte transformation by streptococcal type M1 protein: Relationship to HL-A antigens, *J. Immunol.* **109**:97.

Perrin, L.H., Zinkernagel, R.M., and Oldstone, M.B.A., 1977, Immune response in humans after vaccination with vaccinia virus: Generation of a virus-specific cytotoxic activity by human peripheral lymphocytes, *J. Exp. Med.* **146**:949.

Persson, I., Ryder, L.P., Staub-Nielsen, L., and Svejgaard, A., 1975, The HL-A7 histocompatibility antigen in sarcoidosis in relation to tuberculin sensitivity, *Tissue Antigens* **6**:50.

Plate, J.M.D., and McKenzie, I.F.C., 1973, B cell stimulation of allogeneic T cell proliferation in mixed lymphocyte cultures, *Nature (London) New Biol.* **245**:247.

Rapaport, F.T., and Chase, R.M., 1965, Transplantation antigen-like activity of streptococcal cells, in: *Histocompatibility Testing* (H. Balner, F. Cleton, and V. Brenninkmeijer, eds.) pp. 171–176, Munksgaard, Copenhagen.

Reinsmoen, N.L., Noreen, H.J., Greenberg , L.J., and Kersey, J.H., 1978, Stimulatory determinants expressed on B cells which produce specific PLT reactivity, *Transplant. Proc.* **10**:767.

Reinsmoen, N.L., Noreen, H.J., Friend, P.S., Giblett, E.R., Greenberg, L.J., and Kersey, J.H., 1979, Anomalous mixed lymphocyte culture reactivity between HLA-A,B,C and DR identical individuals, *Tissue Antigens* **13**:19.

Sasazuki, T., Kohno, Y., Iwamoto, I., and Tanimura, M., 1978, Association between and HLA haplotype and low responsiveness to tetanus toxoid in man, *Nature (London)* **272**:359.

Schwartz, R.H., David C.S., Sachs, D.H., and Paul W.E., 1976, T lymphocyte enriched peritoneal exudate cells. III. Inhibition of antigen-induced T lymphocyte proliferation with anti-Ia antisera, *J. Immunol.* **117**:531.

Sercarz, E.E., Herzenberg, L.A., and Fox, C.F., 1977, *Immune System: Genetics and Regulation,* Academic Press, New York.

Shreffler, D.C., and David, C.S., 1975, The H-2 major histocompatibility complex and the I immune response region: Genetic variation, function and organization, *Adv. Immunol.* **20**:125.

Snell, G.D., Dausset, J., and Nathenson, S., 1976, *Histocompatibility,* Academic Press, New York.

Spencer, M.J., Cherry, J. D., and Terasaki, P.I., 1976, HL-A antigens and antibody response after influenza A vaccination, *N. Engl. J. Med.* **294**:13.

Spencer, M.J., Cherry, J.D., Powell, K.R., Mickey, M.R., Terasaki, P.I., Marcy, S.M., and Sumaya, C.V., 1977, Antibody responses following rubella immunizations analysed by HLA and ABO types, *Immunogenetics* **4**:365.

Svejgaard, A., Platz, P., Ryder, L.P., Nielsen, L.S., and Thomsen, M., 1975, HL-A and disease association—A survey, *Transplant. Rev.* **22**:3.

Tada, T., and Taniguchi, M., 1976, Characterization of the antigen-specific suppressive T cell factor with special reference to the expression of I region genes, in: *The Role of Products of the Histocompatibility Gene Complex in Immune Responses* (D.H. Katz and B. Benacerraf, eds.), pp. 513–539, Academic Press, New York.

Taussig, M.J., Munro, A.J., and Luzzati, A.L., 1976, I-region gene products in cell cooperation, in: *The Role of Products of the Histocompatibility Gene Complex in Immune Responses* (D.H. Katz and B. Benacerraf, eds.), pp. 553–567, Academic Press, New York.

Terasaki, P.I., Opelz, G., Park, M.S., and Mickey, M.R., 1975, Four new B lymphocyte specificities, in: *Histocompatibility Testing* (F. Kissmeyer-Nielsen, ed.) pp. 657–664, Munksgaard, Copenhagen.

Thomas D.W., Yamashita, U., and Shevach, E.M., 1977, Nature of the antigenic complex recognized by T lymphocytes. IV. Inhibition of antigen-specific T cell proliferation by antibodies to stimulator macrophage Ia antigens, *J. Immunol.* **119**:223.

Tyan, M.L., 1972, Genetically determined immune responses: *In vitro* studies, *J. Immunol.* **108**:65.

Tyan, M.L., and Ness D.B., 1971, Mouse blood leukocytes: *In vitro* primary and secondary responses to two synthetic polypeptides, *J. Immunol.* **106**:289.

van Leeuwen, A., Schuit, H.R.E., and van Rood, J.J., 1973, Typing for MLC (LD). II. The selection of nonstimulator cells by MLC inhibition tests using SD-identical stimulator cells (MISIS) and fluorescein antibody studies, *Transplant. Proc.* **5**:1539.

van Rood, J.J., van Hooff, J.P., and Keuning, J.J., 1975, Disease predisposition, immune responsiveness and the fine structure of the HL-A supergene: A need for reappraisal, *Transplant. Rev.* **22**:75.

Vaz, N.M., and Levine, B.B., 1970, Immune response of inbred mice to repeated low doses of antigen: Relationship of histocompatibility (H-2) type, *Science* **168**:852.

11

Clinical Histocompatibility Testing in Renal Transplantation

Potential Keys to Alloimmune Specificity and Reactivity

Ronald H. Kerman and Barry D. Kahan

1. Introduction

Allograft rejection is due to recipient sensitization to foreign, donor histocompatibility antigens resulting in activation of multiple immunological vectors of tissue destruction (Medawar, 1944; Stiller and Sinclair, 1979; Carpenter and Morris, 1979). Due to the functional reserve of the kidney, signs of rejection are frequently evident only after extensive damage to the allografted tissue. The clinical diagnosis of renal-allograft rejection is based on patient symptoms and signs, namely, fever, weight gain, swelling, pain, or hypertension. Laboratory evidences of reduced renal function include elevated serum creatinine and blood urea nitrogen, decreased creatinine clearance, increased albumin clearance, and lymphocyturia. Tissue typing and cross-matching procedures attempt to minimize the tissue incompatibility and avert grafting into presensitized hosts. Since the signs, symptoms, and laboratory evidences of rejection are late events, immunological evidences of recipient activation of a primary immune response may alert the clinician, thereby affording the possibility for prompt initiation of immunosuppressive therapy to minimize the extent of tissue damage. However, due to the variety of

Ronald H. Kerman and Barry D. Kahan • Division of Organ Transplantation, Department of Surgery, The University of Texas Medical School at Houston, Houston, Texas 77030.

antibody and cell-mediated components of immune mechanisms documented in rejection (Busch et al., 1976, 1977) recipient immune activation cannot always be documented. Indeed, there is no known test that is immunologically specific, sensitive, predictive, or at least confirmatory, and associated with few false-positive reactions.

In addition to their potential clinical import, immunological monitoring tests might elucidate the antigenic specificities and host responses determining graft rejection or acceptance. Two types of tests have been performed pre- and posttransplantation: those that reveal specific host antidonor reactivity and those that reflect nonspecific recipient immunocompetence. The data presented herein demonstrated that whereas specific antidonor cross-match tests are critical prior to transplantation, nonspecific immune tests are at present more predictive or confirmatory of rejection episodes following allografting. The apparent lack of correlation between the results of tests reflecting specific antidonor reactivity and allograft rejection may relate to: (1) the circumstance that the present assays, which detect HLA antigens only, incompletely reflect reactivity toward other antigenic systems critical to allograft survival; (2) relevant determinants not being expressed on lymphocytes, the target utilized in the donor-specific assays; (3) depletion of the vectors of antidonor immune activity from peripheral blood due to sequestration at the actual site of reaction, namely, the engrafted organ; and finally (4) limitations of present in vitro technology to mimic in vivo conditions encountered during graft rejection. Since nonspecific assays do not depend on identification or demonstration of reactivity against donor antigens, as do the specific in vitro assays, they may reveal immunity in more situations. Presumably, the nonspecific assays reflect fluxes in populations responsive to lymphokines or mediators of allograft rejection. Also, since nonspecific assays demand only simple technology, are reproducible, and permit daily measurements, they are at present more useful in monitoring allograft recipients.

2. Pretransplant Immunological Assessment

2.1. Donor-Specific Resistance

While HLA-A and -B tissue typing has proven invaluable in the choice of the living related donor, it has had significantly less impact in cadaveric transplantation (Dausset et al., 1974; Opelz and Terasaki, 1976; Terasaki et al., 1978; G.M. Williams, 1979). The major application of the lymphocytotoxic antibody technique has been as a visual cross-match to avert previous sensitization. There has been a marked reduction in the incidence of hyperacute rejection (Stiller et al., 1976) since the application of this technique to detect complement-dependent cytotoxic antibody (CDA) against donor peripheral-blood lymphocytes (PBL). Detection of antibody in the visual cross-match is generally regarded as an absolute contraindication to transplantation. Some recent data claim that it is preferable to perform visual CDA cross-matches against separated donor T and B cells at both warm and cold temperatures, to discriminate deleterious antibodies, namely, those directed against HLA-A, -B, and -C antigens, from potentially enhancing antibodies, possibly directed against Ia or DRw antigens (Stiller and Sinclair, 1979; Carpenter and Morris, 1979; Iwaki et al., 1979).

Approximately 10–20% of transplant recipients undergo early, irreversible, accelerated allograft rejection, a presensitized response, despite negative visual CDA results (Collaborative report of the Scanditransplant, 1975). Thus, although the visual cross-match test has reduced the incidence of hyperacute rejection, it is unable to detect a significant number of presensitized patients (Kissmeyer-Nielson et al., 1966; G.M. Williams et al., 1968). Therefore, in addition to the standard procedure of matching ABO, HLA-A, -B, and DRw antigens, and of obtaining negative visual cross-match tests, additional assays should be employed to detect complement-dependent antibody (CDA), lymphocyte-dependent antibody (LDA), K-cell activity, and lymphocyte-mediated cytotoxicity (LMC). This battery of tests to detect antidonor immune responses is denoted as a "comprehensive immune analysis," and employs chromium-51-labeled donor target cells, which afford greater sensitivity. While some investigators have failed to correlate positive pretransplantation CDA, LDA, LMC, or K-cell tests with subsequent rejection (Stiller and Sinclair, 1979), most workers note a good correlation between early, irreversible rejection episodes and positive pretransplant donor-specific assays (Dossetor and Myburgh, 1978; Stiller and Sinclair, 1979; Carpenter and Morris 1979). Our retrospective blinded analysis demonstrated the benefit of a pretransplant comprehensive study: pretransplant-positive LDA, LMC, or CDA tests correlated with occurrence of accelerated rejection episodes and graft loss.

Method of Comprehensive Immune Analysis. Donor target cells obtained from peripheral blood or lymph nodes are purified on a Ficoll–Hypaque gradient, washed in Dulbecco's phosphate-buffered saline (PBS), pH 7.3, and brought to a final concentration of $5-10 \times 10^6$ cells/ml in medium and incubated with 50–400 mCi/ml of radioactive $Na_2^{51}CrO_4$(AmerSham/Searle). Following a 30-min incubation, cells are washed three times, resuspended, and adjusted to 10^6/ml for targets in all assays. In the *LMC* test, potential recipient lymphocytes serve as effectors to kill donor target cells in the absence of complement. For the assay, 10^6 recipient effector cells (200 μl) are incubated with 25 $\times$ 10^3 donor ^{51}Cr-labeled target cells (25 μl) and 25 μl media in round-bottom Linbro microtiter tray wells in triplicate for 4 hr at 37°C. Thereafter, they are centrifuged at 500g for 5 min; 200 μl of supernatant is carefully withdrawn into a plastic tube for measurement in a gamma counter to determine mean test counts per minute (cpm). Negative controls consist of 25 $\times$ 10^3 labeled target cells incubated with 10^6 unlabeled target cells and medium to determine spontaneous chromium release. Positive controls consist of targets incubated with citrimide, a penetrant leading to osmotic lysis of the cell. The experimental test mean cpm are converted to the percentage ^{51}Cr release by the following equation:

$$\frac{\text{Test cpm} - \text{spontaneous cpm}}{\text{Citrimide cpm} - \text{spontaneous cpm}} \times 100$$

Tests resulting in 8% release greater than controls are considered positive.

The *CDA* is performed using potential recipient sera demonstrated to contain cytotoxic antibodies by screening against a 100-cell panel, as well as the most recent serum sample. To determine the specificity of recipient antibody, samples are preabsorbed with donor platelets or lymphocytes or both, and assayed against target cells. In addition, autolymphocytotoxic reactions are excluded by autologous absorptions of the recipient's sera with his own lymphocytes or platelets or both. For the test, 25 μl serum is mixed with 25 μl of labeled target cells (25 $\times$ 10^3 PBL) and 25 μl rabbit complement. Following a 4-hr incubation at 37°C, the reaction is terminated by adding 200 μl cold medium. The trays are centrifuged and 200 μl supernatant counted in a gamma well apparatus. A positive immune control using antilymphocyte sera is incubated with target cells. The percentage ^{51}Cr release is calculated as above by comparing release in the presence of unabsorbed and absorbed sera.

The *LDA assay* detects the binding of patient antibody to donor targets by the capacity of normal K lymphocytes to trigger lysis of coated cells. For the test, 25 μl of target cells (25 $\times$ 10^3 cells) are incubated with 25 μl of unabsorbed or platelet- or lymphocyte-absorbed recipient serum at 37°C for 30 min; 10^6 normal effector cells are added for a 4-hr further incubation at 37°C. The percentage ^{51}Cr release is calculated as described above. In addition, an assay is performed to quantitate the recipient K-cell activity as effectors in the LDA test. The test is performed as described for the LDA, except that the targets (25 $\times$ 10^3 cells in 25 μl) are preincubated with a known positive antibody, ALS (25 μl), and 200

μl (10^6) recipient effector cells. Patient ^{51}Cr release is compared to that obtained in parallel tests using a panel of effector K-cell populations.

The results of our retrospective study are seen in Tables 1 and 2. Table 1 reveals a positive correlation ($p < 0.001$) between the presence of LDA in pretransplant, platelet-absorbed sera from 13 patients suffering from accelerated rejection compared to 17 patients not displaying this phenomenon, namely, 5 acute, 5 chronic, and 7 no rejection. Since LDA activity was present after platelet absorption of the sera, the LDA reactivity appeared to be directed against alloantigens other than HLA-A, -B, or -C. Table 2 shows the correlation ($p < 0.01$) between elevated pretransplant K-cell activity against antibody-coated donor cells and accelerated rejection.

Following this retrospective study, an initial "blinded" series of allografts was performed. The LDA, CDA, LMC, and K-cell results were not considered in the choice of transplant recipients. However, the occurrence of two positive pretransplant immune comprehensive tests (one LMC and one LDA), both attended by accelerated rejection and graft loss, led to the termination of the double-blinded series after 12 cases. None of the 10 patients who had displayed negative cross-match tests experienced accelerated rejection ($p < 0.01$).

TABLE 1. Correlation of the Presence of LDA in Pretransplant Sera with Accelerated Rejection[a]

Finding	Accelerated rejection	Nonaccelerated rejection
+ LDA	13	1
− LDA	0	16

[a] Correlation: $p < 0.001$.

TABLE 2. Correlation of Pretransplant K-Cell Activity with Accelerated Rejection

Finding	Accelerated rejection[a]	Nonaccelerated rejection	p Value[b]
+ K cell	7	22	
			< 0.01
− K cell	0	30	

[a] Accelerated rejection with graft loss in 2 weeks.
[b] Chi-square analysis of accelerated vs. non-accelerated rejection.

Table 3 shows the prospective cross-match data of a patient who underwent renal transplantation and had excellent initial graft function. However, at the 5th postoperative day, accelerated rejection appeared, requiring transplant nephrectomy on the 8th postoperative day. Histological examination revealed hemorrhagic and ischemic damage. The results of the prospective, blinded cross-match revealed negative CDA and LDA results, but a positive (81%) ^{51}Cr release from the donor targets, but not from third-party or self targets, in the LMC assays, a finding consistent with those reported by Garovoy et al. (1973a). These data suggest that a positive pretransplant immune comprehensive test is a contraindication to allografting. However, a negative result on this battery does not guarantee immunological virginity toward the allograft donor.

New antigen systems expressed on human endothelial cells have been recently described. The endothelial antigens differ from previously known HLA antigens, as well as the Ia-like antigens on B lymphocytes. Stastny and co-workers (Moraes and Stastny, 1977) described a cytotoxicity assay using blood monocytes, which appear to share the antigenic determinants with endothelial cells. Cerilli et al. (1977) detected presensitization to antigens on endothelial cells using an immunofluorescence assay. Thus, endothelial antigens may constitute a new system of human allodeterminants that should be subjected to pretransplant matching and cross-matching.

2.2. General (Nonspecific) Host Immune Competence

Of the many factors other than histocompatibility that influence the outcome of cadaveric allograft survival, the level of recipient immuno-

TABLE 3. Prospective Cross-Match Data in a Patient Experiencing Accelerated Rejection

System	Recipient lymphs	Recipient serum	Target	^{51}Cr (%)
LMC	+	None	Donor	81
	+	None	Third-party	2
	+	None	Recipient	12.2
CDA	None	+	Donor	33
	None	+	Third-party	20
	None	+	Recipient	N.D.
LDA[a]	+	+	Donor	18
	+	+	Third-party	5
	+	+	Recipient	17

[a] LDA was performed with an effector pool, since the recipient was LMC-positive.

competence may be the most important. The hypothesis that a given recipient has a genetically inherited capacity for immune responsiveness toward antigens has been proven in animal models (Katz et al., 1970a,b; R.M. Williams and Benacerraf, 1972). Thus, groups of animals are normal, hypo- or hyperresponders to given antigens. Of interest is the fact that the immune-response genes are inherited in linkage dysequilibrium with the major histocompatibility complex (MHC). Preliminary data suggest that this concept may apply to human allograft recipients. Graft survival in chronic renal failure patients appears to correlate with pretransplantation results of an immune profile consisting of nonspecific parameters, namely, total T and active T-rosette-forming cells (T-RFC) (Kerman et al., 1977) or cutaneous hypersensitivity to microbial antigens and sensitization to dinitrochlorobenzene (DNCB) (Rolley et al., 1978). Renal-failure patients who failed to display recall to microbial antigens or primary sensitization to DNCB had significantly prolonged allograft survival compared to responsive individuals ($p < 0.01$) (Rolley et al., 1978). Patients with a low percentage of active T-RFC (A-T-RFC) prior to transplantation had 83% 1-year graft survival compared to 50% survival in individuals with a higher percentage of A-T-RFC (Kerman et al., 1977). Thus, strong immune responders have a poorer chance of 1-year graft survival independent of the degree of HLA compatibility. The concept that immune responsiveness correlates with graft survival, irrespective of HLA, may have important implications not only for patient selection but also for tailoring immunosuppressive regimens. For example, transplantation might be restricted to patients who are weak responders. Alternatively, high-responder individuals might be particularly selected for intensive immunosuppressive therapy with antithymocyte globulin (ATG), total body or nodal irradiation, or newer modes of nonspecific chemical suppression (Rapaport et al., 1972, 1979; Cosimi et al., 1976; Strober et al., 1979; Starzl et al., 1979; Salaman and Miller, 1979).

We have developed a pretransplant battery of tests to identify weak responders likely to have prolonged graft survival. The duration of cadaveric allograft survival in chronic-renal-failure patients correlated with values below the median in percentage of A-T-RFC, in cpm [^{3}H]thymidine incorporated during spontaneous blastogenesis or during mixed-lymphocyte response (MLR) to a stimulation panel of three to five unrelated donors, and to a negative recall response to antigens eliciting cutaneous hypersensitivity to purified protein derivative, mumps, Streptokinase-Streptodornase, dermatophytin, and dermatophytin-O.

Method of Nonspecific Immune Analysis. Briefly, peripheral-blood lymphocytes (PBL) are separated on a Ficoll–Hypaque gradient, washed in Dulbecco's phosphate buffered saline (PBS), pH 7.3, and brought to a final concentration of 2×10^6 PBL/ml in PBS. For the *total T-RFC* assay, 0.25 ml (5×10^5 PBL) are mixed with 0.25 ml 0.5% washed unsensitized sheep red blood cells (SRBC), centrifuged at 200g for 5 min at room temperature, and then incubated in an ice-water bath (4–8°C) for 60 min. After the cell pellets are gently resuspended, a drop of the suspension is placed onto a hemocytometer. The number of rosettes (three or more SRBC surrounding a lymphocyte) are counted. All tests are performed in duplicate; 200 or more PBL are counted to determine the percentage of total T-RFC. For the A-T-RFC, 0.25 ml (5×10^5 PBL) is mixed with 0.25 ml 0.5% washed unsensitized SRBC and centrifuged at 200g for 5 min at room temperature. Cell pellets are gently resuspended and the A-T-RFC counted immediately (without a 60-min 4–8°C ice-water incubation). For the *in vitro* studies of PBL stimulation with *phytohemagglutinin* (PHA), *concanavalin A* (Con A), *pokeweed mitogen* (PWM), or *alloantigen stimulation* in a *panel MLR*, PBL are isolated and brought to a concentration of 1×10^6 PBL/ml. For the assays, 1×10^5 PBL in medium (RPMI 1640, glutamine, pen/strep, Hepes, and 15% inactivated AB plasma) are seeded into microtiter plate wells and incubated with either three concentrations of each mitogen or with 1×10^5 donor-panel stimulation cells (previously inactivated with mitomycin-C) in triplicate in a humidified chamber containing 95% air and 5% CO_2 at 37°C for 96 hr. The lymphocyte response to stimulation is determined by measuring the incorporation of [^{3}H]thymidine into DNA. At 18–24 hr before the cultures are harvested, 1 μCi [^{3}H]thymidine (specific activity 48 Ci/mM, ICN) is added to each well. Incubations are terminated using a Multiple Automatic Sample Harvester (MASH); [^{3}H]thymidine incorporation is measured by liquid scintillation counting. Results are expressed as counts per minute (cpm). *Spontaneous blastogenesis* (SB) is performed in triplicate by adding 50 μl [^{3}H]thymidine (specific activity 48 Ci/mM) to 50 μl heparinized whole blood diluted with 200 μl medium. The mixture is incubated for 2 hr at 37°C in a 5% CO_2 incubator prior to harvesting using a MASH unit. The filter strips are dried and counted in a liquid scintillation system.

Skin-test antigen responses are elicited by intradermal inoculation of 0.1 ml dermatophytin (1:30), dermatophytin-O (1:100) (Hollister-Steir Labs), Streptokinase-Streptodornase (50 units SK/SD, Lederle Labs), mumps (Eli Lilly and Co.), and intermediate-strength tuberculin antigen (Parke, Davis and Co.). Reactions are measured at right angles (mm) at 24 and 48 hr for the average dimension of induration and erythema. Induration greater than 5 mm is considered positive. DNCB was used as a nonspecific measure of leukocyte mobilization by observing the spontaneous flare reaction that occurred at the application site. Doses were 2000 μg to the upper arm and 50 μg to the forearm. A flare after 14 days was scored 4+ at the 2000-μg site only, 3+ at the 50-μg site only. If neither site developed a flare after 14 days, a challenge of 50 μg was applied to the opposite forearm. A cutaneous hypersensitivity reaction at this new site within 48 hr was scored as 2+. An equivocal reaction that required biopsy for confirmation counted 1+ if the histological features of delayed cutaneous hypersensitivity were seen. In practice, reactions of 4+ or 3+ were considered normal and positive; below these values, abnormal or negative to DNCB without further testing (Kerman and Stefani, 1976; Kerman *et al.*, 1979).

The median values for the pretransplant immunological assessment among 41 cadaveric renal allograft recipients were: 55% total T-RFC, 34% A-T-RFC; 12,079 cpm SB, 21,470 cpm (or 5.7 stimulation ratio) on panel MLR; 103,725 cpm response to PHA, 77,030 cpm response to Con A, and 134,249 cpm response to PWM. Patients were considered positive responders if they reacted to one or more microbial antigens or positively to DNCB. Prolonged graft survival correlated with patients having pretransplant values below the group median for three of the four *in vitro* immune assessment tests: A-T-RFC less than 34% ($p < 0.05$); *in vitro* lymphocyte SB less than 12,079 cpm ($p < 0.01$); panel MLR less than 21,470 cpm ($p < 0.01$), and negative response to all microbial skin-test antigens ($p < 0.04$) (Table 4). *De novo* response to DNCB, percentage total T-RFC, and lymphocyte response on stimulation with mitogens were not prognostic of graft survival.

Patients with strong pretransplant immune responses in the four relevant tests displayed an earlier onset of rejection, reduced mean survival time (MST), and requirement for larger steroid doses to dampen rejection events (Table 5). It is of interest that a preliminary study of

TABLE 4. Mean Survival Time of 41 Cadaveric Renal Allografts Based on Pretransplant Nonspecific Immune Assessment

Assay	MST (days)[a]		p Value[b]
Active T-rosette-forming cells (%)	< 34%[c]	> 34%[c]	
	228 ± 68	100 ± 69	< 0.05
Spontaneous blastogenesis	< 12,079 cpm[c]	> 12,079 cpm[c]	
	255 ± 36	70 ± 61	< 0.01
Panel mixed-Lymphocyte response	< 21,470 cpm[c]	> 21,470 cpm[c]	
	255 ± 47	78 ± 51	< 0.01
Microbial skin-test antigens	Anergic	Positive[d]	
	239 ± 42	115 ± 41	< 0.04

[a] Mean survival time in days ± S.D.
[b] Data were analyzed by the two-tailed Wilcoxon test.
[c] Median value for the test.
[d] Positive response to one or more microbial skin-test antigens.

TABLE 5. Cadaveric Graft Survival Based on Pretransplant Immune Response[a]

Finding	Immune response		
	Weak[b]	Strong	p Value[c]
Mean survival time (days)	386 ± 78	111 ± 86	< 0.01
Number of rejection episodes (first 30 days)	1.1 ± 0.4	1.5 ± 0.28	N.S.
Day of rejection onset	17 ± 4.9	8.5 ± 7.0	< 0.05
Mean grams Solu-Medrol/PT (first 30 days)	4.45 ± 1.05	6.65 ± 2.6	< 0.05

[a] Data are presented as means ± S.D. There were no significant differences in *HLA* mismatches between groups.
[b] Weak responses: < 34% A-T-RFC; (−) skin tests; low SB; low panel MLR.
[c] Two-tailed Wilcoxon test.

equine antithymocyte globulin [(ATG) UpJohn Co.] (used as an adjunctive immunosuppressive drug) revealed the drug to have a marked effect to prolong the survival of grafts in patients with strong pretransplant immunocompetence to survival times displayed by weak responders, who showed no benefit of drug treatment (Table 6).

3. Posttransplantation Immunological Assessment

3.1. Donor-Specific Immune Monitoring

The raison d'être of immune monitoring is twofold: first, to establish or confirm the diagnosis of rejection; second, to provide evidence for initiation of early intensified immunosuppressive treatment in an attempt to improve the prognosis of rejection, particularly if instituted prior to

TABLE 6. Renal Allograft Mean Survival Time (Days) Based on Pretransplant Immune Parameters: ATG Study

Assay		Patients		
		Non-ATG	ATG	p Value[a]
Microbial skin test[b]	+	115	207	< 0.05
	−	239	217	N.S.
Active T-rosette-forming cells (%)[c]	> 34%	100	208	< 0.05
	< 34%	228	228	N.S.
Spontaneous blastogenesis[c]	> 12,079 cpm	70	154	< 0.05
	< 12,079 cpm	225	267	N.S.

[a] Data were analyzed by the two-tailed Wilcoxon test.
[b] Patients were considered positive responders if they reacted to one or more microbial skin-test antigens.
[c] Median value of 34% A-T-RFC and 12,079 cpm SB.

clinical evidences of rejection, which represent a late point in the temporal course of events (Kerman and Geis, 1978). Immunological monitoring assays may be important probes, since initial activation of immunocompetent cells probably precedes full expression of a rejection crisis by days to weeks.

The correlation of posttransplant measurement of complement-dependent antibody (CDA), lymphocyte-dependent antibody (LDA), lymphocyte-mediated cytotoxicity (LMC), and K-cell reactivity against ^{51}Cr-labeled donor target cells and rejection is controversial. A positive CDA against donor targets has been associated with rejection and a poor prognosis (Stiller et al., 1976; Gailiunas et al., 1978). However, in some cases the CDA remains positive long after the rejection episode is over, and has therefore been suspected to be of little clinical significance (Stiller et al., 1976). Some workers report positive CDA and LDA reactions during rejection in the absence of LMC reactivity (Gailiunas et al., 1978; Stiller and Sinclair, 1979; Carpenter and Morris, 1979). There are reports of an excellent correlation between LMC and rejection (Garovoy et al., 1973a; Stiller et al., 1976). In fact, positive LMC assays have been claimed to predict impending rejection, although other workers disagree (Kovithavongs et al., 1978). These differences may be due to the variable use of mitogen-stimulated vs. nonstimulated target cells, and of long (16-hr) vs. short (4-hr) incubation periods, which may result in false-positive and false-negative test results (Kovithavongs et al., 1978). There is considerable disagreement concerning the association between LDA and rejection. Some reports show no correlation, others a degree of association with the absence of rejection, and still others a strong association with the presence of rejection (Gailiunas et al., 1978; Kovithavongs et al., 1978; F. Thomas et al., 1978; Stiller and Sinclair, 1979; Carpenter and Morris, 1979). Some investigators suggest that a positive LDA reflects a state of immune enhancement (Descamps et al., 1975; Kovithavongs et al., 1978). On the other hand, it has been claimed that positive LDA tests are associated with chronic rejection in long-surviving renal allografts (d'Apice and Morris, 1974; J. Thomas et al., 1976). The discordant results may be due to the lack of comparable techniques among laboratories. Unfortunately, too few of the studies specify whether or not the antibody was absorbable with platelets, a possible differential index of various biological effect (Table 7).

Preliminary results in our initial group of 47 patients who experienced 63 rejection episodes during the first 30 postoperative days did not clarify the relationship between donor-specific immunity detected in vitro and in vivo rejection. A total of 97 batteries of LDA, CDA, LMC, and K-cell assays were performed against donor targets. If at least one of the four tests was positive, the patient was considered to be immune. The

TABLE 7. Posttransplant Donor-Specific Assays

Assay	Target[a]	Incubation	Correlation with rejection	Reference
CDA	DSpC PHA ^{51}Cr	4 hr	Good	Stiller *et al.* (1976)
	DSpC ^{51}Cr	2 hr	Good; however, CDA was detected in the absence of rejection in some cases.	Gailiunas *et al.* (1978)
	DPBL or SpC PHA ^{51}Cr	4 hr	Good	Kovithavongs *et al.* (1978)
LDA	DPBL or SpC ^{51}Cr	4–6 hr	Poor	Kovithavongs *et al.* (1978)
	DPBL or SpC PHA ^{51}Cr	4 hr	Associated with absence of rejection	Stiller *et al.* (1976)
	DPBL or SpC ^{51}Cr	4 hr	Good	Gailiunas *et al.* (1978)
	DSpC PHA ^{51}Cr	4 hr	Good	F. Thomas *et al.* (1978)
LMC	DPBL ^{51}Cr	4 hr	Good	Garovoy *et al.* (1973a)
	DSpC PHA ^{51}Cr	16–18 hr	Good (predictive of rejection)	Gailiunas *et al.* (1978)
	DPBL or SpC PHA ^{51}Cr	4 hr	Not good	Kovithavongs *et al.* (1978)
	DPBL or SpC ^{51}Cr	18 hr	Good, but not predictive of rejection	Kovithavongs *et al.* (1978)

[a] (D) Donor; (SpC) spleen cell; (^{51}Cr) target cell labeled with ^{51}Cr; (PHA) PHA-treated donor target cells; (PBL) peripheral-blood lymphocytes.

positive reaction was considered to correlate with rejection if it was observed 5 days before or after a clinical episode (Table 8). There were 38 positive and 56 negative batteries. A positive response in one donor-specific assay correlated with rejection in 28/38 (74%) of instances. However, 32 other donor-specific batteries were completely negative during documented rejection episodes. These apparently false-negative tests may be due to (1) mediation of rejection by immune elements present in peripheral blood but not reflected by these assays; (2) the transient presence of elements immunoreactive in these tests at times other than during the performance of the assays; or (3) rapid depletion of reactive elements by absorption to or consumption within the graft.

TABLE 8. Lack of Correlation of Positive Donor-Specific Immune Assays and Rejection

	Comprehensive immune response[a]	
	(+)	(−)
Rejection[b]	28	32
No rejection	10	24 ($p > 0.5$)

[a] A (+) comprehensive immune response refers to any one or more of the four donor-specific assays being positive (LDA, CDA, LMC, or K cell).
[b] A total of 63 rejection episodes were observed, but no immune testing was done during 3 of the rejections.

There were 10/38 positive assays unassociated with documented rejection, suggesting a 26% rate of false-positive tests. Of the 10 false-positive batteries, 7 were associated with the presence of CDA, possibly reflecting cold B (protective) antibody (Iwaki et al., 1979). Chi-square analysis of the raw data did not suggest a significant correlation ($p > 0.5$) between the detection of donor-specific responses in vitro and allograft rejection in vivo (Table 8).

Other tests have been reported to reflect specific host antidonor activity, including: the leukocyte aggregation test, which measures host-cell adherence to donor-kidney-cell targets; the mixed-lymphocyte culture (MLC) responses, measuring proliferation by host cells; release of migration-inhibition factor (MIF) a lymphokine from sensitized cells; presence of warm B-cell antibodies; and finally elicitation of delayed cutaneous hypersensitivity following intradermal challenge of renal allograft recipients with soluble donor-type antigen.

Adherence of sensitized lymphocytes to target cells is a prerequisite for cellular cytotoxicity (Wilson, 1965). Utilizing this principle, Kahan and co-workers (Tom et al., 1974; Kahan et al., 1974, 1975) applied a leukocyte adherence test (LAT) to detect emergence of cellular immunity in renal-transplant patients. The assay sought immunospecific adherence and aggregation of recipient leukocytes onto cultured donor kidney cells. Recipient peripheral-blood leukocytes were reacted with donor kidney cells maintained in tissue culture. Immune adhesion of recipient immunocompetent lymphocytes onto donor targets induced clumping of other leukocytic cells. In the absence of immunoreactive lymphocytes, leukocytes uniformly spread over the culture. The LAT is a rapid, specific test requiring only small amounts of patient material. It has been shown to (1) diagnose rejection episodes 2–15 days before patients display clinical or chemical signs of rejection; (2) differentiate between rejection and other causes of graft failure; (3) detect host presensitization by specific reactivity toward a battery of kidney targets; and (4) predict sensitivity to bolus methylprednisolone therapy. The drawbacks to the LAT assay are the requirement for tissue-culture technology and the limited amount of available donor material, precluding daily tests.

When lymphocytes from two individuals incompatible at the MHC are coincubated in an MLC, they undergo proliferation (Bain and Lowenstein, 1964). If donor lymphocytes are prevented from undergoing division, by the use of a metabolic inhibitor such as mitomycin C, they become pure stimulator elements allowing one to assess the degree of cell division, and presumably histoincompatibility, by "responder" recipient cells (Bach and Voynow, 1966). Thus, proliferation in a one-way culture is the positive response, reflecting recipient recognition of disparate antigens. Several investigators have reported that long-term patients with excellent renal function are specifically unresponsive to donor but normally responsive to third-party control cells in one-way MLC (Garovoy *et al.*, 1973b; Suciu-Foca *et al.*, 1974).

Miller and colleagues (Hattler *et al.*, 1972; Miller *et al.*, 1973) reported in both dogs and man that recipient peripheral blood lymphocytes (PBL) displayed decreased MLC reactivity at the time of allograft rejection. They attributed this paradoxical observation to entrapment of immunoreactive cells in the graft, and thus out of the circulation that is sampled for the test. Resolution of the rejection episode was accompanied by reappearance of MLC-responsive cells. Unfortunately, this hyporesponsiveness was not diagnostic of rejection, since it was present during cytomegalovirus infection and obscured by production of a cytophilic antibody that blocked recognition by responding cells (Miller *et al.*, 1976). In a retrospective correlative study, Stiller *et al.* (1976) performed MLC reactions between lymphocytes of cadaveric recipients and stimulating cells from donor spleen. There were 17 positive and 10 negative MLC responses at the time of rejection; there were 16 positive and 16 negative MLC responses in the absence of rejection.

While the MLC is not useful to predict the onset of rejection, it may contribute to an understanding of host adaptation to allografts. The presence of humoral factors that block MLC reactions may be associated with a favorable posttransplant course (Miller *et al.*, 1975, 1976; Rashid *et al.*, 1975). Miller and colleagues tested the stimulatory capacity of donor cells with third-party cells in an MLC in the presence and absence of recipient serum. The presence of a high-avidity, cytotoxic antibody in recipient serum was associated with a rejection episode. On resolution, this immune response evolved to an antibody that blocked MLC activity and could be removed by washing the cells (Rashid *et al.*, 1975). Since other studies have suggested that MLC-blocking factors are associated with acute and with chronic rejection episodes (Buda *et al.*, 1975), the clinical significance of blocking factors is uncertain.

Recently, Miller *et al.* (1978) utilized the "secondary MLC" reaction [primed MLC or primed-lymphocyte test (PLT)] for immune monitoring posttransplantation. To perform a secondary MLC, recipient cells are initially cultivated with donor cells for 9 days, then exposed to fresh donor cells and pulse-labeled at 48 hr. An accelerated, secondary MLC response, detected by high levels of [^{3}H]thymidine incorporation at this early time, was associated with rejection. In contrast to the one-way MLC, the secondary MLC assay did not appear to be affected by viral infection. However, the test is not clinically useful for the prospective diagnosis of rejection, since it requires 12 days to perform.

In the presence of specific antigen, sensitized lymphocytes release lymphokines including MIFs (Phillips *et al.*, 1972). Tests that detect MIF depend on the observation that leukocytes tend to migrate spontaneously unless inhibited by the presence of this lymphokine. The assays observe the emigration from a capillary tube onto a flat surface of either recipient leukocytes admixed with donor antigen (Falk *et al.*, 1972) or indicator guinea pig macrophages exposed to the supernatant generated by the interaction of recipient lymphocytes with donor antigen. Extracts of donor kidney, spleen, neonatal kidney, or PBL (David *et al.*, 1964; Weeke *et al.*, 1970; Dormont *et al.*, 1972; R.J. Williams *et al.*, 1974) have been used as antigen sources. Regardless of the methodology or source of the antigen, the results have been remarkably consistent. MIF release either accompanies or precedes 80–90% of acute rejection episodes, with few false-positive or false-negative results (Weeke *et al.*, 1970; R.J. Williams *et al.*, 1974).

Recently, Iwaki *et al.* (1979) suggested that antibodies directed against antigens on donor B cells are more important than those on T cells. Early graft failure was associated with the presence of anti-B-cell antibodies more frequently than with the presence of anti-T-cell antibodies: of 26 graft failures, 22 had positive anti-B donor-specific reactions, while only 4 of 31 patients with functioning grafts displayed such antibodies (Soulillon *et al.*, 1979). The presence of B warm (37°C) antibodies was related to rejection in 6 out of 6 cases, while B cold (5°) antibodies were not (Iwaki *et al.*, 1979). However, other workers report that anti-B-cell antibodies are common in patient sera posttransplantation regardless of the clinical outcome (Carpenter and Morris, 1979). Further analysis of the nature, specificity, and distribution of B-cell antibodies detected by dye exclusion is clearly needed to assess their relevance to allografting.

Kahan *et al.* (1973) reported that specific cutaneous hypersensitivity can be elicited in transplanted patients by intradermal challenge with soluble donor HLA-type antigens. Specificity of immune reactions for HLA A2 and A3 was demonstrated by cross-challenge tests: only allograft recipients challenged with soluble antigens prepared from a lymphoblastoid line that contained disparate donor specificities elicited delayed cutaneous hypersensitivity reactions. Further, the corresponding soluble antigen specifically inhibited the cytotoxic reaction of recipient alloantibody *in vitro*. Since transplantation antigens are the focus of the host's response, soluble donor antigen may afford an immunological probe to dissect patient reactivity. The application of this assay as a cross-match test would require appropriate soluble donor antigen reagents prior to transplantation, an impossibility at present due to the 72-hr period required to prepare, administer, and observe the effects of the soluble material compared to the currently limited time of organ storage. Furthermore, immunological monitoring by repeated skin-testing of renal-allograft recipients to detect specific antidonor responses is probably not practical, since it might promote host sensitization. However, donor-specific soluble antigens might be useful for *in vitro* immune monitoring (Kerman *et al.*, 1978).

Thus, although donor-specific assays should potentially provide the most incisive information about the mechanisms of allograft rejection and the prognosis of the host response, these tests are at present of limited utility. First, the requirement for tremendous quantities of recipient blood restricts the frequency of assays to weekly or biweekly. This problem is exacerbated in lymphopenic patients, particularly those treated with antilymphocyte serum. Second, the number of obtainable, viable donor lymphocytes, particularly from cadaveric sources, is limited. Third, the assays do not always reflect *in vivo* events. There is a high incidence of false negatives, possibly due to compartmentalization of recipient immune cells or antibodies in the graft. In this regard, it would be of interest to perform the tests with fresh urinary lymphocytes as effectors. Furthermore, rejection episodes occurring in the presence of false-negative reactions might reflect recipient reactivity against organ-specific antigens not present on indicator donor lymphocytes. Therefore, at present, evaluation of nonspecific reactivity, rather than specific antidonor reactivity, represents a more feasible approach to detect *in vitro* correlates of *in vivo* immune events in allograft recipients.

3.2. Nonspecific Immune Monitoring

Two nonspecific immunological monitoring assays appear to detect emerging host reactivity: enumeration of the percentage active T-rosette-forming cells (A-T-RFC) and measurement of spontaneous blastogenesis (SB) (Hersh *et al.*, 1971; Kerman and Geis, 1976, 1978; Morris *et al.*, 1978; Kerman *et al.*, 1979). Since cellular allograft rejection is probably mediated by T cells, numerous investigators have monitored their numbers (Kerman and Geis, 1976, 1978; Buckingham *et al.*, 1977; Thomas *et al.*, 1978). Two T-cell populations can be identified on the basis of their differential ability to bind sheep red blood cells (SRBC) in rosette configurations (Wybran and Fudenberg, 1973; Fudenberg *et al.*, 1975; Kerman *et al.*, 1976). Total T-RFC are enumerated after incubation of PBL and SRBC in an ice-water bath for at least 1 hr. The total T-RFC presumably represent all T cells in the peripheral blood. A second population, termed the active T-RFC (A-T-RFC), is detected by rosette formation immediately after incubation of PBL and SRBC. The A-T-RFC has been proposed to be a subpopulation of the total T-RFC with surveillance properties more closely reflecting cell-mediated immune events than the total T-RFC (Wybran and Fudenberg, 1973; Fudenberg *et al.*, 1975; Kerman and Stefani, 1976; Kerman and Geis, 1978).

There have been contradictory reports of the diagnostic value of the total T-RFC after renal transplantation. F. Thomas *et al.* (1978) claimed a good correlation between high levels of total T-RFC and acute rejection episodes: more than 80% of recipients demonstrating acute rejection had a total T-RFC level above 20% of normal (360 T-RFC/mm³). In contrast, the majority of patients not having acute rejection appeared to have total T-RFC levels below 20%. These authors claimed that when the total T-RFC levels were maintained below 20% in the early post-cadaveric-transplant period, acute rejecion was a rare event. In 85% of cases, they found the onset of acute rejection to be heralded by a rise in the level of total T-RFC. However, T-cell levels also rose above 20% in the absence of acute rejection, especially after the first transplant month. Buckingham *et al.* (1977) failed to confirm these findings.

An evaluation of total T and A-T-RFC levels in transplant recipients by Kerman and Geis (1976, 1978) demonstrated no association between rejection episodes and total T-RFC, but a good correlation with a decreased percentage of A-T-RFC. The absolute numbers of either T-cell population did not discriminate rejection; rather, the important index was the degree of change. In a recent report applying the same tests at an entirely different transplant center, Kerman *et al.* (1979) confirmed the diagnostic value of serial monitoring of A-T-RFC in renal-allograft recipients. Clinically apparent rejection episodes were always associated with decreased A-T-RFC. Episodes of decreased A-T-RFC, which were not associated with clinically apparent rejection episodes and might therefore have been interpreted as false-positive reactions, were usually associated with increased spontaneous blastogenesis (SB) and impaired renal handling of radionuclides, two sensitive measures of modest, subclinical events. All patients subsequently experienced clinically evident rejection episodes within 5–10 days.

The nonspecific A-T-RFC assay is easy to perform on a daily basis, since it does not require donor cells or large volumes of recipient blood. The decrease in A-T-RFC prior to the onset of a clinically detected rejection episode presumably reflects specific host anti-donor-T-cell immune sensitization, leading to the release of lymphokines that attract and hold T cells in the attack on the end organ. Alternatively, donor alloantigens may activate T-RFC, causing increased expression or activity of the T-RFC receptor and resulting in active emigration of these cells from the peripheral blood to recognize and attack the renal allograft (Kerman *et al.*, 1978).

The SB activity of peripheral blood mononuclear cells from renal-allograft recipients presumably reflects the presence of circulating blastoid cells possibly due to an *in vivo* mixed-lymphocyte response on allogeneic stimulation. Transformed blasts capable of incorporating thymidine appear in the lymph draining transplanted kidneys. Significant increases in DNA or RNA synthesis occur prior to, or concomitant with, clinical signs of rejection in both renal and cardiac transplantation (Hersh et al., 1971; Morris et al., 1978). The studies presented herein confirm the prognostic value of the SB test (Kerman et al., 1979).

The two nonspecific immune monitoring assays, A-T-RFC and SB, were used to monitor patients thrice weekly after renal allotransplantation. The immune parameters were correlated with: (1) glomerular and tubular function tests and (2) serial measurements of kidney function by radionuclide studies of glomerular function utilizing [^{99m}Tc]diethylemetriaminepentaacetic acid (DTPA) and of tubular function with [^{131}I]Hippuran. The radionuclide studies were processed using an MDS-Trinary 32 K computer and graded on a scale of 30 to yield kidney/aorta ratios (normal = 5, score = 0.8), kidney/background DTPA concentration ratios (normal = 5, score = 3.0), DTPA bladder-appearance time (normal = 5.0, score = < 4.49 min), Hippuran kidney/background ratio (normal = 5, score = > 3.5), Hippuran bladder-appearance time (normal = 5, score $^-$ < 4.49 min), and peak Hippuran renogram (normal = 5, score = < 4.49 min). Immunological and radionuclide studies were performed and interpreted blindly by individuals unaware of the patient's clinical course.

The following sequence of events was consistently observed in 63 acute cellular rejection episodes (no hyperacute rejections occurred) displayed by 47 renal allograft recipients during their first 30 postoperative days: (1) an initial immediate increase in SB and decrease in A-T-RFC following transplantation surgery; (2) an increase in SB prior to (76%) or at the same time as (24%) clinical evidences of rejection; (3) a decrease in A-T-RFC concomitant with or shortly after increased SB; (4) a decrease in SB and increase in A-T-RFC with resolution of rejection. Clinically apparent rejection episodes were significantly associated (p < 0.01) with abnormal radionuclide studies of kidney function, that is, a 5- to 6-point (or 25%) decrease in the combined computer-analyzed scores. The results of the immunological and radionuclide monitoring displayed an excellent correlation (p < 0.001) with graft rejection.

During the first 30 postoperative days of 47 renal allograft recipients who experienced 63 acute rejection episodes, there occurred 121 immune events (increased SB and decreased A-T-RFC) and 102 abnormal (decreased) radionuclide scans (Table 9). There were 63 immune events and 58 cases of decreased radionuclide scans; that is, 5 rejection episodes occurred in the absence of a prior decreased radionuclide scan (Table 9, Line 1). The 58 remaining immune events, which occurred in the absence of clinical rejection, were associated with impaired renal function by the radionuclide scan in 44 cases (Table 9, Line 2). There were 14 remaining extra immune events in the absence of either clinical rejection or an

TABLE 9. Immunological and Radionuclide Results of 63
Treated Rejection Episodes during the First 30 Postoperative
Days in 47 Non-ATG-Treated Patients

	Concomitant findings			
	↓ % Active T-RFC	↑ Spontaneous blastogenesis	↓ Radionuclide scans	Clinical rejection
Line 1	63	63	58	63
Line 2	58	58	44	0
Line 3	14^a	14^a	0	0
Line 4	4^b	4^b	0	0

^{a} 14/121 = 11.5% False-positive immune events.
^{b} 14 Extra ↓ A-T-RFC and ↑ SB minus 10 infection-related events = 4; 4/121 = 3.3%
  false-positive immune events.

impaired radionuclide scan (Table 9, Line 3). That these 14 episodes do
not represent an 11.5% rate of false-positive results was concluded from
documentation of 10 infectious episodes occurring at these times. Thus,
10 of the 14 paradoxical immune events may have been due to infection.
Thus, the false-positive rate is 3.3% (4/121) (Table 9, Line 4).

The application of serial immune monitoring with these two nonspecific assays and radionuclide scanning is illustrated in Fig. 1 and 2.
Figure 1 shows the immunological monitoring data following transplantation of a cadaveric kidney HLA-A3, −; B12, Bw35; Cw4, −, into a 33-
year-old recipient (HLA-A29, A31; B12, Bw35; Cw4, −) with renal
failure due to chronic pyelonephritis in crossed ectopic kidneys. Following a modest rejection reaction at day 6 as evidenced by a change in both
immune and radionuclide parameters, there was a return of graft function.
At day 13, increased SB was accompanied by decreased A-T-RFC and
a subsequent decline in handling of radionuclides on day 19, all unassociated with significant clinical changes. This triad might have been a
premonition of a clinical rejection episode. Although there was a modest
decrease in radionuclide handling by the kidney on day 25, accompanied
by changes in immune parameters, chemical and clinical signs of rejection
were not evident until day 28, when therapy was instituted with prompt
restoration of renal function and resolution of the immune parameters.

In Fig. 2, radionuclide handling is divided into three parameters —
(1) perfusion of the graft (kidney/aorta ratio), (2) glomerular handling of
[^{99m}Tc]-DTPA, and (3) tubular handling of [^{131}I]-Hippurate—which are
summated to express the overall nuclide score. In Fig. 2, a cadaveric
graft (HLA-A3, A24; B40, B27; Cw3, −) was placed into a 33-year-old
woman (HLA-A2, A9; Bw35, B40; Cw3, −) with quiescent immune
complex nephritis. Chemical and clinical signs of rejection at day 9 were

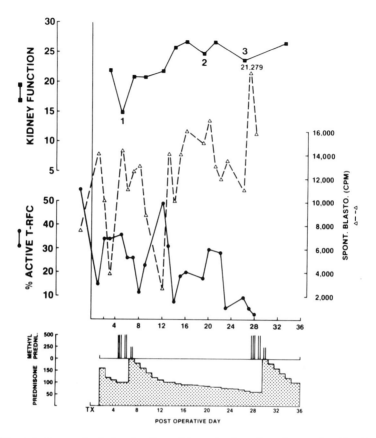

Figure 1. Immunological and radionuclide evaluation of renal transplant No. 21.

preceded by a fall in A-T-RFC and increased SB beginning at day 6. Following successful treatment, a rise in SB and a fall in A-T-RFC were associated with a plateau of radionuclide function at days 20–22, which spontaneously resolved. The immunological changes of rejection evident by day 34 were followed by a decrease in renal function detected by radionuclides at day 44 and responsive to a second course of pulse therapy.

These data suggest that alterations in two nonspecific immune assays, when coupled with computerized radionuclide scans, afford early indices of rejection. Immune events always occurred prior to clinical detection of rejection. Resolution of the A-T-RFC fall without institution of additional immunosuppressive therapy may be due to (1) internal homeostatic regulation, such as spontaneous activation of suppressor cells; (2) entrapment in the organ followed by a second wave of release

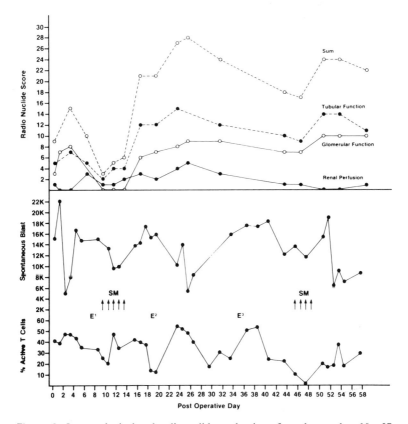

Figure 2. Immunological and radionuclide evaluation of renal transplant No. 27.

of additional cells; (3) a possible cellular role of the A-T-RFC to activate other T-cell subpopulations or antibody production, leading to subsequent attack on the end organ; or (4) effects of humoral antibody or chemotactic factors on cellular homing or traffic patterns. The trigger and the control of these T-cell fluxes are unclear.

4. Summary

Immunological monitoring has evoked considerable interest as an early diagnostic key to the events leading to allograft rejection. Presumably, sophisticated analysis should reveal and dissect the antigenic determinants eliciting alloimmunity. However, since rejection is mediated by a complex interplay of cellular and humoral effector mechanisms, it is unlikely that any single test will provide the crucial data in every case. Indeed, the failure of available techniques to detect alloimmune reactions precipitating clinical rejection underlines the limited utility of tissue typing for HLA-A and -B antigens. It is uncertain whether matching for the DRw antigens, which may represent the serologically identified analogue of the *HLA-D* locus, will improve cadaveric allograft survival. Of potentially great import is the application of nonspecific immune evaluation of potential allograft recipients prior to transplantation. Preliminary data suggest that intrinsic immune competence may be an important determinant of the potential for graft loss. Patients with weak immune responsiveness as determined by low numbers of active T-rosette-forming cells (A-T-RFC), anergy to microbial skin test antigens, low spontaneous blastogenesis (SB), and poor response to allogeneic stimulation from a panel of unrelated lymphocytes displayed prolonged graft survival compared to strong responders.

One cannot be assured of compatibility based on present typing techniques. A pretransplant evaluation of specific host antidonor reactivity must be performed to assess potential presensitization. We recommend a battery of lymphocyte-dependent antibody (LDA), complement-dependent antibody (CDA), lymphocyte-mediated cytotoxicity (LMC), and K-cell assays using recipient materials directed against ^{51}Cr-labeled donor targets, in addition to the visual cross-match technique. Patients with positive pretransplant reactivity experienced accelerated or early acute rejection and a high incidence of graft loss. However, this battery of assays may not delineate recipient presensitization against all relevant antigens, since it is directed only against peripheral blood lymphocytes as target cells, and does not reflect potentially important determinants on kidney or endothelial cells.

Since the major cause of renal-allograft loss is rejection, immunological monitoring assays may be important probes to detect emerging recipient sensitization and afford indices for prompt therapy. Immune reactions against donor lymphocytes in CDA, LDA, LMC, or K-cell assays do not correlate with clinically defined rejection episodes. Indeed, documented episodes were not accompanied by demonstrable immunity, presumably due to (1) use of inappropriate target cells (i.e. lymphocytes) as target antigens; (2) infrequency of testing; or (3) compartmentalization of recipient elements into the allograft and therefore inaccessibility in the peripheral blood. Since the relevant antigens or immune reactions mediating rejection are variable and not entirely established, it appears more feasible at present to monitor nonspecific cellular assays. Combined alterations in two tests, the percentage A-T-RFC and SB, correlated with renal functional changes presenting subclinically as altered handling of radionuclides or clinically as rejection. Furthermore, when alterations in the two nonspecific immune assays were combined with changes in the computerized radionuclide tests, one obtained a more reliable index to diagnose rejection than the currently available donor-specific assays. The present success of nonspecific methods should be regarded only as an impetus for dissection of the actual antigen provoking renal-allograft immunity, to obtain scientific and diagnostic skills to detect the evolution of specific host immunity.

References

Bach, F., and Voynow, N., 1966, One-way stimulation in mixed leucocyte cultures, *Science* **153**:545.

Bain, B., and Lowenstein, L., 1964, A reaction between leukocytes in mixed peripheral blood cultures, *Science* **145**:1315.

Buckingham J.M., Ritts, R.E., Woods, J.E., and Ilstrup, D.M., 1977, An assessment of cell-mediated immunity in acute allograft rejection in man, *Mayo Clin. Proc.* **52**:101.

Buda, J., Jacob, G., Lattes, C., Stevens, L., Sotelo, J., Suciu-Foca, N., Weil, R., and Reemstma, K., 1975, Prediction of humoral rejection in renal allograft recipients by MLC inhibition, *Transplant. Proc.* **7**:671.

Busch, G.J., Schamberg, J.F., and Moretz, R.C., 1976, T and B cell patterns in irreversibly rejected human renal allografts, *Lab. Invest.* **35**:272.

Busch, G.J., Schamberg, J.F., Strom, T.B., Tilney, N.L., and Carpenter, C.B., 1977, Four patterns of human renal allograft rejection: A cytologic and *in vitro* analysis of the infiltrate in 24 irreversibly rejected kidneys, *Transplant. Proc.* **9**:37.

Carpenter, C.B., and Morris, P.J., 1979, Immunologic monitoring of transplant patients, *Transplant. Proc.* **11**:1153.

Cerilli, J., Holliday, J.E., and Fesperman, D.P., 1977, Role of antivascular endothelial antibody in predicting renal allograft rejection, *Transplant. Proc.* **9**:771.

Collaborative report of the Scanditransplant, 1975, *Lancet* **1**:240.

Cosimi, A.B., Wortis, H.H., Delmonico, F.L., and Russell, P.S., 1976, Randomized clinical trial of antithymocyte globulin in cadaver renal allograft recipients: Importance of T cell monitoring, *Surgery* **80**:155.

d'Apice, A.J., and Morris, P.J., 1974, The role of antibody-dependent mediated cytotoxicity in renal allograft rejection, *Transplantation* **18**:20.

Dausset, J., Hors, J., and Busson, M.N., 1974, Serologically defined HLA antigens and long term survival of cadaver kidney transplants, *N. Engl. J. Med.* **290**:979.

David, J.R., Al-Askari, S., Lawrence, H.W., and Thomas, L., 1964, The specificity of inhibition of cell migration by antigen, *J. Immunol.* **93**:264.

Descamps, B., Gagnon, R., Debray-Sachs, M., Barbanel, C., and Crosnier, J., 1975, Lymphocyte-dependent and complement-dependent antibodies in human renal allograft recipients, *Transplant. Proc.* **7**:635.

Dormont, J., Sobel, A., Galanand, P., Crevon, M.C., and Colombani, J., 1972, Leucocyte migration inhibition with spleen extracts and other antigens in patients with renal allografts, *Transplant. Proc.* **4**:265.

Dossetor, J.B., and Myburgh, J.A., 1978, Posttransplant immunologic monitoring: Summation, *Transplant. Proc.* **10**:661.

Falk, R.E., Guttman, R.D., and Falk, J.A., 1972, A study of cell mediated immunity to transplantation antigens in human renal allograft recipients, *Transplant. Proc.* **4**:271.

Fudenberg, H.H., Wybran, J., and Robbins, O., 1975, T-rosette forming cells, cellular immunity and cancer, *N. Engl. J. Med.* **292**:475.

Gailiunas, P., Suthanthiran, M., Person, A., Strom, T.B., Carpenter, C.B., and Garavoy, M.R., 1978, Posttransplant immunologic monitoring of the renal allograft recipient, *Transplant. Proc.* **10**:609.

Garovoy, M.R., Franco, V., Zschaeck, D., Strom, T., Carpenter, C.B., and Merrill, J.P., 1973a, Direct lymphocyte-mediated cytotoxicity as an assay of presensitization, *Lancet* **1**:573.

Garovoy, M.R., Phillips, S.M., Carpenter, C.B., and Merrill, J.P., 1973b, Antibody modulation of cellular reactivity post renal transplantation, *Transplant. Proc.* **5**:129.

Hattler, B.G., Miller, J., and Johnson, M.C., 1972, Cellular and humoral factors governing canine mixed lymphocyte cultures after renal transplantation, *Transplantation* **14**:47.

Hersh, E.M., Butler, W.T., Rossen, R., Morgan, R.O., and Suki, W., 1971, *In vitro* studies of the human response to organ allografts: Appearance and detection of circulating activation lymphocytes, *J. Immunol.* **107**:571.

Iwaki, Y., Terasaki, P.I., Weil, T., Koep, L., and Starzl, T., 1979, Retrospective tests of B-cold lymphocytotoxins and transplant survival at a single center, *Transplant. Proc.* **11**:941.

Kahan, B.D., Mittal, K.K., Reisfeld, R., Terasaki, P.I., and Bergan, J.J., 1973, The antigenic stimulus in human transplantation, *Surgery* **74**:153.

Kahan, B.D., Tom, B.H., Mittal, K.K., and Bergan, J.J., 1974, An immunodiagnostic test for transplant rejection, *Lancet* **1**:37.

Kahan, B.D., Krumlovsky, F., Ivanovitch, P., Greenwald, J., Firlit, C., Bergan, J.J., and Tom, B.H., 1975, Immunodiagnostic and immunotherapeutic applications of the leucocyte aggregation test, *Arch. Surg.* **110**:984.

Katz, D., Paul, W., Goidl, E.A., and Benacerraf, B., 1970a, Carrier function in anti-hapten immune responses, *J. Exp. Med.* **132**:261.

Katz, D., Paul, W., Goidl, E.A., and Bennacerraf, B., 1970b, Stimulation of antibody synthesis and facilitation of hapten specific antibody responses by GVH reactions, *J. Exp. Med.* **133**:169.

Kerman, R.H., and Geis, W.P., 1976, Total and active T cell kinetics in renal allograft recipients, *Surgery* **79**:398.

Kerman, R.H., and Geis, W.P., 1978, T-RFC monitoring of CMI events in renal allograft recipients, *Transplant. Proc.* **10**:633.

Kerman, R., and Stefani, S., 1976, Immunological evaluation of patients with solid tumors before and after radiotherapy, in: *Neoplasms Immunity: Mechanisms* (R.G. Crispen, ed.), pp. 109–120, University of Illinois Press, Chicago.

Kerman, R.H., Smith, R., Ezdinli, E., and Stefani, S., 1976, Unification and technical aspects of total T, active T and B lymphocyte rosette assays, *Immunol. Commun.* **5**:685.

Kerman, R.H., Ing, T.S., Hano, J.E., and Geis, W.P., 1977, Prognostic significance of the active T-RFC in renal allograft survival, *Surgery* **82**:607.

Kerman, R.H., Roesler, H., and Kahan, B.D., 1978, Specific stimulation of active T-rosette forming cells by 3M KCl solubilized antigen, *Fed. Proc. Fed. Am. Soc. Exp. Biol.* **37**:1686.

Kerman, R.H., Floyd, M., Conner, W., McConnell, B.J., McConnell, R., Van Buren, C.T., and Kahan, B.D., 1979, Combined immunological and radionuclide techniques to monitor renal allograft rejection, *Transplant. Proc.* **11**:1229.

Kissmeyer-Nielson, F., Olsen, S., Peterson, V., and Fjeldborg, O., 1966, Hyperacute rejection of kidney allografts associated with pre-existing antibodies against donor cells, *Lancet* **2**:663.

Kovithavongs, T., Schlant, J., Pazdaka, V., Lao, V., Pazderka, F., Bettcher, K.B., and Dossetor, J.B., 1978, Posttransplant immunologic monitoring with special consideration of technique and interpretation of LMC, *Transplant. Proc.* **10**:547.

Medawar, P.B., 1944, The behavior and fate of skin autografts and skin homografts in rabbits, *J. Anat. (London)* **78**:176.

Miller, J., Howard, R.J., Hattler, B.G., and Najarian, J.S., 1973, Correlation of MLC reactivity after experimental and clinical transplantation—Virus and cytophilic antibody: Source of false negatives, *Transplant. Proc.* **5**:1771.

Miller, J., Lifton, J., Rood, F., and Hattler, B., 1975, Blocking vs. cytotoxic antibody in HLA and mixed lymphocyte culture identical and nonidentical human renal transplant recipients, *Transplantation* **20**:53.

Miller, J., Lifton, J., DeWolf, W.C., Stevens, B.J., and Wilcox, C., 1976, Adaptation to human and animal organ allografts: Reconsideration of a hypothesis, *Transplant. Proc.* **8**:217.

Miller, J., Lifton, J., and Wilcox, C., 1978, The use of second-generation assays in pre- and posttransplant monitoring: The primed or second-degree MLC, *Transplant. Proc.* **10**:573.

Moraes, J.R., and Stastny, P., 1977, A new antigen system expressed in human endothelial cells, *J. Clin. Invest.* **60**:449.

Morris, R.E., Dong, E., Struthers, C.M., Griepp, R.B., and Stinson, E.B., 1978, Immunologic monitoring of cardiac transplant recipients by a modified reactive leucocyte blastogenesis assay, *Transplant. Proc.* **10**:585.

Opelz, G., and Terasaki, P.I., 1976, Recipient selection for renal retransplantation, *Transplantation* **21**:483.

Phillips, S.M., Carpenter, C.B., and Merrill, S.P., 1972, Cellular immunity in the mouse: Correlation of *in-vivo* and *in-vitro* phenomena, *Cell. Immunol.* **5**:249.

Rapaport, F.T., Watanabe, K., and Cannon, F.D., 1972, Histocompatibility studies in a closely bred colony of dogs, *J. Exp. Med.* **136**:1080.

Rapaport, F.T., Bachvaroff, R.C., Dicke, K., and Santos, G., 1979, Total body irradiation and host reconstitution with stored autologous marrow: An experimental model for the induction of allogeneic unresponsiveness in large mammals, *Transplant. Proc.* **11**:1028.

Rashid, A., Sengar, D.P.S., and Harris, T.E., 1975, Role of mixed-leucocyte-culture blocking factor activity in human kidney transplants, *Transplant. Proc.* **7**:667.

Rolley, R.T., Widman, D.G., Parks, L.C., Sterioff, S., and Williams, G.M., 1978, Monitoring of responsiveness in dialysis–transplant patients by delayed-cutaneous hypersensitivity tests, *Transplant. Proc.* **10**:505.

Salaman, J.R., and Miller, J.J., 1979, Nonspecific chemical immunosuppression, *Transplant. Proc.* **11**:845.

Soulillon, J.P., Mouton, A. de, Reyrat, M.A., and Guenell, J., 1979, Role of anti-donor B lymphocyte antibodies in definitive allograft rejection, *Transplant. Proc.* **11**:770.

Starzl, T.E., Koep, J., Weil, R., Halgrimson, C.G., and Franks, J.J., 1979, Thoracic duct drainage in organ transplantation: Will it permit better immunosuppression?, *Transplant. Proc.* **11**:276.

Stiller, C.R., Sinclair, St.C., Abrahams, S., McGirr, D., Singh, H., Howson, W.T., and Ulan, R.A., 1976, Anti-donor immune responses in prediction of transplant rejection, *N. Engl. J. Med.* **294**:979.

Stiller, C.R., and Sinclair, N.R. St.C., 1979, Monitoring of rejection, *Transplant. Proc.* **11**:343.

Strober, S., Slavin, S., Fuks, Z., Kaplan, H.S., Gottlieb, M., Bieber, C., Hoppe, R.T., and Brumet, F.C., 1979, Transplantation tolerance after total lymphoid irradiation, *Transplant. Proc.* **11**:1032.

Suciu-Foca, N., Buda, J.A., Thiem, S., and Reemstma, K., 1974, Evaluation of the immune status of transplant recipients by mixed lymphocyte culture, *Clin. Immunol. Immunopathol.* **2**:530.

Terasaki, P.I., Opelz, G., and Mickey, M.R., 1978, Summary of kidney transplant data, 1977: Factors affecting graft outcome, *Transplant. Proc.* **10**:417.

Thomas, F., Mendez-Picon, G., Thomas, J., Lee, H.M., and Lowe, R., 1978, Effective monitoring and modulation of recipient immune reactivity to prevent rejection in early posttransplant period, *Transplant. Proc.* **10**:537.

Thomas, J., Thomas, F., and Kaplan, A., 1976, Antibody-dependent cellular cytotoxicity and chronic renal allograft rejection, *Transplantation* **22**:94.

Tom, B.H., Jakstys, M.M., and Kahan, B.D., 1974, Leukocyte aggregation: An *in-vitro* assay for cell-mediated immunity, *J. Immunol.* **113**:1288.

Weeke, E., Weeke, B., and Bendixen, G., 1970, Organ specific, anti-renal cellular hypersensitivity after kidney transplantation, *Acta Med. Scand.* **188**:307.

Williams, G.M., 1979, Progress in clinical renal transplantation, *Transplant. Proc.* **11**:4.

Williams, G.M., Hume, D.M., Hudson, R.P., Morris, P.J., Kano, K., and Milgrom, F., 1968, Hyperacute renal-homograft rejection in man, *N. Engl. J. Med.* **279**:611.

Williams, R.J., Mallick, N.P., Taylor, G., and Orr, W.M., 1974, The early diagnosis of rejection by the leucocyte migration test in cadaveric renal transplantation, *Clin. Nephrol.* **2**:100.

Williams, R.M., and Benacerraf, B., 1972, Genetic control of thymus-derived cell function, *J. Exp. Med.* **135**:1279.

Wilson, D.B., 1965, Quantitative studies on the behavior of sensitized lymphocytes *in vitro*, *J. Exp. Med.* **122**:143.

Wybran, J., and Fudenberg, H.H., 1973, Thymus-derived rosette-forming cells, *N. Engl. J. Med.* **288**:1072.

12

Human Ia-like Alloantigens and Their Medical Significances

Faramarz Naeim and Roy L. Walford

1. Introduction

The major histocompatibility complex (MHC) represents one of the so-called multigene families, and as such is characterized by multiplicity, close linkage, sequence homology, and related or overlapping phenotypic functions. Multigene families are thought to be composed of units of chromosomal organization encompassing a number of genes coding for simple and complex but related traits (Hood *et al.*, 1975). The MHCs in all vertebrate species so far investigated are strikingly homologous and involved in controlling a wide array of biological activities, including allograft survival, immune responsiveness, and susceptibility to disease. The mouse MHC, the *H-2* system, has been extensively studied and more completely mapped than the corresponding *HLA* system in man, largely because of availability of congenic strains differing only in the MHC region.

McDevitt and Tyan (1968) demonstrated that specific genes concerned with regulation of the immune response to certain antigens are located in a region (the *I* region) between the *K* and *D* loci of the *H-2* system. These immune-response *(Ir)* genes are primarily concerned with T-dependent immune responses. Some evidence suggests that *I*-region genes may code for those T-cell products needed for interaction of T cells with B cells and macrophages (Benacerraf and McDevitt, 1972; Katz and Benacerraf, 1975; Benacerraf and Germain, 1978; Shevach *et*

Faramarz Naeim and Roy L. Walford • Department of Pathology, University of California, Los Angeles, California 90024.

al., 1973, 1977; Taussing *et al.*, 1975; Shevach, 1976). Investigators utilizing alloantibodies directed against determinants coded for by the *I*-region genes (David *et al.*, 1973; Hämmerling *et al.*, 1974; Klein *et al.*, 1974) have also defined a new class of antigens that are expressed on the surfaces of most B cells, a high percentage of macrophages (Hämmerling *et al.*, 1975; Dorf and Unanue, 1977), and a small fraction of T lymphocytes (David *et al.*, 1976; Murphy *et al.*, 1976). These antigens are called immune-associated (Ia) antigens. The B-cell population in the mouse can probably be divided into two subpopulations on the basis of whether they carry Ia antigens or not (McDevitt *et al.*, 1976). Ia (+) B cells have the potential to give rise to IgG antibody, while Ia (−) B cells can produce only IgM. The subgroup of T cells that bear Fc receptors or function as suppressor cells appear to be Ia (+), while those T cells that respond in the mixed-lymphocyte reaction (MLR) are Ia (−) (McDevitt *et al.*, 1976). The Ia antigens have also been reported to be expressed on spermatocytes, epidermal cells, and fetal liver cells (Hämmerling *et al.*, 1974; Klein, 1975).

Many other genes exist within the *H-2* supergene system, for example, genes for controlling the expression of theta-antigen (Mickova and Ivanyi, 1973); the development of specific suppressor cells (Debre *et al.*, 1976); the MLR and the cell-mediated lymphocytotoxicity reaction (Sollinger and Bach, 1976); susceptibility to a number of spontaneous malignancies including lymphomas and cancers of the breast, lungs, and liver (G.S. Smith and Walford, 1978); susceptibility to a number of nonmalignant diseases (Doherty and Zinkernagel, 1975); levels of plasma testosterone and testosterone-binding protein (Ivanyi *et al.*, 1972); and probably the age-related maturation rate of some immune-response capacities (Meredith and Walford, 1979). The *H-2* system influences a wide variety of physiological and immunological processes in the mouse.

2. Human Ia-like Alloantigens

The human *HLA* supergene region demonstrates a striking homology with the *H-2* system of the mouse (Klein, 1975), and human lymphocytes possess alloantigens that show many features similar to the Ia antigens of mice (Arbeit *et al.*, 1975; Wernet, 1976). These include:

1. Antibodies against Ia-like antigens in humans are often contained within antisera raised against other antigens controlled by the MHC region.
2. The Ia-like antigens are expressed predominantly on B lymphocytes, as well as on macrophages, epidermal cells, and spermatozoa.

3. Prior incubation of lymphocytes with the antisera may inhibit the MLR and the secondary immune response.

4. Anti-Ia antibodies in the mouse and their homologous antibodies in humans inhibit the binding of heat-aggregated immunoglobulin complexes to Fc receptors, whereas antibodies to the *H-2K* and *D* regions of the mouse or the *HLA-A* and *-B* regions of human lymphocytes fail to do so.

The first serological studies in defining what are now recognized to be "B-cell" or Ia-like antigenic systems in the human were done with chronic lymphocytic leukemia (CLL) cells by Walford *et al.* (1971a,b, 1973), with cultured lymphoblastoid-cell lines (LCL) by Dick *et al.* (1972, 1973), and with unfractionated peripheral-blood lymphocytes by van Rood's group (van Leeuwen *et al.*, 1973), who were attempting to demonstrate HLA-D determinants by serological instead of the more cumbersome cellular reactions. The work with CLL cells by Walford and associates led to the identification of an Ia-like alloantigenic system referred to eventually as the *Merrit* system (Walford *et al.*, 1973; Gossett *et al.*, 1975). Van Leeuwen *et al.* (1975) and Winchester *et al.* (1975a,c) demonstrated that antibodies of this nature react selectively with B as opposed to T lymphocytes in complement-dependent lymphocytotoxicity assays. This observation was promptly extended and confirmed by different laboratories (Arbeit *et al.*, 1975; Bodmer *et al.*, 1975a,b; Fellous *et al.*, 1975; Ferrone *et al.*, 1975; Gossett *et al.*, 1975; Klouda and Reeves, 1975; Legrand and Dausset, 1975a,b; Mann *et al.*, 1975a,b; van Rood *et al.*, 1975a,b, 1976; Wernet *et al.*, 1975). These investigations resulted in alloantigenic systems of "B-cell" (Ia-like) specificities being defined independently by Terasaki *et al.* (1975), van Rood *et al.* (1975a,b, 1976), Mann *et al.* (1975a,b, 1976), Bodmer *et al.* (1975b), Ferrone *et al.* (1975), Thompson *et al.* (1975), and Legrand and Dausset (1975a,b).

3. Merrit Alloantigenic System

The work with CLL cells in our laboratory was stimulated by the observation that some of the *HLA*-typing antisera that with normal peripheral lymphocytes appeared to be monospecific showed with CLL cells "extra" reactions that were not demonstrated by other *HLA*-typing sera of the same specificity. Several possibilities were entertained to explain these extra reactions, including cross-reaction with known HLA antigens, reactions with immunoglobulin subgroups that might be present on the surface of CLL cells (Walford *et al.*, 1973), leukemia-associated alloantigens (Walford *et al.*, 1973), T- or B-cell alloantigens (Walford *et al.*, 1971b, 1973), and MLR determinants and the products of *Ir* genes

(Walford *et al.*, 1973). A series of studies eventually ruled out all but the last two categories. On the basis of cross-absorption studies, seven alloantigenic specificities were described, detectable by sera from which HLA antibodies had been absorbed, and considered to define an *HLA*-linked but distinct system (Walford *et al.*, 1973). Later, absorption experiments with separated T- and B-lymphocyte suspensions (Gossett *et al.*, 1975) indicated that the system was represented preferentially on B cells, at which point it was referred to as the *Merrit* system, after the first serum donor whose "extra" reactions prompted the investigations (Walford *et al.*, 1971b).

Based on the use of serum batteries and chi-square testing (van Rood and van Leeuwen, 1963), up to 24 specificities have so far been defined in the Merrit alloantigenic system (Walford *et al.*, 1977; Gossett *et al.*, 1977; Naeim *et al.*, 1978c). Many of these could be arranged into two segregant series. In addition to CLL cells, the Merrit alloantigens were shown to be present on T-depleted peripheral mononuclear (TDPM) cells, B-type human LCL, and blast cells of a high proportion of acute myeloid and lymphoid leukemias (Walford *et al.*, 1977; Naeim *et al.*, 1977a,b, 1978c,d).

4. Relationship of Ia-like Alloantigenic Systems to the *HLA* Complex

Family studies by Mann *et al.* (1975b), Jones *et al.*, (1975), and Wernet (1976) all indicated segregation of the Ia-like alloantigens with the *HLA* system, with the exception of system Ly-Co (Legrand and Dausset, 1975b), which segregated independently. Analysis of LCL derived from a single family in our laboratory showed segregation of Merrit alloantigens with *HLA*. Additional evidence of association of Ia-like antigens with the *HLA* system was the demonstration by Jones *et al.* (1975) that the only clone from among six clones of somatic-cell hybrids positive for the Ia-like ("B-cell") alloantigens detected by serum P1530B was the one containing chromosome 6, which carries the *HLA* system.

The *HLA*-linked Ia-like antigens appear to be distinct from HLA-A, -B, and -C antigens (Ferrone *et al.*, 1975; Wernet *et al.*, 1975b). The latter are present on all nucleated cells, whereas the tissue distribution of the former is more restricted. HLA but not "B-cell" alloantibodies can be readily absorbed with platelets. Variant cell lines such as Daudi, which do not express HLA antigens on their surfaces and lack β_2-microglobulins, nevertheless react with B-cell typing sera (Pious *et al.*, 1974; Jones *et al.*, 1975). HLA membrane antigens are shed into culture medium only after treatment with antibody and complement, whereas B-cell alloantigens are shed spontaneously even in the absence of specific antibody (Wernet *et al.*, 1975b). There may be a degree of linkage dysequilibrium between HLA-A, -B, -C, and Ia-like alloantigens (Mann *et al.*, 1975a,b; Walford *et al.*, 1976; Thompson *et al.*, 1977). In the Second B-cell Workshop of the Americas (Thompson *et al.*, 1977), 5 of the 120 sera showing negative reactions with T cells gave B-cell patterns correlating with HLA-B13 and were themselves part of a cluster related to Merrit group 13. Correlations with *HLA-B* were shown by the reaction patterns of 10 antisera of the workshop, but with *HLA-A* or -*C* by only one serum.

In contrast to the situation with *HLA-A*, -*B*, and -*C*, early studies showed strong linkage dysequilibrium between HLA-D determinants and many of the Ia-like alloantigens (Bodmer *et al.*, 1975b; van Rood *et al.*, 1975a,b, 1976; Solheim *et al.*, 1975). For example, Merrit 1 correlated with HLA-Dw1 and -2, and Merrit 13, a rather high-frequency antigen, included HLA-Dw3 and -6 (Walford *et al.*, 1977). Van Rood's B cell sera *Mo* and *Be* reacted with determinants strongly correlated with and possibly identical to Dw3, his serum *Pl* was strongly correlated with but still probably separate from Dw6, his serum Ag recognized a locus clearly separate from *HLA-D* [probably between *HLA-B* and -*A* (van Rood, personal communication)], and serum *Ko* showed no relationship at all to HLA-A, -B, -C or -D determinants. Serum *Po* appeared to recognize Dw 2 + 6, and *Si* gave an almost perfect fit with LD-107. Sera Nos. 58 and 77 of Winchester *et al.* (1975a) correlated strongly with Dw3, whereas Nos. 57 and 265 showed no correlation with *HLA-D* (although they would inhibit stimulator function). Serum *SØW* of Solheim *et al.* (1975) was highly associated with Dw2 ($P < .0001$), and serum *TH* was much broader than but completely included Dw3. Among the B-cell groups described by Bodmer *et al.* (1975b), *OX1* included Dw4 and Dw5 plus additional reactions, *OX2* included Dw3, *OX3* included Dw1, and *OX5* included Dw5.

The strong correlation between Ia-like alloantigens and some, albeit clearly not all, of the HLA-D determinants provoked considerable interest among investigators seeking to find serological methods to replace the more cumbersome MLR tests for *HLA-D* typing.

5. Seventh International Histocompatibility Workshop and HLA-DRw Specificities

The 7th IHW (Oxford, September 1977) was primarily devoted to the study and definition of human Ia-like antigens and their relationship to HLA-D determinants (Bodmer, 1978). The Ia-like alloantigenic systems reported previously by several investigators were compared and correlated in this workshop by using 180 "Ia" sera against TDPM cells, LCL, and CLL cells. Study of a large number of unrelated individuals in the workshop revealed a significant association between seven Ia-like antigenic groups and HLA-D determinants, indicating that these Ia-like antigens are closely linked to or perhaps identical to antigens of the *HLA-D* region. These Ia-like antigens officially were called HLA-DRw (HLA-D-related workshop) antigens, and demonstrated patterns of cross-reactions. In this regard, two subgroups were identified: DRw 1,2,3,6 and DRw 4,7,5,8 (Bodmer, 1978). Correlations of some of the *Merrit groups* with HLA-DRw antigens are as follows: *Merrit-ℓ* (Gossett *et al.*, 1975) ≈ HLA-DRw1, *Merrit*-1 [Merrit-C (Walford *et al.*, 1971b)] ≈ HLA-DRw2, *Merrit*-4 [Ev-i (Walford *et al.*, 1973)] ≈ HLA-DRw7, *Merrit*-8 ≈ HLA-DRw3, *Merrit*-9 ≈ HLA-DRw4, and *Merrit*-10 ≈ HLA-DRw4 (Bodmer, 1978). In addition to the HLA-DRw specificities, reaction patterns of some of the 7th IHW "Ia" sera with TDPM and CLL cells demonstrated several antigenic groups with no significant chi-square correlation with HLA-D determinants, suggesting the existence of specificities probably distinct from HLA-D determinants. This matter will be discussed later.

Population analysis of HLA-DRw antigens in the 7th IHW revealed a virtual absence of DRw3 and 7 in Japanese and lower frequencies of DRw4 (4×7) and DRw7 in African blacks. Also, in contrast to the pattern in American Caucasians, HLA-DRw1 and 5 were absent in Navajo Indians, while antigen *JA*, an Eskimo antigen, was found in the Navajo. Table 1 demonstrates antigen frequencies of HLA-DRw specificities for

TABLE 1. Frequencies of HLA-DRw Antigens for CLL and for American Caucasian and Navajo Indian TDPM Cells[a]

HLA	CLL ($N = 87$)	American Caucasian ($N = 47$)	Navajo Indian ($N = 49$)
DRw1	13%	9%	0
DRw2	21%	32%	14%
DRw3	21%	15%	21%
DRw4	24%	15%	53%
DRw5	16%	26%	0
DRw6	21%	26%	?
DRw7	18%	28%	9%
WIA8	1%	13%	44%
WIAA	2%	80%	?

[a] Adapted from Gossett *et al.* (1978a).

CLL cells and for Caucasian and Navajo Indian TDPM cells (Gossett *et al.*, 1978a; Troup *et al.*, 1978).

One of the problems encountered in analyzing the 7th IHW data was the lack of reproducibility, in part due to the insufficient experience of a number of laboratories in "Ia" serology. According to the 7th IHW report (Bodmer, 1978), only 41% of the participating laboratories produced results with a reproducibility based on unknown duplicates of greater than 75%.

A satisfactory typing of T-depleted lymphoid cells with "Ia" (DRw) sera requires nonspecific sera, reactive but nontoxic complement, and substantial depletion of the T cells from the peripheral-mononuclear-cell suspension. TDPM cells carry HLA-A,B,C antigens as well as Ia-like determinants. Thus, it is also essential that the typing sera contain no HLA-A,B,C antibodies. Reactivity to HLA-A,B,C antigens can be absorbed out by platelets or other cells, or blocked (for example, by anti-β_2-macroglobulins). The most practical approach is absorption with platelets, which carry HLA-A,B,C but not "Ia" antigens and are stable for a long period of time if kept in a refrigerator. It is important to select a proper proportion of packed platelets to serum to avoid incomplete as well as nonspecific absorptions (Naeim *et al.*, 1977a). For example, in the 7th IHW report, about 12% of the sera used for HLA-DRw typing reacted with more than 8% of T-cell suspensions, indicating incomplete removal of the HLA-A,B,C antibodies (Bodmer, 1978).

A significant number of "Ia" sera submitted to the 7th IHW reacted with more than one HLA-DRw specificity. Patterns of reactivities in some of these sera suggested cross-reactions. For example, a highly significant excess of sera reacting with DRw1+2, DRw1+6, DRw2+6, and DRw3+6 determinants was observed.

Absorption studies may be quite helpful in analyzing multispecific Ia-like antisera. B-type LCL represent a valuable resource for absorption, since large quantities of cells may be needed (Naeim *et al.*, 1977a,b). Table 2 demonstrates splitting of HLA-DRw activities of two sera, "Merrit" and "Evans" by means of absorption. Platelet-absorbed Merrit serum, found to initially react with both HLA-DRw1 and 2, could be "split" by absorption with cell line LG-27 and CLL cells La; Merrit serum absorbed with LG-27 demonstrated good HLA-DRw1 activity without DRw2, and conversely Merrit absorbed with La showed HLA-DRw2 activity without DRw1. Similarly, serum Evans absorbed with Et red cells (to remove anti-Le^A activity) and CLL cells Br possessed good HLA-DRw7 activity, while the same serum after absorption with Et and cell line Pa reacted with the HLA-DRw5 antigen.

For satisfactory typing, the complement should be active but not toxic to the cells. Toxic effects of rabbit serum as complement source

TABLE 2. Splitting of the Anti-HLA-DRw Activities of Merrit and Evans Sera by Absorption[a]

Sera	DRw2								DRw1			
7th IHW serum No.	13	14	15	16	17	18	60	9	42	120	128	152
Merrit abs.[b] La	0.85	0.61	0.81	0.73	0.84	0.62	0.65	0.18	0.18	0.03	0.09	0.07
Merrit abs. Lg-27	0.22	0.10	0.12	0.15	0.09	0.17	0.08	0.72	0.56	0.64	0.45	0.64

	DRw7					DRw5	
7th IHW serum No.	51	52	53	54	149	74	155
Evans abs. Et + Br	0.70	0.70	0.64	0.68	0.50	-0.02	-0.03
Evans abs. Et + Pa	-0.20	-0.19	0.08	-0.25	-0.23	0.72	0.78

[a] Adapted from Gosset et al. (1978). The values given are the r values of Merrit or Evans sera compared to individual 7th IHW sera.
[b] (Abs.), Absorbed with.

are more frequently observed in typing cell lines, acute leukemia cells, and TDPM cells than with unfractionated peripheral lymphocytes. This toxic effect appears to be due to heteroantibodies in normal rabbit serum. The effect increases if the cells are washed in saline or balanced salt solutions devoid of protein or sugars (Gossett *et al.*, 1978b). Toxicity due to heteroantibodies appears to involve activation of the classic complement pathway rather than the alternate pathway. This activation is inhibited by addition of 2-mercaptoethanol, implying that IgM and not other immunoglobulin subclasses are involved. The heteroantibodies present in normal rabbit serum lose their toxicity for human lymphoid cells when the serum is incubated at 50°C for 15 min, or when it is diluted with human or fetal calf serum (Gossett *et al.*, 1978b; Naeim *et al.*, 1977a,b). Not all rabbit sera are toxic for TDPM cells. By screening different lots of rabbit serum, one can find a complement source with minimal cytotoxic effects on TDPM cells. In our experience, most available rabbit sera are toxic for LCL and the majority of acute leukemia cells.

6. Correlation between *HLA-D* and DRw

The relationship between HLA-D determinants and DRw specificities was examined in the 7th IHW. For certain specificities such as DRw1 and 2, the correlation with the corresponding HLA-Dw (1 and 2) was excellent, suggesting that some *DR* alleles may be either identical to or closely linked with *Dw* alleles. Other possible associations, such as Dw4 with DRw4, Dw6 with DRw6, and Dw8 with WIA8, were not convincingly shown. Discrepancies also existed between HLA-DRw typing of the homozygous typing cells (HTC) and their HLA-Dw determinants (Bodmer, 1978).

In our studies on 31 B-type LCL derived from *HLA-D*-homozygous individuals (Fig. 1), the highest correlation was found between HLA-DRw2 and -Dw2, and HLA-DRw3 and -Dw3 (Naeim *et al.*, 1978c). Nevertheless, some discrepancies were noted. Three homozygous cell lines typed as DRw7 were known to be Dw5, 10, and 11, respectively. Cell line LG 28, which reacted with HLA-DRw6 sera, was known to be HLA-Dw3. None of the homozygous cell lines typed as HLA-DRw4 was unequivocally -Dw4, and some cell lines derived from members of a family typed serologically as HLA-DRw7 but with HTC as HLA-Dw11. Further investigations (Gatti *et al.*, 1979) demonstrated that an antiserum to HLA-DRw7 could suppress proliferation of all 6 -DRw7 (+) but none of 12 -DRw7 (−) cell lines. This suppressor activity could be removed by absorptions with three HLA-DRw7 (+) cell lines, each representing a

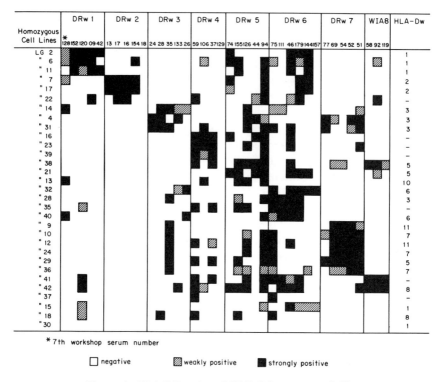

*7th workshop serum number

□ negative   ▨ weakly positive   ■ strongly positive

Figure 1. *HLA-DR* typing of *HLD-D*-homozygous LCL.

different *HLA-Dw* allele, namely, -Dw7, -Dw10, and -Dw11. These studies accord with results of family studies by Suciu-Foca *et al.* (1978) indicating that HLA-D and -DR determinants are controlled by closely linked but nevertheless distinct genes.

By *HLA-D* and -*DR* typing of randomly selected Navajo Indians, Troup, *et al.* (1978) demonstrated a highly significant correlation between DRw7/Dw7 and WIA8/Dw8, but no correlation at all between DRw2/ Dw2, DRw3/Dw3, and Dw4/DRw4. Studies of Festenstein (1978) on a recombinant family suggested crossover between *HLA-D* and -*DR* in the father. Reinsmoen *et al.* (1978) recently presented a family showing positive mixed-lymphocyte culture reactivity (MLR) between *HLA-A,B,C-* and *DR*-identical siblings. This might be taken as further evidence that *HLA-D* and -*DR* are nonidentical.

It appears that reactivity observed in the primed-lymphocyte test (PLT) may be more closely associated with *HLA-DR* typing than with HLA-D determinants (Sasportes *et al.*, 1978; Fradelizi *et al.*, 1978; Reinsmoen *et al.*, 1978). This concept was supported by absorption studies (De Wolf *et al.*, 1978) in which the capacity of the cells to restimulate in the PLT was blocked both by DRw alloantisera and by the p29, 34 fraction of heteroantiserum. The inhibition was specific: the PLT stimulation by HLA-DRw1 (+) cells was blocked by anti-HLA-DRw1 serum, but not by anti-DRw2, -DRw3, or control sera.

7. Ia-like Alloantigenic Segregants Distinct from *HLA-DR*

Evidence for more than one locus in the *HLA*-linked Ia-like alloantigenic system has been presented by several groups (Mann *et al.*, 1975a, 1976; Walford *et al.*, 1975, 1976; Terasaki *et al.*, 1975; van Rood *et al.*, 1977). Analyzing family crossover data, Mann and his associates (Mann *et al.*, 1976; Abelson and Mann, 1978) concluded that the "B-cell" (Ia-like) alloantigens reflected at least two loci, one more closely associated with the *HLA-A* and the other with the *HLA-B* locus. The reaction pattern of one serum in several crossover families led van Rood *et al.* (1977) to postulate the existence of two *Ia*-like loci, one near *HLA-D* and a second on the *A* side of the *HLA* complex. These conclusions are consistent with the population analysis of Walford *et al.* (1976), who demonstrated linkage dysequilibrium between *HLA-A*, *-B*, and certain Merrit specificities, suggesting the presence of two *Ia*-like loci. Recent studies by Park *et al.* (1978) based on population analysis and using cells from 635 American Caucasians, 115 Japanese, and 73 American blacks suggested the existence of two "Ia"-like alloantigenic groups, referred to as T-E21 and T-E22. These two allelic groups seemed distinct from *HLA-DR* but located on the *HLA-B* side of chromosome 6.

Our typing results of *HLA-D*-homozygous cell lines by 7th IHW "Ia" sera revealed four antigenic groups, Merrit 5, 13, 23, and 24, with mutually high r values (Naeim *et al.*, 1978c) (Fig. 2) that showed no significant correlation with HLA-A, -B, -C, -DR, or -D specificities. Similar results were obtained when TDPM, CLL, and acute leukemia cells were used as target cells. This study is in line with our previous results and suggests that Merrit groups 5, 13, 23, and 24 may represent Ia-like specificities distinct from *HLA-D* or *-DR* region(s).

8. Leukemia Cells and Ia-like Alloantigens

The presence of Ia-like alloantigens on CLL cells was first described by Walford *et al.* (1973, 1975, 1976, 1977). Results from a total of 475 CLL donor cells in the 7th IHW revealed a higher frequency of HLA-DRw3, 4, 5, and 6 among the CLL patients than among controls (Lawler

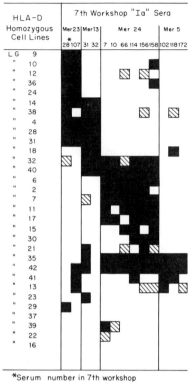

Figure 2. Ia-like segregant series distinct from *HLA-DR*.

and Jones, 1978). However, it was postulated that this difference might reflect merely technical problems rather than dysequilibrium of HLA-DRw antigens in CLL. According to our studies, one of the workshop Ia-like specificities (WIAA) defined by workshop sera Nos. 85 and 86 was detected in only 2% of CLL patients compared to 80% of normal controls (Gossett *et al.*, 1978a). Now, in routine preparation of TDPM cells from normal persons, a significant proportion of the cells (between 40 and 60%) are monocytes; we considered whether the difference in WIAA frequency between normal and CLL donors might be related to the monocytes. This possibility was further supported by the reactivity pattern of normal TDPM cells, LCL, and various leukemic cells against selected groups of 7th IHW "Ia" sera, including sera Nos. 85 and 86 (WIAA). As demonstrated in Table 3, peripheral-cell suspensions containing large numbers of monocyte or myelomonocytic elements, such as TDPM cells and cells from patients with acute myelogenous leukemia (AML), showed a higher frequency of reactions with these sera than suspensions with only a few monocytes. Either WIAA antigens are manifested more strongly on monocytes or their detection in cytotoxicity tests is potentiated by the presence of monocytes (Naeim et al., 1978c).

CLL is not a homogenous lymphoproliferative disorder; although in most cases CLL appears to result from clonal proliferation of abnormal B lymphocytes, a small percentage of CLL cases are of T-cell origin (Brouet et al., 1975 Uchiyama et al., 1977). In addition, subsets of chronic lymphoproliferative disorders exist that in some aspects resemble classic CLL, yet are distinct entities. These include "hairy-cell" leukemia (leukemic reticuloendotheliosis), prolymphocytic leukemia, Sézary syndrome, and the leukemic phase of lymphomas (lymphosarcoma-cell leukemia). Each of these entities may be heterogeneous by itself. For example, B- and T-type prolymphocytic leukemias have been described (Catovsky et al., 1973), circulating abnormal lymphoid cells in Sézary syndrome (leukemic phase of a T-cell cutaneous lymphoma) may share characteristics of helper T cells or suppressor T cells (Broder et al., 1976; Kansu and Hauptman, 1977), and "hairy-cell" leukemia is heterogeneous (Naeim et al., 1978a).

Results of testing mononuclear cells from 11 patients with "hairy-cell" leukemia against 7th IHW "Ia" sera are presented in Fig. 3. The cells from 1 patient showed over 80% spontaneous rosetting with sheep erythrocytes, only 2% of the cells were positive for surface-membrane immunoglobulins (SmIg's), and they did not react with any workshop "Ia" sera. Most cells from the remaining 10 patients were SmIg (+) and reacted with workshop "Ia" sera (Fig. 3); however, the reactions were less strong and less frequent than with CLL cells.

Our preliminary results indicate the presence of Ia-like as well as other HLA alloantigens on malignant lymphoid cells from patients with lymphoma and lymphosarcoma-cell leukemia. *HLA* typing of lymphoma

TABLE 3. Frequency of Reactivity of Normal and Leukemic White Blood Cells with Certain 7th IHW "Ia" Sera[a]

Cells[b]	Number of cases	7th IHW Serum No.						
		18	85	86	87	92	98	112
TDPM	47	31%	70%	68%	53%	23%	19%	13%
AML	43	18%	12%	16%	30%	23%	14%	9%
ALL	34	3%	9%	9%	3%	6%	6%	3%
CLL	87	11%	2%	2%	1%	6%	4%	0
LCL	45	0	4%	4%	6%	10%	2%	2%

[a] The values given are the percentages of positive reactions.
[b] (TDPM) T-depleted peripheral mononuclear; (AML) acute myelogenous leukemia; (ALL) acute lymphoid leukemias and lymphosarcoma-cell leukemias; (CLL) chronic lymphocytic leukemia; (LCL) lymphoblastoid cell lines.

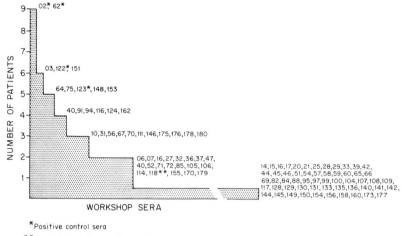

Figure 3. Reactivity of 7th IIIW "Ia" sera with peripheral mononuclear cells from patients with hairy-cell leukemia.

patients along with proper subclassification and "homogenization" of the diseases might ultimately show correlation with HLA antigens.

Acute leukemia cells of both lymphoid and nonlymphoid types carry HLA antigens including Ia-like determinants (Billing *et al.*, 1976a,b; Walford *et al.*, 1977; Kadin and Billing, 1977, 1978). Evidence suggests that Ia-like antigens present on certain less than mature hematopoietic elements may disappear during the process of maturation. For example, segmented granulocytes, platelets, and plasma cells, all end stages of respective maturation sequences, are devoid of surface Ia-like antigens (Drew *et al.*, 1978b; Kadin and Billing, 1978; Halper *et al.*, 1978). At least most of the circulating T lymphocytes also do not express Ia-like antigens, while T cells primed against allogeneic lymphocytes in MLR react with anti-DRw sera in a pattern identical to B cells from the same donor (Suciu-Foca *et al.*, 1978a). Ia determinants are expressed on the hematopoietin-sensitive erythroid precursors and become undetectable during subsequent stages of differentiation (Winchester *et al.*, 1978). The presence of Ia-like antigens on circulating monocytes is well documented (Moraes *et al.*, 1977; Drew *et al.*, 1978a; Stastny, 1978a; Colbaugh and Stastny, 1978; Cicciarelli *et al.*, 1978), but it is not clear whether histiocytes and multinucleated giant cells, which are apparently more mature than monocytes, contain Ia-like antigens. Studies of possible correlation between Ia-like antigens and acute leukemias are few. Billing *et al.* (1976a) reported the absence of group B of Terasaki Ia-like alloantigenic groups from leukemia cells and LCL, but further investigations revealed that reactivities represented by Terasaki B group are due to cold autoantibodies. Our preliminary studies concerning HLA-DRw specificities for AML cells are summarized in Table 4. HLA-DRw2, 5, and 6 were more frequent in TDPM cells from 47 normal individuals than in blast cells from 40 AML patients. However, no significant differences were noted in distribution of HLA-DR antigens among subsets of AML classified as proposed by the French–American–British Group (Bennett *et al.*, 1976). Of the AML patients, 19 had received similar therapy with 6-thioquanine, cytosine arabinoside, and daunomycin. No significant correlation was found between the HLA-DR antigens and remission, duration, or survival time (Naeim *et al.*, 1978d).

9. Ia-like Alloantigens and Nonmalignant-Disease Associations

Experimental proof of involvement of *H-2*-linked antigens in Gross-virus-leukemia susceptibility was first demonstrated by Lilly (1966) and Lilly *et al.* (1964). The responsible gene was called *Rgv-1*. In subsequent studies, *Rgv-1* appeared to be associated with the *Ir-1* loci at the *K* end of the *H-2* complex. Since then, susceptibility to several other viruses has been shown to be linked to *H-2*.

Numerous diseases in man are associated with different alleles of the *HLA* complex. In autoimmune disorders, this association is primarily with alleles of the *B–D,DR* segment of the complex—in short, the area homologous to the *I* region of the *H-2* system.

As part of a multigene family (Hood *et al.*, 1975), the *B–D,DR* segment in *HLA* may represent a chromosomal organization "unit" primarily involved in immune responsiveness and self–nonself recogni-

TABLE 4. Frequency of HLA-DR Antigens for TDPM Cells from 47 Controls and for AML Cells from 40 Patients

HLA-DRw	TDPM cells	AML cells	
1	9%	15%	
2	32%	17.5%	$(P > 0.1)$
3	15%	5%	
4	15%	17.5%	
5	26%	0	$(P < 0.001)$
6	26%	0	$(P < 0.001)$
7	28%	25%	

tion. This view is supported by the demonstration of a significant correlation between HLA-B8, -DRw3, and levels of anti-acetylcholine-receptor antibodies in myasthenia gravis (MG) (Naeim et al., 1978d).

The possibility that MG is an autoimmune disorder was proposed by Smithers (1959), Nastuk et al. (1960), and Simpson (1960). The high rate of thymic abnormalities (Castleman, 1966), the often favorable response to thymectomy, and the association of MG with other autoimmune disease (Simpson, 1960) accord with this view. Patrick and Lindstrom (1973) produced experimental autoimmunity against acetylcholine receptors (AChR) in rabbits. This was characterized by muscular weakness and respiratory insufficiency, which were improved after treatment with anticholinesterase agents. Anti-AChR antibodies have subsequently been demonstrated in the sera of MG patients (Almon et al., 1974; Bender et al., 1975; Appel et al., 1975; Lindstrom et al., 1976).

Although the target in MG appears to be AChR, clinicopathological differences exist among patients with the disease. These differences tend to be associated with different frequencies of HLA antigens in subgroups of MG patients. Young females with hyperplasia of thymic germinal centers show an excessively high prevalence of HLA-B8 (Fritz et al., 1974, 1976; Feltkamp et al., 1974; Priskanen et al., 1972; Priskanen, 1976). In contrast, HLA-B8 is uncommon in older males and in patients with thymoma, who, according to Fritz et al. (1974, 1976), demonstrate a high frequency of HLA-A3 compared with normal controls. Among 82 Caucasoid MG patients studied at the UCLA Medical Center (Keesey et al., unpublished data), the titer of anti-AChR antibodies correlated with sex and distribution of HLA antigens, but not with activity or severity of the disease. Of the 68 nonthymoma patients, 21 (31%) were HLA-B8 (+). Among those with elevated anti-AChR titers, 93% of females and only 20% of males were HLA-B8 (+) ($p < 0.01$). No correlation was found between HLA-B8 and MG in the thymoma group, and the average anti-AChR titer was higher than in the nonthymoma group. Among 23 nonthymoma MG patients typed for HLA-DRw antigens in addition to HLA-A, -B, and -C (Naeim et al., 1978b), the frequency of both HLA-B8 and -DRw3 was significantly higher than normal. Most patients with elevated anti-AChR titers were positive for HLA-B8 or -DRw3, or both, whereas most HLA-B8- and/or -DRw3-negative patients showed antibody titers below average (Table 5). In contrast to these results, Smith et al. (1978) found no correlation between HLA-B8 and titer of AChR antibodies in MG.

The association between autoimmune diseases and Ia-like alloantigens is further supported by the fact that Type 1 (insulin-dependent, juvenile-onset) diabetes mellitus, irrespective of age of onset, shows an increased relative risk of development in subjects who are HLA-DRw3

TABLE 5. Correlation between HLA Antigens and
the Average Serum Anti-AChR Titers of 23 MG
Patients without Thymoma

| HLA | Anti-AChR titer[a] | | χ^2 | P Values |
| | < 28[b] | > 28 | | |
	Number of patients	Number of patients		
B8+	4	6	7.304	< 0.01
B8-	12	1		
DRw3+	2	6	11.507	< 0.001
DRw3-	14	1		

[a] Concentration of 10^{-9} mol receptor bound per liter of serum.
[b] Average titer of anti-AChR in the MG patients without thymoma.

(+), with secondary associations with HLA-A1, -B8, or -B18, and in subjects who are HLA-DRw4 or -Dw4 (+), with secondary associations with HLA-A2, -B15, -B40, and -CW3 (Jeannet et al., 1977; Mayr et al., 1977; Batchelor and Morris, 1978; Cudworth and Festenstein, 1978). The secondary associations are probably due to linkage dysequilibrium among the various HLA loci. Results of the 7th IHW (Batchelor and Morris, 1978) demonstrated that a significant proportion of Type 1 diabetic patients who were positive for pancreatic-islet-cell antibodies typed as HLA-B8, -DRw3 or -DRw4. A study of 110 newly diagnosed diabetic patients (Cudworth and Festenstein, 1978) demonstrated that the HLA-B8-, -15-positive patients had elevated antibody titers to Coxsackie B 1–4 variants compared with HLA-B8- or -15-negative patients. Although HLA-DRw antigens were not reported in that study, the strong dysequilibrium between HLA-B8 and -DRw3 is consistent with the idea that HLA-B-linked "Ia" genes may enhance specific immune responsiveness in diabetic patients.

Associations between Ia-like alloantigens and other diseases with altered immune conditions have also been reported. A high correlation exists between chronic active hepatitis and HLA-B8, -DRw3 (Batchelor and Morris, 1978); patients with Goodpasture's syndrome reveal a high frequency of HLA-DRw2, with a relative risk of 15.9 (Rees et al., 1978). HLA-DRw4 is increased in frequency in adult rheumatoid arthritis (Batchelor and Morris, 1978; Stastny, 1978b), and patients with positive tests for both HLA-DRw4 and rheumatoid factor tend to have a more severe form of the disease (Roitt et al., 1978). The frequencies of HLA-DRw2 and 3 are significantly higher in patients with systemic lupus erythematosus than in controls (Reinertsen *et al.*, 1978; Gibofsky *et al.*, 1978).

There is evidence suggesting *HLA*-linked genetic control of host response to exogenous agents. In leprosy, de Vries *et al.* (1979) demonstrated that HLA-DRw2 may be a genetic marker for susceptibility to the tuberculoid form (in an endemic area in India), whereas HLA-DRw6 correlated with resistance. In individuals whose lymphocytes were tested for lymphocyte transformation to vaccinia virus 3–4 weeks after primary vaccination, de Vries (1979) reported an association of HLA-Cw3 and -DRw4 with low lymphocyte response. Association with HLA-DRw4 was thought to be secondary to linkage dysequilibrium with HLA-Cw3. Coeliac disease, which results from gluten sensitivity, shows increased frequencies of HLA-B8, -DRw3, and -Dw3 (Keuning *et al.*, 1976; Solheim *et al.*, 1976; Mackintosh and Asquith, 1978). Increased frequencies of HLA-B7, -DRw2, and -Dw2 in multiple sclerosis have been reported in Caucasoid populations (Jersild *et al.*, 1972; Naito *et al.*, 1972; Terasaki *et al.*, 1976; Batchelor and Morris, 1978). It has been suggested that multiple sclerosis results from an *HLA*-linked abnormal immune response initially provoked by exogenous agent(s) (Batchelor *et al.*, 1978; Compston *et al.*, 1976; Winchester *et al.*, 1975b).

10. HLA and Cancer: New Considerations

Except for Hodgkin's disease (Amiel, 1967), acute lymphatic leukemia (Walford *et al.*, 1971b), and particularly nasopharyngeal carcinoma (Simons *et al.*, 1975), attempts to find correlation between *HLA* types and human malignancy have been disappointing, especially in view of the known association of *H-2* with leukemia in mice (Lilly, 1966). It might be thought that the association in mice is only with induced, and particularly virally induced, malignancies, but in fact the incidence of various spontaneous malignancies in mice is also highly *H-2*-influenced. In a life-span study of 14 strains of mice congenic at *H-2* and on three different backgrounds, Smith and Walford (1977) noted that within each background, the *H-2* type markedly influenced both incidence and types of malignancies. A portion of their data is shown in Table 6. It is clear that both the strain background and the *H-2* type influence the malignancies. For example, on the BL/10 background (strains 1–7 in Table 6), all strains displayed a high incidence of lymphoma, but some much higher than others. Pulmonary-tumor incidence among strains congenic on the BL/10 background varied from 0 to 18%, and on the A-strain background from 4 to 29%. Other variations are evident from the table. Now, it seems probable that if all strains of mice shown in Table 6 were allowed

TABLE 6. Incidences (%) and Mean Ages of Death (Weeks) from Lymphomas, Hepatomas, and Lung and Mammary Tumors of Male and Female Congenic Mice at the H-2 Chromosomal Region and on Three Different Backgrounds[a]

Strain	H-2 allele	Lymphoma		Hepatoma		Lung tumors		Mammary tumors	
		Male	Female	Male	Female	Male	Female	Male	Female
1. B10.AKM	m	53 (92)	77 (103)	5 (113)	2 (108)	0	4 (119)	0	0
2. B10.BR/Sg	k	35 (103)	33 (125)	2 (141)	2 (159)	14 (131)	7 (139)	0	0
3. B10.PL	u	24 (125)	48 (113)	2 (124)	2 (139)	7 (125)	2 (139)	0	0
4. B10.A/Sg	a	20 (109)	36 (126)	3 (139)	0	18 (139)	7 (133)	0	0
5. B10.D2/n	d	42 (116)	42 (128)	2 (108)	2 (155)	2 (121)	0	0	0
6. C57BL/10	b	29 (127)	36 (108)	2 (132)	0	3 (145)	2 (118)	0	0
7. B10.RIII	r	23 (127)	52 (133)	0	0	10 (141)	2 (143)	0	0
8. A.BY	b	10 (90)	13 (103)	2 (79)	0	10 (105)	4 (125)	0	0
9. A.SW	s	3 (100)	12 (93)	2 (89)	0	18 (100)	9 (113)	0	0
10. A.CA	f	0	6 (117)	14 (105)	4 (95)	29 (96)	22 (108)	0	0
11. A/Wy	a	13 (101)	10 (120)	15 (108)	2 (136)	26 (110)	17 (122)	0	0
12. C3H/HeDi	k	5 (111)	7 (112)	51 (97)	3 (102)	10 (123)	3 (106)	0	43 (88)
13. C3H.JK	j	3 (108)	7 (117)	50 (104)	15 (112)	14 (124)	3 (112)	0	23 (111)
14. C3H.SW	b	3 (141)	8 (118)	38 (108)	7 (120)	0	3 (130)	0	3 (135)

[a] Adapted from Smith and Walford (1977). Incidences of the tumors in percentage are given first, and mean ages of death of tumor-bearing animals in parentheses. All values are rounded to the nearer whole number.

to interbreed freely, producing a randomly outbred strain, and *H-2*/tumor correlations were sought on this outbred strain, the actual or potential *H-2* influence would be quite obscured by the concomitant influence of diverse non-*H-2* genes from the intermingled primary strains. Such a situation in the outbred human species might well exist.

It is also possible, as another alternative, that genes associated with increased susceptibility to cancer may be linked to *HLA* but not show linkage dysequilibrium with known *HLA* factors. We suggest that such genes exist and that they may be concerned with DNA repair efficiency. In the next section, we shall present direct evidence for linkage of some form(s) of DNA repair with the MHC. Suffice it to note here that an increase of *HLA* haploidentity among afflicted siblings has been found in a number of families in which xeroderma pigmentosum was segregating (Giraldo *et al.*, 1977). Furthermore, a suggestion of homozygosity at the *HLA-A* locus has been reported in aplastic anemia and in Fanconi's anemia (Dausset, 1977). Xeroderma pigmentosum and Fanconi's anemia, both of which are characterized by increased rates of malignancy, are well-known examples of diseases with faulty DNA-repair mechanisms. Recent evidence has also suggested that aplastic anemia, which at times eventuates in acute leukemia, may be associated with faulty DNA-repair mechanisms (Morley *et al.*, 1978).

11. Major Histocompatibility Complex, Aging, and DNA Repair

As a critical test of the immunological theory of aging (Walford, 1969), evidence was presented elsewhere that the MHC has a striking influence on the rate of biological aging (Smith and Walford, 1977). This was adduced by comparing mean and 10th-decile survivorship within different sets of mice congenic at *H-2* on three specific backgrounds, specifically BL/10, C3H, and A. Experiments by other workers, conceptually unrelated to the aforementioned work, demonstrated a remarkable correlation between maximum life-span in a number of mammalian species and the rate of DNA-excision repair as measured by unscheduled DNA synthesis (Hart and Setlow, 1974). Beighlie and Teplitz (1975) presented evidence for decreased DNA-excision-repair capacity in systemic lupus erythematosus, and a number of separate groups of investigators, including our own, have reported dysequilibrium of the *HLA* system in relation to this disease (Waters *et al.*, 1971; Nies *et al.*, 1974; Kissmeyer-Nielsen *et al.*, 1975; Ivanyi *et al.*, 1976; Goldberg *et al.*, 1976; Rigby *et al.*, 1978; Gibofsky *et al.*, 1978).

TABLE 7. Unscheduled DNA Synthesis in UV-Irradiated vs. Nonirradiated Lymphocytes from Mice Congenic at *H-2* on Three Backgrounds[a]

Congenic strains	*H-2* allele	Number tested	Ratio of ^{3}H uptake in UV-irrad./nonirrad. cells ($\pm$ S.E.)
C57 BL/10	*b*	8	3.9 ($\pm$ 0.30)
B10. BR	*k*	5	2.2 ($\pm$ 0.17)
B10. AKM	*m*	7	2.7 ($\pm$ 0.15)
C3H/Sw	*b*	7	2.1 ($\pm$ 0.20)
C3H/He	*k*	7	1.7 ($\pm$ 0.15)

[a] Adapted from Walford and Bergmann (1979).

While no direct studies had been reported in which major histocompatibility alleles were specifically known or determined at the same time DNA-excision-repair capacity was estimated, we inferred from the aforementioned studies as well as other information, including that given in the previous section, that genes associated with the MHC might influence DNA-repair mechanisms, and that a relationship might exist among the MHC, maximum life-span potential, and DNA-repair efficiency (Walford, 1979). In a recent investigation (Walford and Bergmann, 1979), we therefore selected long-lived and short-lived strains of mice from among congenics previously studied (Smith and Walford, 1977). DNA-excision-repair capacity was assessed in spleen-cell populations from individual mice of these strains by measuring unscheduled DNA synthesis following ultraviolet radiation and in the presence of hydroxyurea. DNA repair was found to vary significantly in some instances with the *HLA* type of the congenic mice on each particular background (Table 7). This study provided the first direct evidence that genes associated with the MHC influence DNA-excision-repair mechanisms. Preliminary additional studies of repair of bleomycin-induced DNA damage in congenic mice support this evidence. While the matter requires both further confirmation—including segregation analysis of F_2 progeny (in progress)—and detailed insightful investigations at the molecular level, we believe that a linkage association of DNA-repair mechanisms with the MHC does exist and that this may have important implications for both gerontology and cancer research.

ACKNOWLEDGMENT. This research was supported by USPHS Research Grant AI-10088.

References

Abelson, L.D., and Mann, D.L., 1978, Genetic control of B-cell alloantigens: Evidence for gene(s) linked to the HLA-A locus, *Tissue Antigens* **11**:295.

Almon, R.R., Andrew, C.G., and Appel, S.H., 1974, Serum globulin in myasthenia gravis: Inhibition of α-bungarotoxin binding to acetylcholine receptors, *Science* **186**:55.

Amiel, J.L., 1967, Study of the leucocyte phanotypes in Hodgkin's disease, in: *Histocompatibility Testing 1967* (E.S. Curtoni, P.L. Mattinz, and R.M. Tosi, eds.), p. 79, Williams and Wilkins, Baltimore.

Appel, S.H., Almon, R.R., and Levy, N. 1975, Acetylcholine receptor antibodies in myasthenia gravis, *N. Engl. J. Med.* **293**:760.

Arbeit, R.D., Sachs, D.H., Amos, D.B., and Dickler, H.B., 1975, Human lymphocyte alloantigen(s) similar to murine Ir region-associated (Ia) antigens, *J. Immunol.* **115**:1173.

Batchelor, J.R., Compston, A., and McDonald, W.I., 1978, The significance of the association between HLA and multiple sclerosis, *Br. Med. Bull.* **34**:279.

Batchelor, J.R., and Morris, P.J., 1978, HLA and disease, in: *Histocompatibility Testing* (W.F. Bodmer, J.R. Batchelor, J.G. Bodmer, H. Festenstein, and P.J. Morris, eds.), p. 205, Munksgaard, Copenhagen.

Beighlie, D.J., and Teplitz, RL., 1975, Repair of UV damaged DNA in systemic lupus erythematosus, *J. Rheum.* **2**:149.

Benacerraf, B., and Germain, R.N., 1978, The immune response genes of the major histocompatibility complex, *Transplant. Rev.* **38**:70.

Benacerraf, B., and McDevitt, H.O., 1972, The histocompatibility-linked immune response genes, *Science* **175**:273.

Bender, A.N., Ringel, S.P., Engel, W.K., Daniels, M.P., and Zvi, O., 1975, Myasthenia gravis: A serum factor blocking acethylcholine receptors of the human neuromuscular junction, *Lancet* **1**:607.

Bennett, J.M., Catovsky, D., Flandrin, D.M., Galton, D.A.G., Gralnick H.R., and Sultan, C., 1976, Proposals for the classification of the acute leukemias, *Br. J. Haematol.* **33**:451.

Billing, J., Honig, R., Terasaki, P.I., and Peterson, P., 1976a, Leukaemia cells and lymphoblastoid cell lines, *Lancet* **1**:1365.

Billing, R., Rafizadh, B., Drew, I., Hartman, H., Gale, R., and Terasaki, P., 1976b, Human B-lymphocyte antigens expressed by lymphocytic and myelocytic leukemia cells. I. Detection by rabbit antisera, *J. Exp. Med.* **144**:167.

Bodmer, W.F., 1978, Summary and conclusions; Ia serology, in: *Histocompatibility Testing 1977* (J.G. Bodmer, H. Festenstein, and P.J. Morris, eds.), p. 351, Munksgaard, Copenhagen.

Bodmer, W.F., Bodmer, J.G., Cullen, P.R., Dick, H.M., Gelsthorpe, K., Harris, R., Lawler, S.D., McKintosh, P., and Morris, P.J., 1975a, Ia antigens on chronic lymphocytic leukemic lymphocytes? Association between the reactions of VI Workshop sera on CLL and lymphoid line cells, in: *Histocompatibility Testing 1977* (F. Kissmeyer-Nielsen, ed.), p. 685, Munksgaard, Copenhagen.

Bodmer, W.F., Jones, E.A., Young, D., Godfellow, P.N., Bodmer, J.G., Dick, H.M., and Steal, C.M., 1975b, Serology of Human Ia type antigens detected on lymphoid lines: An analysis of the VI Workshop sera, in: *Histocompatibility Testing 1977* (F. Kissmeyer-Nielsen, ed.), p. 677, Munksgaard, Copenhagen.

Broder, S., Edelson, R.L., Lutzner, M.A., Nelson, D.L., MacDermott, R.P., Durm, M.E., and Goldman, C.K., 1976, The Sézary syndrome: A malignant proliferation of helper T-cells, *J. Clin. Invest.* **58**:1297.

Brouet, J.C., Flandrin, G., Sasportes, M., Flandrin, G., Preud'Homme, J.-L., and
Seligmann, M., 1975, Chronic lymphocytic leukemia of T-cell origin: Immunological
and clinical evaluation in 11 patients, *Lancet* **2**:890.

Castleman, B., 1966, The pathology of the thymus gland in myasthenia gravis, *Ann. N.Y.
Acad. Sci.* **135**:496.

Catovsky, D., Galetto, J., Okos, A., Galton, D.A., Wiltshaw, E., and Stathopoulas, G.,
1973, Prolymphocytic leukemia of B and T cell type, *Lancet* **2**:232.

Cicciarelli, J.C., Berkoco, D., Terasaki, P.I., and Shirahama, S., 1978, Studies of HLA-A,
-B,-C, and -D antigens on monocytes, *Transplant. Proc.* **10**:863.

Colbaugh, P., and Stastny P., 1978, Antigens in human monocytes. III. Use of monocytes
in typing for HLA-D related (DR) antigens, *Transplant. Proc.* **10**:871.

Compston, D.A., Batchelor, J.R., and McDonald, W.K., 1976, B-lymphocyte alloantigens
associated with multiple sclerosis, *Lancet* **2**:1261.

Cudworth, A.G., and Festenstein, H., 1978, HLA genetic heterogeneity in diabetes
mellitus, *Br. Med. Bull.* **34**:285.

Dausset, J., 1977, HLA and association with malignancy: A critical view, in: *HLA and
Malignancy* (G.P. Murphy, E. Cohen, J.E. Fitzpatrick, and D. Pressman, eds.), p.
131, Alan R. Liss, New York.

David, C.S., Shreffler, D.S., and Frelinger, J.A., 1973, New lymphocyte antigen system
(Lna) controlled by the Ir region of the mouse H-2 complex, *Proc. Natl. Acad. Sci.
U.S.A.* **70**:2509.

David, C.S., Meo, T., McCormick, J., and Shreffler, D., 1976, Expression of individual Ia
specificities on T and B cells. I. Studies with mitogen-induced blast cells, *J. Exp.
Med.* **143**:218.

Debre, P., Waltenbaugh, C., Dorf, M.E., and Benacerraf, B., 1976, Genetic control of
specific immune suppression. III. Mapping of H-2 complex complementing genes
controlling immune suppression by the random copolymer L-glutamic acid-L-tyrosine
(GT), *J.Exp. Med.* **144**:272.

de Vries, R.R.P. (ed.), 1979, *The HLA System and Infectious Disease,* J.H. Pasmans, The
Hague.

de Vries, R.R.P., Mehra, N.K., Vaidya, M.C., Gupte, M.D., Meera-Khan, P., and van
Rood, J.J., 1979, HLA-linked genetic control of host response to mycobacterium
leprae, in: *The HLA System and Infectious Disease* (R. de Vries, ed.) p. 24, J.H.
Pasmans, The Hague.

DeWolf, W.C., Carroll, P.G., and Yunis, E.J., 1978, Genetic studies of the HLA-DR region
by the primed lymphocyte test, *Transplant. Proc.* **10**:775.

Dick, H.M., Steel, C.M., and Crichton, W.B., 1972, HLA-A typing of cultured peripheral
lymphoblastoid cells, *Tissue Antigens* **2**:85.

Dick, H.M., Steel, C.M., Crichton, W.B., and Hutton, M.M., 1973, Anomalous
reactivity of some HL-A typing sera, in: *Immunobiological Standardization,* International Symposium on Standardization of HL-A Reagents, p. 116, S. Karger,
Basel.

Doherty, P.C., and Zinkernagel, R.M., 1975, A biological role for the major histocompatibility antigens, *Lancet* **1**:1406.

Dorf, M.E., and Unanue, E.R., 1977, Subpopulations of peritoneal macrophages identified
with anti-Ia sera, in: *Ir Genes and Ia Antigens,* Proceedings of the Third Ir Genes
Workshop (H.O. McDevitt, ed.), p. 171, Academic Press, New York.

Drew, S.I., Carter, B.M., Nathanson, D.S., Terasaki, P.I., Naeim, F., and Billing, R.,
1978a, Serological characterization of human monocytes for HLA, B-lymphocyte and
granulocyte antigens, *Tissue Antigens* **11**:385.

Drew, S.I., Carter, B.M., Terasaki, P.I., Naeim, F., Nathanson, D.S., Abromowitz, B., and Gale, R.P., 1978b, Cell surface antigens detected on mature and leukemic granulocytic population by cytotoxicity testing, *Tissue Antigens* 12:75.

Fellous, M., Mortchelewicz, F., Kamoun, M., and Dausset, J., 1975, The use of a lymphoid cell line to define new B lymphocyte specificities, probably controlled by the MHC region, in: *Histocompatibility Testing 1975* (F. Kissmeyer-Nielsen, ed.), p. 708, Munksgaard, Copenhagen. Feltkamp, T.E., van den Berg-Loonen, P.M., Nijenhuis, L.E., Engelfriet, C.P., van Rossum, A.L., van Loghem, J.J., and Oosterhuis, H.J.G.H., 1974, Myasthenia gravis, autoantibodies and HL-A antigens, *Br. Med. J.* 1:131.

Ferrone, S., Reisfeld, R.A., Terasaki, P.I., and Pellegrino, M.A., 1975, The use of cultured human lymphoid cells to detect cytotoxic antibodies to B lymphoid cell antigens, in: *The First HLA Workshop of the Americas* (R.J. DuGuesnoy and T.C. Fuller, eds.), p. 199, DHEW Publ. No. (NIH) 76-1064.

Festenstein, H., 1978, Summary and conclusions: Cellular typing, in: *Histocompatibility Testing 1977* (W.F. Bodmer, J.R. Batchelor, J.G. Bodmer, H. Festenstein, and P.J. Morris, eds.), p. 358, Munksgaard, Copenhagen.

Fradelizi, D., Nuñez-Roldan, A., and Sasportes, M., 1978, Human Ia-like DRw lymphocyte antigens stimulating activity in primary mixed lymphocyte reaction, *Eur. J. Immunol.* 8:88.

Fritz, D., Herrmann, C., Jr., Nacim, F., Smith, G., and Walford, R.L., 1974, HL-A antigens in myasthenia gravis, *Lancet* 1:240.

Fritz, D., Herrmann, C., Jr., Naeim, F., Smith, G., Zeller, E., and Walford, R.L., 1976, The biologic significance of HLA antigen markers in myasthenia gravis, *Ann. N. Y. Acad. Sci.* 274:440.

Gatti, R.A., Cousineau, M., Naeim, F., and Leibold, W., 1979, Suppression of lymphoblastoid cell line proliferation by antisera to HL-DR and other HLA antigens, *Tissue Antigens* 14:213.

Gibofsky, A., Winchester, R.J., Patarroyo, M., Fotino, M., and Kunkel, H.G., 1978, Disease association of the Ia-like human alloantigens; contrasting patterns in rheumatoid arthritis and systemic lupus erythematosus, *J. Exp. Med.* 148:1728.

Giraldo, G., Degos, L., Beth, E., Gharbi, R.M., Day, N.K., Dastot, H., Haus, M., Robonl, M., and Schmid, M., 1977, HLA antigens in 16 families with scleroderma pigmentosum, *Tissue Antigens* 9:167.

Goldberg, M.A., Arnett, F.C., Bias, W.B., and Shulman, L.E., 1976, Histocompatibility antigens in systemic lupus erythematosus, *Arthritis Rheum.* 19:129.

Gossett, T., Walford, R.L., Smith, G.S., Robins, A., and Ferrara, G.B., 1975, The Merrit alloantigenic system of human lymphocytes, in: *Histocompatibility Testing 1975* (F. Kissmeyer-Nielsen, ed.), p. 687, Munksgaard, Copenhagen.

Gossett, T., Walford, R.L., and Gatti, R.A., 1977, Distribution of HLA-A,B,C, and Merrit B-cell alloantigen specificitites in chronic lymphotic leukemia, in: *HLA and Malignancy* (G.P. Murphy, E. Choeh, J.E. Fitzpatrick, and D. Pressman, eds.), p. 55, Alan R. Liss, New York.

Gossett, T., Braun, W.E., Collins, Z., Gatti, R.A., Leibold, W., Naeim, F., Shaw, J.F., Thompson, J.S., Troup, G., and Walford, L., 1978a, B-cell antigens expressed on normal B-lymphocytes, chronic lymphocytic leukemia cells, and lymphoblastoid cell lines, in: *Histocompatibility Testing 1977* (W.F. Bodmer, J.R. Batchelor, J.G. Bodmer, H. Festenstein, and P.J. Morris, eds.), p. 587, Munksgaard, Copenhagen.

Gossett, T., Naeim, F., Zeller, E., and Johns, S., 1978b, Activation of the complement pathway by naturally occurring heteroantibodies in normal rabbit serum: Effect on subpopulations of human lymphoid cells, *Tissue Antigens* 12:330.

Halper, J., Fu, S.M., Wang, R., Winchester, R., and Kunkel, H.G., 1978, Patterns of expression of human "Ia-like" antigens during the terminal stages of B cell development, *J. Immunol.* **120**:1480.

Hämmerling, G.J., Deak, B.D., Mauve, G., Hämmerling, V., and McDevitt, H.O., 1974, B lymphocyte alloantigens controlled by the I region of major histocompatibility complex in mice, *Immunogenetics* **1**:68.

Hämmerling, G.J., Mauve, G., Goldberg, E., and McDevitt, H.O., 1975, Tissue distribution of Ia antigens on spermatozoa, macrophages, and epidermal cells, *J. Immunol* **1**:1.

Hart, R.W., and Setlow, R.B., 1974, Correlation between deoxyribonucleic acid excision repair and lifespan in number of mammalian species, *Proc. Natl. Acad. Sci. U.S.A.* **71**:2169.

Hood, L., Campbell, J.H., and Elgin, S.C.R., 1975, The organization, expression and evolution of antibody genes and other multigen families, in: *Ann. Rev. Genetics,* Vol. 9 (H.L. Roman, ed.), p. 309, Annual Review, Inc., Palo Alto.

Ivanyi, P., Dorstal, C., and Miklas, L., 1976, HLA-B8 in systemic lupus erythematosus, *Tissue Antigens* **8**:91.

Ivanyi, P., Hampl, R., Starka, L., and Mickova, M., 1972, Genetic association between H-2 gene and testosterone metabolism in mice, *Nature (London) New Biol.* **238**:280.

Jeannet, M., Raffour, C., Moeroloose, P. de, Debry, G., Bally, C., Streiff, F., and Sisonenko, P., 1977, HLA and Ia-like antigens in juvenile-onset diabetes, *Tissue Antigens* **10**:196 (abstract).

Jersild, C., Svejgaard, A., and Fog, T., 1972, HL-A antigens and multiple sclerosis, *Lancet* **1**:1240 (letter).

Jones, E.A., Goodfellow, P.N., Bodmer, J.G., and Bodmer, W.F., 1975, Serological identification of HLA linked human "Ia-type" antigens, *Nature (London)* **256**:650.

Kadin, M.E., and Billing, R.J., 1977, Immunofluorescent method for positive identification of null cell type acute lymphocytic leukemias: Use of heterologous antiserum, *Blood* **50**:771.

Kadin, M.E., and Billing, R.J., 1978, B lymphocyte antigens in the differential diagnosis of human neoplasia, *Blood* **51**:813.

Katz, D.H., and Benacerraf, B., 1975, The function and inter-relations of T-cell receptors: Ir genes and other histocompatibility gene products, *Transplant. Rev.* **22**:175.

Kansu, E., and Hauptman, J., 1977, Suppressor cell activity in Sézary syndrome, *Blood* **50**(Suppl. 1):221.

Keuning, J.J., Pena, A.S., van Leeuwen, A., van Hooff, J.P., and van Rood, J.J., 1976, HLA-Dw3 associated with coeliac disease, *Lancet* **1**:506.

Kissmeyer-Nielsen, F., Kjerbye, K.E., Anderson, E., and Halberg, P., 1975, HL-A antigens in systemic lupus erythematosus, *Transplant. Rev.* **22**:164.

Klein, J., 1975, *Biology of the Mouse Histocompatibility-2 Complex,* Springer-Verlag, New York.

Klein, J., Hauptfeld, M., and Hauptfeld, V., 1974, Evidence for a third Ir-associated histocompatibility region in the H-2 complex of the mouse, *Immunogenetics* **1**:45.

Klouda, P.T., and Reeves, B.R., 1975, Serial studies of the reactivity of CLL cells with anti-CLL sera, in: *Histocompatibility Testing 1975* (F. Kissmeyer-Nielson, ed.), p. 697, Munksgaard, Copenhagen.

Lawler, S., and Jones, E.H., 1978, HLA and disease; leukemia, in: *Histocompatibility Testing 1977* (W.F. Bodmer, J.R. Batchelor, J.G. Bodmer, H. Festenstein, and P.J. Morris, eds.), p. 232, Munsgaard, Copenhagen.

Legrand, L., and Dausset, J., 1975a, A second lymphocyte system (Ly-Li), in: *Histocompatibility Testing 1975* (F. Kissmeyer-Nielsen, ed.), p. 665, Munskgaard, Copenhagen.

Legrand, L., and Dausset, J., 1975b, Immunogenetics of a new lymphocyte system, *Transplant. Proc.* **7**(Suppl. 1):5–8.

Lilly, F., 1966, The H-2 locus and susceptibility to tumor induction, *Natl. Cancer Inst. Monogr.* **22**:631.

Lilly, F., Boyse, E.A., and Old, L.J., 1964, Genetic basis of susceptibility to viral leukemogenesis, *Lancet* **2**:1207.

Lindstrom, J.M., Seybold, M.E., Lennon, V.A., Whittingham, S., and Duane, D.D., 1976, Antibody to acetylcholine receptor in myasthenia gravis: Prevalence, clinical correlates and diagnostic value, *Neurology (Minneapolis)* **26**:1054.

Mackintosh, P., and Asquith, P., 1978, HLA and coeliac disease, *Br. Med. Bull.* **34**:291.

Mann, D.L., Abelson, L., Harris, S., and Amos, D.B., 1975a, Detection of antigens specific for B-lymphoid culture cell lines with human alloantisera, *J. Exp. Med.* **142**:84.

Mann, D.L., Abelson, L., Henkart, P., Harris, S.D., and Amos, D.B., 1975b, Specific human B lymphocyte alloantigens linked to HL-A, *Proc. Natl. Acad. Sci. U.S.A.* **72**:5103.

Mann, D.L., Adelson, L., Harris, S., and Amos, D.B., 1976, Second genetic locus in the HL-A region for human B-cell alloantigens, *Nature (London)* **259**:143.

Mayr, W.R., Schernthaner, G., Ludwig, H., Pausch,V., and Dub, E., 1977, Ia type alloantigens in insulin-dependent diabetes mellitus, *Tissue Antigens* **10**:194 (abstract).

McDevitt, H.O., and Tyan, M.L., 1968, Genetic control of the antibody response in inbred mice: Transfer of response by spleen cells and linkage to the major histocompatibility (H-2) locus, *J. Exp. Med.* **128**:1–11.

McDevitt, H.O., Delovitch, T.L., Press, J.L., and Murphy, D.B., 1976, Genetic and functional analysis of the Ia antigens: Their possible role in regulating the immune response, *Transplant. Rev.* **30**:197.

Meredith, P., and Walford, R.L., 1979, Autoimmunity, histocompatibility, and aging, *Mech. Ageing Dev.* **9**:61.

Mickova, M., and Ivanyi, P., 1973, Genetic differences in the manifestation of G-C3H-antigen association with the H-2 system, *Transplant. Proc.* **5**:1421.

Moraes, M.E., Sittler, S., and Stastny, P., 1977, Characterization of cell population used for studies of antibodies to I-region products, *Transplant. Proc* **9**(Suppl.):137.

Morley, A., Seshadri, R., Trainor, K., and Sorrell, J., 1978, Is aplastic anemia due to abnormality of DNA?, *Lancet* **2**:9.

Murphy, D.B., Herzenberg, L.A., Okumura, K., and McDevitt, H.O., 1976, A new subregion (I-J) marked by a locus (Ia-4) controlling surface determinants on suppressor T-lymphocytes, *J. Exp. Med.* **144**:699.

Naeim, F., Gregg, B., Gatti, R.A., Leibold, W., and Walford, R.L., 1977a, Simplification of B-cell antisera of the Merrit system with platelets and lymphoblastoid cell lines, *Transplant. Proc.* **9**:439.

Naeim, F., Leibold, W., Gatti, R.A., and Walford, R.L., 1977b, Reactivity of alloantibodies of the Merrit B-cell system with leukemic cells and lymphoblastoid cell lines, *Transplant. Proc.* **9**(Suppl. 1):151.

Naeim, F., Gatti, R.A., Johnson, C.E., Jr., Gossett, T., and Walford, R.L., 1978a, "Hairy cell" leukemia: A heterogenous chronic lymphoproliferative disorder, *Am. J. Med.* **65**:479.

Naeim, F., Keesey, J.C., Herrmann, C., Jr., Lindstrom, J., Zeller, E., and Walford, R.L., 1978b, Association of HLA-B8, DRw3 and anti-acetylcholine receptor antibodies in myasthenia gravis, *Tissue Antigens* **12**:381.

Naeim, F., Leibold, W., Gatti, R.A., Ferrara, G.B., Johns, S., and Walford, R.L., 1978c, Ia-like segregant series probably distinct from HLA-DRw: A study of lymphoblastoid cell lines and leukemic cells with evidence for a class of cytotoxic antibodies requiring the presence of monocytes, *Transplant. Proc.* **10**:815.

Naeim, F., Zighelboim, J., Foon, K., Gale, R., and Walford, R.L., 1978d, Acute myelogenous leukemia and HLA-DR antigens, *Blood* **52**(Suppl. 1):266.

Naito, S., Namerow, N., Mickey, M.R., and Terasaki, P.I., 1972, Multiple sclerosis: Association with HL-A 3, *Tissue Antigens* **2**:1.

Nastuk, W.L., Plescia, O.J., and Osserman, K.E., 1960, Changes in serum complement activity in patients with myasthenia gravis, *Proc. Soc. Exp. Biol Med.* **105**:177.

Nies, K.M., Brown, J.C., Dubois, E.L., Quismoris, F.P., Fricu, G.J., and Terasaki, P.I., 1974, Histocompatibility (HL-A) antigens and lymphocytotoxic antibodies in systemic lupus erythematosus (SLE), *Arthritis Rheum.* **17**:397.

Park, M.S., Terasaki, P.I., Bernoco, D., and Iwaki, Y., 1978, Evidence for a second B-cell locus separate from the DR locus, *Transplant. Proc.* **10**:823.

Patrick, J., and Lindstrom, J., 1973, Autoimmune response to acetylcholine receptor, *Science* **180**:871.

Pious, D., Bodmer, J., and Bodmer, W., 1974, Antigenic expression and cross reactions in HL-A variants of lymphoid cell lines, *Tissue Antigens* **4**:247.

Priskanen, R., 1976, On the significance of HL-A and LD antigens in myasthenia gravis, *Ann. N. Y. Acad. Sci.* **274**:451.

Priskanen, R., Tillikainen, A., and Hokkanen, E., 1972, Histocompatibility (HL-A) antigens associated with myasthenia gravis, *Ann. Clin. Res.* **4**:304.

Rees, A.D., Peters, D.K., Compston, D.A.S., and Batchelor, J.R., 1978, Strong association between HLA-DRw2 and antibody-mediated Goodpasture's syndrome, *Lancet* **1**:966.

Reinertsen, J.L., Klippel, J.H., Johnson, A.H., Steinberg, A.D., Decker, J.L., and Mann, D.L., 1978, B-lymphocyte alloantigens associated with systemic lupus erythematosus, *N. Engl. J. Med.* **299**:515.

Reinsmoen, N.L., Noreen, H.J., Friend, P.S., Giblett, E.R., Greenberg, L.J., and Kersey, J.H., 1978, Positive mixed lymphocyte culture reactivity between HLA-DR identical siblings, *Transplant. Proc.* **10**:793.

Rigby, R.J., Dawkins, R.L., and Wetherall, J.D., 1978, HLA in systemic lupus erythematosus: Influence on severity, *Tissue Antigens* **12**:255.

Roitt, I.M., Corbett, M., Festenstein, H., Jaraquemada, D., Papasteriadis C., Hay, F.C., and Nineham, L.J., 1978, HLA-DRw4 and prognosis in rheumatoid arthritis, *Lancet* **1**:990.

Sasportes, M., Fradelizi, D., and Dausset, J., 1978, HLA-DR-specific suppressor cells after repeated allogeneic sensitizations of human lymphocytes *in vitro*, *Transplant. Proc.* **10**:905.

Shevach, E.M., 1976, The function of macrophages in antigen recognition by guinea pig T lymphocytes. III. Genetic analysis of the antigens mediating macrophage–T lymphocytes interaction, *J. Immunol.* **5**:1482.

Shevach, E.M., Lundquist, M.L., Geczy, A.F., and Schwartz, B.D., 1977, The guinea pig I region. II. Functional analysis, *J. Exp. Med.* **146**:561.

Shevach, E.M., Rosenthal, D.L., and Green, I., 1973, The distribution of histocompatibility antigens on T and B cells in the guinea pig, *Transplantation* **16**:126.

Simons, M.J., Chan, S.H., Ho, J.H.C., Chau, J.C.W., and Day, N.E., de The G.B., 1975, A Singapore 2-associated LD antigen in Chinese patients with nasopharyngeal carcinoma, in: *Histocompatibility Testing 1975* (F. Kissmeyer-Nielsen, ed.), p. 809, Munksgaard, Copenhagen.

Simpson, J.A., 1960, Myasthenia gravis: A new hypothesis, *Scott. Med. J.* **5**:419.

Smith, C.I.E., Hammarstrom, L., Moller, E., Lefvert, A.K., and Matell, G., 1978, Correlation of HLA-B8 and amount of antibodies directed to acetylcholine receptor protein in patients with myasthenia gravis, *Tissue Antigens* **12**:387.

Smith, G.S., and Walford, R.L., 1977, Influence of the main histocompatibility complex on aging in mice, *Nature (London)* **270**:727.

Smith, G.S., and Walford, R.L., 1978, Influence of the H-2 and H-1 histocompatibility systems upon life-span and spontaneous cancer incidences in congenic mice, in: *Genetic Effects on Aging; Birth Defects, Orig. Artic. Ser.* **14**:281.

Smithers, D.W., 1959, Tumors of the thyroid gland in relation to some general concepts of neoplasia, *J. Facult. Radiol.* **10**:3.

Solheim, B.G., Bratlie, A., Winther, N., and Thorsby, E., 1975, LD typing with antisera produced by planned immunization, in: *Histocompatibility Testing 1975* (F. Kissmeyer-Nielsen, ed.), p. 713, Munksgaard, Copenhagen.

Solheim, B.G., Ek, K., Thune, P.O., Baklein, K., Bratlie, A., Rankin, B., Thoresen, A.B., and Thorsby, E., 1976, HLA antigen in dermatitis herpetiformis and coeliac disease, *Tissue Antigens,* **7**:57.

Sollinger, H.W., and Bach, F.H., 1976, Collaboration between *in vivo* responses to LD and SD antigens of major histocompatibility complex, *Nature (London)* **259**:487.

Stastny, P., 1978a, Antigens in human monocytes. I. Ia antigens detected in monocytes using Seventh Workshop sera, in: *Histocompatibility Testing 1977* (W.F. Bodmer, J.R. Batchelor, J.G. Bodmer, H. Festenstein, and P.J. Morris, eds.), p. 566, Munksgaard, Copenhagen.

Stastny, P., 1978b, Association of the B-cell alloantigen DRw4 with rheumatoid arthritis, *N. Engl. J. Med.* **298**:869.

Suciu-Foca, N., Susinno, E., McKiernan, P. Rohowsky, C., Weiner, J., and Rubinstein, P., 1978a, DRw determinants on human T cells primed against allogeneic lymphocytes, *Transplant. Proc.* **10**:845.

Suciu-Foca, N., Weiner, J., Rohowsky, C., McKiernan, P., Susinno, E., and Rubinstein, P., 1978b, Indication that Dw and DRw determinants are controlled by distinct (but closely linked) genes, *Transplant. Proc.* **10**:799.

Taussing, M.J., Munro, A.J., Campbell, R., David, C.S., and Stains, N., 1975, Antigen specific T cell factor in cell cooperation, mapping with the I region of the H-2 complex and ability to cooperate across antigenic barriers, *J. Exp. Med.* **142**:694.

Terasaki, P., Opelz, G., Park, M.S., and Mickey, M.R., 1975, Four new B lymphocyte specificities, in: *Histocompatibility Testing 1975* (F. Kissmeyer-Nielsen, ed.), p. 713, Munksgaard, Copenhagen.

Terasaki, P.I., Park, M.S., Opelz, G., and Ting, A., 1976, Multiple sclerosis and high incidence of a B lymphocyte antigen, *Science* **193**:1245.

Thompson, J.S., Blaschke, J.W., Severson, C.D., Ferrone, S., and Walford, R.L., 1975, Identification of antisera detecting unique specificities on lymphocytes of the B-type, in: *The First HLA Workshop of the Americas* (R.J. DuGuesnoy and T.C. Fuller, eds.), p. 215, DHEW Publ. No. (NIH) 76-1064.

Thompson, J.S., Braun, W.E., Carpenter, C.B., Dossetor, J.B., Dupont, B., Falk, J.A., Ferrone, S., Johnson, A.U., Shaw, J.F., Signal, D.P., Terasaki, P.I., Troup, G.M., and Walford, R.L., 1977, Report on the Second New World B-cell Workshop, *Transplant. Proc.* **1**(Suppl. 1):9.

Troup, G.M., Jameson, J., Thomsen, M., Svejgaard, A., and Walford, R.L., 1978, Studies of HLA alloantigens of Navajo Indians of North America. I. Variance of association between HLA-DRw (WIA) and HLA-Dw specificities, *Tissue Antigens* **12**:44.

Uchiyama, T., Yodoi, J., Sagawa, K., Takatsuki, K., and Uchino, H., 1977, Adult T-cell leukemia; clinical and hematologic features of 16 cases, *Blood* **50**:481.

van Leeuwen, A., Schuit, H.R.E., and van Rood, J.J., 1973, Typing for MLC (LD) II: The selection of non-stimulator cells by MLC inhibition tests using SD-identical simulator cells (MISIS) and fluorescence antibody studies, *Transplant. Proc.* **5**:1539.

van Leeuwen, A., Winchester, R.J., and van Rood, J.J., 1975, Serotyping for MLC II: Technical aspects, *Ann. N. Y. Acad. Sci.* **254**:289.

van Rood, J.J., and van Leeuwen, A.V., 1963, Leukocyte grouping: A method and its application, *J. Clin. Invest.* **42**:1382.

van Rood, J.J., van Leeuwen, A.V., Keuning, J.J., and van Oud-Aeblas, A.B., 1975a, The serological recognition of the human MLC determinants using a modified cytotoxicity technique, *Tissue Antigens* **5**:73.

van Rood, J.J., van Leeuwen, A., Parlevliet, J., Termijtelen, A., and Keuning, J.J., 1975b, LD typing by serology. IV. Description of a new locus with three alleles, in: *Histocompatibility Testing 1975* (F. Kissmeyer-Nielsen, ed.), p. 629, Munksgaard, Copenhagen.

van Rood, J.J., van Leeuwen, A., Termijtelen, A., and Keuning, J.J., 1976, B-cell antibodies, Ia-like determinants, and their relation to MLC determinants in man, *Transplant. Rev.* **30**:122.

van Rood, J.J., van Leeuwen, A., Keuning, J.J., and Termijtelen, A., 1977, Evidence for two series of B-cell antigens in man and their comparison with HLA-D, *Scand. J. Immunol.* **6**:373.

Walford, R.L., 1969, *The Immunology Therapy of Aging,* Munksgaard, Copenhagen.

Walford, R.L., 1979, Multigene familes, histocompatibility systems, transformation, meiosis, stem cells, and DNA repair, *Mech. Ageing Dev.* **9**:19.

Walford, R.L., and Bergmann, K., 1979, Influence of genes associated with the main histocompatibility complex on deoxyribonucleic acid excision repair in mice, *Tissue Antigens* **14**:336.

Walford, R.L., Smith, G.S., and Waters, H., 1971a, Histocompatibility systems and disease states with particular reference to cancer, *Transplant. Rev.* **7**:78.

Walford, R.L., Zeller, E., Combs, L., and Konrad, P., 1971b, HI-A specificities in acute and chronic lymphatic leukemia, *Transplant. Proc.* **3**:1297.

Walford, R.L., Waters, H.W., Smith, G.S., and Sturgeon, P., 1973, Anomalous reactivity of certain HL-A typing sera with leukemic lymphocytes, *Tissue Antigens* **3**:222.

Walford, R.L., Gossett, T., Smith, G.S., Zeller, E., and Wilkinson, J., 1975, A new alloantigenic system on human lymphocytes, *Tissue Antigens* **5**:196.

Walford, R.L., Gossett, T., Troup, G.M., Gatti, R.A., Mittal, K.K., Robins, A., Ferrara, G.B., and Zeller, E., 1976, The Merrit alloantigenic system of human B lymphocytes: Evidence for thirteen possible factors including one six-member segregant series, *J. Immunol.* **6**:1704.

Walford, R.L., Ferrara, G.B., Gatti, R.A., Leibold, W., Thompson, J.S., Mercuriali, F., Gossett, T., and Naeim, F., 1977, New groups and segregant series among B-cell alloantigens of the Merrit system, *Scand. J. Immunol.* **6**:393.

Waters, H., Konrad, P., and Walford, R.L., 1971, The distribution of HL-A histocompatibility factors and genes in patients with systemic lupus erythematosus, *Tissue Antigens* **1**:68.

Wernet, P., 1976, Human Ia-type alloantigens: Methods of detection, aspects of chemistry and biology, markers for disease states, *Transplant. Rev.* **30**:271.

Wernet, P., Winchester, R.J., Dupont, B., and Kunkel, H.G., 1975, Serological aspects of a human alloantigen system with restricted tissue distribution: The equivalent of the murine Ia-system?, in: *Histocompatibility Testing 1975* (F. Kissmeyer-Nielsen, ed.), p. 637, Munksgaard, Copenhagen.

Winchester, R.J., Dupont, B., Wernet, P., Fu, S.M., Hansen, A., Laursen, N., and Kunkel, H.G., 1975a, Studies on HL-B, a system of non-HL-A alloantigens selectively expressed on B lymphocytes and its relation to LD determinants, in: *Histocompatibility Testing 1975* (F. Kissmeyer-Nielsen, ed.), p. 651, Munksgaard, Copenhagen.

Winchester, R.J., Ebers, G., Fu, S.M., Espinosa, L., Zabriskie, J., and Kunkel, H.G., 1975b, B-cell alloantigen Ag 7a in multiple sclerosis, *Lancet* **2:**814 (letter).

Winchester, R.J., Fu, S.M., Wernet, P., Kunkel, H., Dupont, B., and Jersild, C., 1975c, Recognition by pregnancy serums of non-HL-A alloantigens selectively expressed on B lymphocytes, *J. Exp. Med.* **141:**924.

Winchester, R.J., Meyers, P.A., Broxmeyer, H.E., Wang, C.Y., Moore, M.A.S., and Kunkel, H.G., 1978, Inhibition of human erythropoietic colony formation in culture by treatment with Ia antisera, *J. Exp. Med.* **148:**613.

13

The Enigma of Good Kidney-Graft Survival in the Face of Poor *HLA* Matches

HLA Matching for Kidney Transplantation Makes Sense

J.J. van Rood, G.G. Persijn, E. Goulmy, and B.A. Bradley

1. Introduction

One of the few facts all those involved in kidney allografting agreed on almost from the beginning is that matching for the HLA system plays an overriding role when donor and recipient are siblings. It was one of the fundamental observations that identified the HLA system as the major histocompatibility complex (MHC).

Although the HLA system is extremely complex, its polymorphism can be considered finite. This implies that unrelated individuals exist who share one or two *HLA* haplotypes. In the parent–child combination, matching for the unrelated haplotype was shown to improve kidney-graft survival (van Rood *et al.,* 1967). On the basis of this observation, it was suggested that to overcome the difficulty of finding good matches between unrelated individuals, a large pool of patients awaiting kidney transplantation should be created (van Rood, 1967). Whenever a kidney donor becomes available, the best-matched recipient is selected from the pool.

Although this proposal, which led to unique international and inter-

J.J. van Rood, E. Goulmy, and B.A. Bradley ● Department of Immunohaematology, University Medical Center, Leiden, The Netherlands.   G.G. Persijn ● Eurotransplant Foundation, University Medical Center, Leiden, The Netherlands.

center medical collaboration, was received well, it took ten years before the consensus was reached that *HLA* matching was helpful in the unrelated donor–recipient combinations (*Transplantation Proceedings,* 1977). In retrospect, this delay can be explained by the following considerations:

1. Many of the early studies had, because of the extreme polymorphism of *HLA,* far too few "good" matches—i.e., *HLA-A-* and -*B-* identical matches—to allow for a meaningful interpretation of the data.
2. The influence of linkage dysequilibrium was insufficiently taken into account in most studies.
3. In the unrelated donor–recipient combination, where complete *HLA* identity is rare, if it occurs at all, helper or suppressor mechanisms, or both, can be activated that make a simplistic interpretation of the number of *HLA-A* and -*B* mismatches redundant.

That *HLA-A* and -*B* matching does improve kidney allografting is illustrated by Fig. 1, which presents the results obtained in the organ-exchange organization Eurotransplant in the period 1972–1977 and concerns over 3000 first cadaveric transplants (Persijn *et al.,* 1979). The data show that 5 years after transplantation, grafts with no *HLA-A* and -*B* mismatches do over 15% better than grafts mismatched for three or four antigens. The difference is statistically significant from 6 months post-transplant onward and meaningful both for the patient and in the context of the cost–benefit aspects of the treatment of end-stage renal failure.

Two further points can be deduced from Fig. 1 as well. The first is that about one third of the transplants fail within the first 3–6 months after transplantation, and the second is that although the grafts mismatched for three or four *HLA-A* and -*B* antigens do on the average less well tban those that were better matched, some of these three- to four-antigen-mismatched grafts do quite well even after 5 years. In other words, even a good *HLA-A* and -*B* match is no guarantee of good function, and by contrast, good graft function can occur vis-à-vis a very poor *HLA* match. It is both of great theoretical importance and of great practical importance to understand the mechanism by which these mismatched grafts are able to survive.

Recently, several variables have been identified that apart from *HLA-A* and -*B* matching *per se* are able to significantly influence kidney graft survival. We will discuss three of these. Blood transfusion and *HLA-DR* matching have a graft-protecting effect, while incompatibility for MHC-restricted and MHC-nonrestricted non-HLA antigens can impair graft survival.

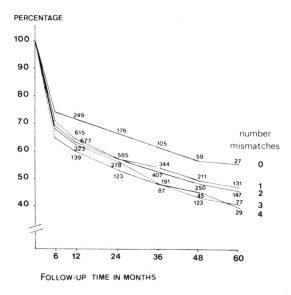

Figure 1. Kidney-graft survival of over 3000 consecutive transplants performed in collaboration with the Eurotransplant organ-exchange organization. Note that after 6 months, there is an 8% difference, and after 60 months a 15% difference, between the best- and poorest-matched grafts. From Persijn *et al.* (1979).

2. Blood Transfusion

Opelz *et al.* (1973) were the first to present significant evidence not only that blood transfusion can cause immunization, which endangers graft survival, but also that it can prolong graft survival. Their observation has been confirmed by most workers, including our own group (Persijn *et al.*, 1977). Furthermore, a randomized prospective study in rhesus monkeys that received five blood transfusions over a 3-month period prior to transplantation and standard immunosuppression after transplantation showed a significant fourfold prolongation of graft survival (Fig. 2) (van Es *et al.*, 1977).

In Leiden, a retrospective study by van Hooff *et al.* (1976) showed that patients who had received one blood transfusion appeared to do better than patients who had received none. Next, Persijn *et al.* (1979) evaluated the role of the number of blood transfusions in kidney-graft survival in 895 patients who had received a kidney transplant between January 1, 1967, and March 1, 1977. The transfusion history was checked by scrutinizing the relevant documents (e.g., medical history, blood bank files, hemodialysis reports) and by personal interviews with the patients or their relatives or both. For female patients, the number of pregnancies

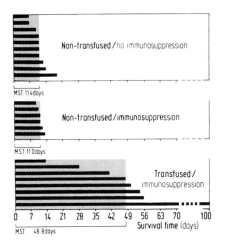

Figure 2. Influence of blood transfusion on kidney-allograft survival in unrelated rhesus monkeys. Solid black bars depict individual survival times; shaded areas indicate the mean survival time (M.S.T.) per experimental group. Immunosuppression consisted of azathioprine (4 mg/kg) and prednisolone (2 mg/kg), given on alternate days. Five blood transfusions were given at biweekly intervals. Transplantation was performed 11–23 days after the last transfusion. From van Es et al. (1977).

and abortions was recorded. In this way, these authors found 68 male and 6 female patients who had never been transfused or been pregnant before transplantation. None of them had preformed leukocyte antibodies in their serum. Similarly, 27 male and 3 never-pregnant female patients were identified who had received only a single blood transfusion, a third of them 1 year or more before transplantation. Some of these patients remembered the exact date of transfusion, and this was checked and confirmed in the blood bank records. None of these patients had detectable antileukocyte antibodies in their sera. The composition of the transfusate (e.g., whole blood, washed erythrocytes, filtered blood) was not taken into account because accurate information on this was not available. All patients in this analysis, except one patient in the nontransfused group, had received blood transfusions during transplantation varying from 1 to more than 5 units. As can be seen in Fig. 3, the patients who had received one blood transfusion did extremely well (80% graft survival at 6 months after transplantation), while those who had received no blood transfusion did very poorly indeed.

On the basis of these findings, a prospective trial was started in Holland in which it was planned to compare the graft-protecting effect of one pretransplant transfusion of leukocyte-poor blood with three such transfusions. The precise way in which the blood was to be prepared was not specified. Most centers gave "washed" leukocyte-poor blood, but a few used cotton-wool-filtered blood, which for all practical purposes is leukocyte-free (Diepenhorst et al., 1972). As is shown in Fig. 3, this prospective study confirmed the retrospective study with respect to the graft-protecting effect of one transfusion of leukocyte-poor blood. In contrast, the patients transfused with cotton-wool-filtered leukocyte-free

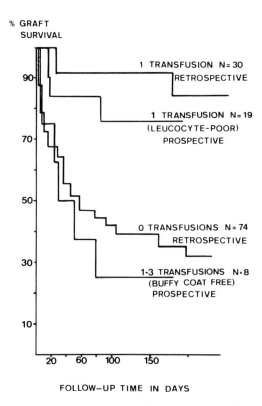

Figure 3. Graft survival in relation to a single pretransplant blood transfusion. Only transfusions of leukocyte-poor blood had a graft-protecting effect. From Persijn *et al.* (1978).

blood did as poorly as the nontransfused patients. We conclude from these data that a small amount of buffycoat cells given once before transplantation induces significant graft protection and that buffycoat-free erythrocytes will not do so. Others have suggested that peroperative blood transfusions without preoperative ones can cause graft facilitation (Stiller *et al.*, 1978). During the last two years, almost all peroperative blood transfusions to the patients shown in Fig. 3 have been leukocyte-free. However, before that date, leukocyte-poor blood was often given. Its effect on graft survival is under study. Because of the very poor overall graft survival in the group of patients who received no blood transfusions before transplantation, it appears unlikely to us that peroperative blood transfusions with leukocyte-poor blood are as effective as preoperative ones.

On two points, our findings are at variance with those of others.

First, although almost all authors agree that patients who had received pretransplant blood transfusions do better than those who did not, most centers find that graft survival in the nontransfused group is not 20–30% as we observed (Fig. 3), but 40–60% at 1 year (Morris *et al.*, 1978; Opelz and Terasaki, 1978). We have no good explanation for this discrepancy. Inadequate inventorying of the blood-transfusion history might be an explanation for some but not for all studies. The poorer graft survival in our nontransfused-patient group is unlikely to be due to poorer *HLA* matches as compared to the other studies. This discrepancy thus focuses our attention on yet another unknown variable determining the outcome of kidney transplantation.

Second, another discrepancy lies in the number of blood transfusions given. Although some centers (Morris, personal communication) have confirmed our finding that one blood transfusion protects graft survival, others have not (Opelz and Terasaki, 1978). This is another unexplained discrepancy. Preliminary findings from our group suggest that one blood transfusion is especially effective in the group of patients who received a one-DR-antigen-mismatched graft (see below). Because Opelz's patient material is racially more heterogeneous than the Dutch material, this observation might be relevant.

The mechanism by which blood transfusion protects graft survival is unknown. In all probability, this mechanism is different when many blood transfusions have been given as compared to the situation in which only one or a few were given. Many blood transfusions will induce cytotoxic HLA antibodies in many patients. Those who do not form cytotoxic HLA-A and -B antibodies are so-called "nonresponders." Graft survival in this group is known to be good. The term nonresponder is a misnomer, because these patients do form antibodies (anti-HLA-DR or other) that might be enhancing (Iwaki *et al.*, 1978; Thompson *et al.*, 1976). Those who have formed cytotoxic anti-HLA antibodies will receive kidneys from donors who lack the corresponding antigens. It is assumed but not proven that such recipients cannot easily form immunity against other HLA antigens, and thus incompatibility for these will not influence graft survival.

This selection phenomenon cannot play a role when only one blood transfusion has been given because in such cases, no antibodies or only weak antibodies in only a few recipients are formed. Whether the improved graft survival is due to the induction of suppressor cells, broad-reacting enhancing antibodies, or another mechanism is as yet unclear.

In conclusion, almost everybody agrees that blood transfusion can improve graft survival, but there is no agreement on the optimal number of blood transfusions to be given, the time interval between blood transfusion and transplantation, or even the way in which the blood should be prepared.

3. *HLA-DR* Matching

Almost from the beginning of clinical kidney allografting, evidence has been accumulating that indicated that a low or negative mixed-lymphocyte culture (MLC) test was indicative for good transplant prognosis. This was in itself an important impetus to develop methods of typing the HLA-D determinants, which are the strongest stimulus in the MLC test (*Transplantation Proceedings,* 1977). The methods all used the basic MLC test or variants of it. However, because the MLC test is so time-consuming, it is suitable only for selection of living donor–recipient pairs.

Thus, a method was developed that would allow rapid identification of *HLA-D*-identical donor–recipient pairs and that could be applied to cadaveric donors. A systematic search for antibodies that could recognize the HLA-D determinants was begun. This effort was successful, and antibodies were identified that allowed the recognition of HLA-D antigens or determinants closely linked to them (Fig. 4) (van Rood *et al.,* 1978). The main topic of the 7th Histocompatibility Workshop was the recognition of these so-called "HLA-DR determinants" (*Histocompatibility Testing 1977*).

To assess the importance of *HLA-DR* matching in kidney transplantation, *DR* typing was performed on peripheral-blood cells of the recipient and frozen spleen cells from the corresponding kidney donor (Persijn *et al.,* 1978). Figure 5A shows the influence of *DR* matching alone and Fig. 5B the influence of *DR* matching combined with (partial) matching for the HLA-A and -B antigens. Although the numbers are small and this is a retrospective study, the study strongly suggests that (1) even matching for one HLA-DR determinant can significantly reduce early graft loss (cf. Fig. 1); and (2) matching for HLA-DR combined with partial matching for the HLA-A and -B antigens might further improve prognosis; and (3) matching for both DR antigens appears to result in good graft survival as well, but here the numbers are too small for meaningful conclusions.

Other groups have done similar studies. A summary of the total of the published European data is presented in Table 1 (Ting and Morris, 1978; Martins-da-Silva *et al.,* 1978; Albrechtsen *et al.,* 1978). It is clear that although the number of *HLA-DR*-identical grafts is small, they give the highest percentage of functioning grafts in all series, and that the

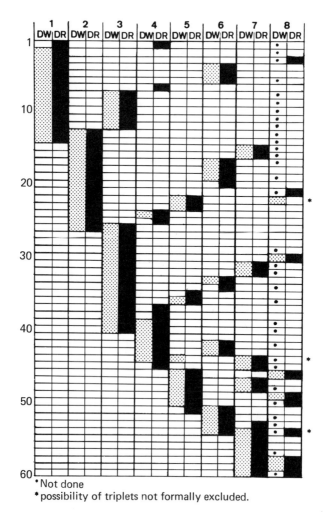

* Not done
** possibility of triplets not formally excluded.

Figure 4. Results of testing of lymphocytes of 60 unrelated donors by homozygous typing cells (HTC) and primed-lymphocyte typing (PLT) recognizing the HLA-D specificities HLA-Dw1–8. Positive results are indicated by the stippled bars. The same panel was tested by sera recognizing HLA-DRw1–7 and HLA-WIA8. Positive results are indicated by the hatched bars. Note the excellent agreement of the results obtained with cellular (HTC and PLT) and serological (*HLA-DR* serology) techniques for determinants 1, 2, 3, and 7. The number of possible triplets is only one for HLA-DR, suggesting that HLA-DR determinants might be coded for by one locus.

percentage of functioning grafts in the two-DR-antigens-mismatched group is the lowest. Problems arise with the one-DR-antigen-mismatched group because it is often unclear from publications of others whether these include potential incompatibilities or not (e.g., an HLA-DRwl/− donor transplanted onto an HLA-DRwl/2 recipient). With this restriction, the available data show that in the majority of transplants performed in Europe, matching for two and also for one HLA-DR antigen improves graft survival significantly. The improvement by matching for two HLA-DR determinants was expected because earlier studies had shown that a low or negative MLC test between parent–child or unrelated donor–recipient pairs improved graft survival (Jeannet, 1970; Hamburger *et al.*, 1971; Cochrum *et al.*, 1973). Although not all *HLA-D*- or -*DR*-identical combinations lead to a negative or low MLC test, the majority do

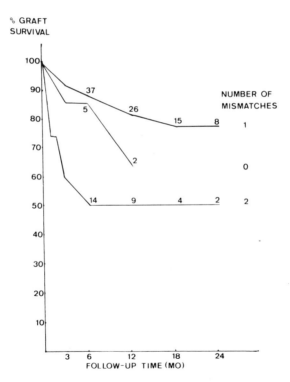

Figure 5A. Kidney-graft survival and matching for HLA-DR antigens alone. The top curve represents grafts with one mismatch at the *DR* locus; the middle curve, *DR*-identical grafts; the bottom curve, grafts with two mismatches at the *DR* locus. The figures above the curves are the numbers of grafts at risk.

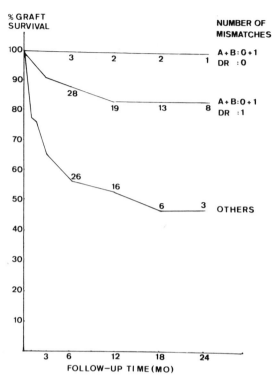

Figure 5B. Kidney-graft survival and matching for HLA-A, -B, and -DR antigens. The top curve represents *DR*-identical grafts with one or fewer mismatches at the *A* or *B* locus; the middle curve, grafts with one or fewer mismatches at the *A* or *B* locus and one mismatch at *DR;* the bottom curve, other grafts. From Persijn *et al.* (1978).

TABLE 1. DR Matching in Europe[a]

Source	Zero DR mismatches	One DR mismatch	Two DR mismatches
	Grafts (functional[b]/total)		
Eurotransplant	6/7	37/42	18/30
Geneva	0/0	22/25	12/23
Oslo	2/2	15/24	14/31
Oxford	4/4	32/40	27/40
TOTALS:	12/13	106/131	71/124
	92%	81%	57%
	$p = 0.60$	$p = 0.0002$	

[a] For references, see van Rood *et al.* (1979).
[b] At 6 months after transplantation.

(Termijtelen *et al.*, 1977), and this could explain the good results in the *HLA-DR*-identical group.

On the other hand, combinations that are mismatched for one HLA-DR determinant are always MLC-positive. Why is it then that grafts mismatched for one HLA-DR antigen do so well? From the point of immunogenetics, this is of course heresy: a difference of an antigen between donor and recipient has always been considered to be dominant over sharing an antigen, and the first question we have to answer is whether our observation that a one-DR-mismatched graft does so well is correct.

Corroboratory evidence was obtained from a study by van Hooff *et al.* (1974), who had already shown that matching between unrelated individuals for an HLA-A and -B antigen combination in strong linkage dysequilibrium with an HLA-DR determinant, such as the HLA-A1,B8,DRw3 combination, was associated with an improved graft survival. The percentage of graft survival exceeded that obtained for the overall survival in patients who were matched for two HLA-A and -B antigens that were not in linkage dysequilibrium. Thus, in this situation, donor and recipient were also matched, although indirectly, for one DR antigen (and mismatched for the other), and this was associated with better graft survival. There also exists corroborating evidence that one-DR-mismatched grafts do well in the parent–child data. They do much better than those differing by two DR antigens; in fact, in Holland they do as well as *HLA*-identical siblings (Persijn, unpublished observations). Others have made similar observations (Thompson *et al.*, 1977a; Oliver *et al.*, 1972; Fotino and Allen, 1972; Cochrum *et al.*, 1973; Belzer *et al.*, 1974; Dausset *et al.*, 1974; Dausset and Hors, personal communications; Hors *et al.*, 1974; Stenzel *et al.*, 1974; Festenstein *et al.*, 1976).

These observations reinforce our finding that matching for only one DR determinant can significantly improve graft survival. It is also clear that the data available are limited and in part retrospective and that prospective trials are indicated. This will be one of the main topics in the forthcoming 8th Histocompatibility Workshop. This is especially urgent because data from Los Angeles (Terasaki) and more recently from European studies have failed to show a significant improvement of graft survival in the one-DR-antigen-mismatched group. We cannot yet exclude, of course, the possibility that it is not *DR* we should match for but another closely linked locus, e.g., *HLA-D*. Interracial transplants will be very useful in evaluating this (Troup *et al.*, 1978).

It should be stressed that with the exception of two individuals, all the recipients in this study who received a kidney mismatched for one DR determinant had been transfused. Although this might be an important prerequisite, conflicting data exist on this point. Swedish workers found that graft survival in parent–child combinations was good only if the recipient had been transfused before transplantation (Brynger *et al.*, 1977). The Dutch data are consistent with this, although a control group of nontransfused recipients is lacking. By contrast, Solheim *et al.* (1977) and Opelz and Terasaki (1978) did not find a graft-protecting effect of blood transfusions in parent–child combinations, and furthermore Morris claims that the beneficial effect of *DR* matching is most clear in the nontransfused group (Morris, personal communications).

In an attempt to clarify the mechanism by which matching for one or two DR determinants overrides the effect of incompatibility for other antigens, we investigated whether these findings on *DR* matching and graft survival had an *in vitro* correlate. Both MLC tests and cell-mediated lymphocytotoxicity (CML) tests (after *in vitro* priming) were studied. Lymphocytes were taken from patients 3–18 months *after* transplantation, and these were reacted with the splenocytes from their specific kidney donor, which had been stored in liquid nitrogen. The lymphocytes of slightly more than half the patients who had functioning grafts had a negative CML test, while they were reactive with lymphocytes from random donors. We could actually show that the CML test changed from positive before transplantation to negative after transplantation (Fig. 6).

Our findings show striking similarity to observations of Thomas *et al.* (1977), who studied CML reactivity in parent–child combinations, and of Wonigeit and Pichlmayr (1977), who studied cadaveric-kidney-transplant recipients. The new data from these longitudinal studies presented here show that the increment of percentage kill against donor as measured in CML can be negative a few weeks and not many years after transplantation. In other words, a decreasing CML may be associated with good survival and an increasing CML with poor survival.

Although our preliminary studies suggested that CML nonreactivity occurred most frequently in the one-DR-mismatched group, our recent, more extensive, data have failed to confirm this. In other words, CML nonreactivity and *DR* matching appear not to be significantly associated.

In summary, the current picture emerges as follows:

1. Matching, for two and for one DR determinant improves graft survival to about 80% at 1 year. It should be stressed that almost three fourths of our patients were grafted with a kidney that carried zero or one *HLA-A* or *-B* mismatch only. Our data suggest that *DR* matching reinforces but does not replace *HLA-A* and *-B* matching.
2. A fall in donor-specific CML develops in at least half the patients following transplantation. The origin of this phenomenon is under study.

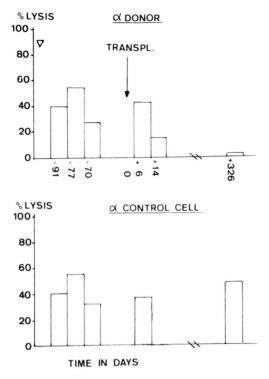

Figure 6. Longitudinal CML study after a planned blood transfusion (▽) and kidney transplantation. *Top:* CML reactivity against the specific kidney donor; *bottom:* percentage lysis against a control cell. The follow-up time in days is on the abscissa.

4. Incompatibility for Non-HLA Determinants

Incompatibilities for determinants outside *HLA* will influence graft survival as well. The first example of this was the deleterious effect of ABO-blood-group incompatibility on graft survival (Starzl *et al.,* 1964). More recently, French workers have noticed that kidneys transplanted in Lewis-blood-group-negative recipients have a poorer prognosis than Lewis-positive recipients, presumably because of incompatibility for the Lewis system (Oriol *et al.,* 1978). This observation could explain why grafts from Caucasoid donors, who have a high frequency of Lewis-positive individuals, do so poorly if transplanted in patients of negroid descent, who are often Lewis-negative.

Very little attention has so far been paid to cell- or tissue-line-specific systems outside that of the HLA-DR antigens. However, Moraes and Stastny (1977) have identified a multiallelic system that occurs on both endothelial cells and monocytes (Table 2). Paul *et al.* (1979) and Claas *et al.* (1979) have independently identified similar antibodies and have shown that these play in all probability an important role in rejection of both kidneys (Table 3) and bone-marrow grafts (Table 4). Little is yet known of the precise conditions under which these antibodies can be formed, but they can arise after repeated transfusions or kidney-graft rejection, or both. It is also uncertain whether the locus or loci coding for the determinants recognized by them lie in or near the *HLA* complex, but Thompson *et al.* (1977b) have identified a polymorphic locus not linked to *HLA* coding for determinants on monocytes, endothelial cells, and neutrophils. Now that the technical difficulties originally met in the recognition of the monocyte antigens have been solved and their clinical relevance has been established, it will not take long before a more complete description of the system will be possible.

Another point that has to be taken into account is that of MHC restriction, which is dealt with more fully in Chapter 3. In brief, MHC restriction implies that incompatibility for a non-MHC determinant will be recognized by the recipient only if donor and recipient share at least part of the HLA-A and -B determinants. To describe this, the term "dual recognition" was coined, by which is meant that both the non-MHC determinant and the self HLA-A or -B antigens have to be recognized on the target cell (Zinkernagel and Doherty, 1974; Shearer, 1974). The dual-recognition phenomenon was first described in the mouse, but it has also been shown to exist in man. The non-MHC determinants concern both intrinsic determinants such as H-Y and extrinsic or acquired antigens such as those of choriomeningitis or influenza virus.

MHC-restricted immunity against H-Y has been shown in the mouse

TABLE 2. Presence of E Antigens in Endothelial (E) Cells and in Adherent Cells from Peripheral Blood[a]

Sera tested	Results of cytotoxicity tests		
	E cells	Adherent monocytes	Nonadherent lymphocytes
Experiment 1			
G.B.	50	60	10
R.G.	70	80	10
W.W.	60	40	10
C.S.	75	80	10
E.W.	90	70	10
V.S.	80	65	10

[a] From Moraes and Stastny (1977).

TABLE 3. Incidence of Circulating
Endothelial Antibodies (CEAb) in 97
Consecutive Allograft Recipients[a]

	CEAb	
Clinical results	Present	Absent
Irreversible vascular rejection in less than 50 days	7	5
Graft survival for more than 50 days	2[b]	74
Nonimmunological failure	0	9
	9	88

[a] Adapted from Paul *et al.* (1979). Two patients are excluded, one because of ABO incompatibility and another because donor kidney tissue was not available.
[b] CEAb present during rejection episodes.

skin-graft model to be a transplantation barrier of medium strength (von Boehmer *et al.*, 1977; Hurme *et al.*, 1978). In man, it has been shown that MHC-restricted anti-H-Y immunity can occur *in vivo* and *in vitro* using an indirect CML assay. It is of interest that so far MHC restriction has been found only for the HLA-A2 and -B7 antigens, which belong to the most immunogenic antigens of the *HLA* system. That this *HLA*-restricted anti-H-Y immunity is of clinical importance is not definitively proven, but suggestive evidence supporting this notion has been presented for both kidney and bone-marrow allografts (Table 5) (Storb *et al.*, 1977; Goulmy *et al.*, 1978). So far, such information is available only for H-Y in man, but it is likely that this will be true for other non-MHC determinants as well, as has been discussed by one of us (Bradley and

TABLE 4. Correlation between the
Presence of Antimonocyte Antibodies
in the Serum and Rejection of the
Bone-Marrow Graft[a]

		Rejection	
		+	−
Antimonocyte antibodies (TCF)[b]	+	3	2
	−	0	11
		$p = 0.02$	

[a] From Claas *et al.* (1979).
[b] (TCF) Two-color fluorescence.

TABLE 5. Two-year Actuarial Cadaveric-Renal-
Graft Survival in Eurotransplant Patients: Sex and
HLA-A2 Data for Male Donors and Female
Recipients[a]

Leukocyte-antibody-*positive* group			
Donor:	A2-positive	A2-negative	
			T p
Recipient:	A2-positive	A2-negative	
	38%	58%	
			1.96 0.05
	N = 48[b]	N = 50[b]	
Leukocyte-antibody-*negative* group			
	57.9%	61.0%	
			0.24 0.8
	N = 53[b]	N = 53[b]	

[a] From Goulmy *et al.* (1978).
[b] At risk after 2 years.

Festenstein, 1978; Bradley, in prep.). An effect on graft survival of these
non-MHC incompatibilities will be present only if donor and recipient
share at least some of the HLA-A or -B determinants. In other words, if
donor and recipient share none of the HLA-A or -B determinants, the
effect of these determinants might be negligible. This could explain why
grafts mismatched for three or four HLA-A and -B antigens sometimes
do relatively well. These individuals, although mismatched for HLA-A
and -B, would suffer no adverse effect from non-HLA incompatibilities
if these show MHC restriction. In contrast, recipients of grafts well
matched for HLA-A and -B would recognize most of the HLA-A- or -B-
restricted minor histocompatibility antigens.

All this concerns dual recognition in which a non-MHC and an
MHC determinant participate. There is, however, no reason to exclude
the possibility that dual recognition could also exist between two different
classes of MHC determinants. A good case in point is the targets of the
CML reaction in *HLA,* the so-called "CD determinants." Preliminary
studies indicate that these are closely associated with the HLA-A and -
B determinants but not identical to them (Fig. 7). That this is indeed a
case of *HLA-B* restriction is suggested by the fact that not a single
positive reaction was found if neither Bw35 nor Bw53 was present. We
assume that to recognize these CD determinants, either Bw35 or Bw53
must be present. The MHC-restricted non-HLA determinants have been
named by Bradley the histocompatibility-associated membrane or (HAM)
minor antigens; the MHC-restricted HLA determinants, the HAM major
antigens (Bradley and Festenstein, 1978).

We have discussed the role of dual recognition in connection with

	HLA antigens		Cytotoxic effector cells	
Panel	Bw53	Bw35	Anti-S1	Anti-S2
1	−	+	43	−2
2	−	+	42	−2
3	−	+	46	
4	−	+	46	0
5	−	+	43	−1
6	−	+	43	−2
7	−	+	8	7
8	−	+	57	2
9	−	+	41	0
10	−	+	34	2
11	−	+	31	2
12	−	+	41	1
13	−	+	40	2
14	−	+	43	1
15	−	+	37	1
16	−	+	39	−2
17	−	+	50	5
18	−	+	48	0
19	−	+	46	1
20	−	+	20	35
21	−	+	50	23
22	−	+	1	19
23	−	+	2	15
24	−	+	7	28
25	−	+	3	22
26	+	+	27	3
27	+	+	45	1
28	+	−	24	2
29	+	−	21	3
30–70	−		0–9	0–5

Figure 7. Non-HLA-B CML killing. Cytotoxic effector cells (anti-S1 and anti-S2) were raised *in vitro* between siblings of one family. It was expected that these cells would react with Bw35-positive individuals. It turned out that they did so only in part. The donors carrying the determinants recognized by anti-S1 and anti-S2 were always Bw35- and/or Bw53-positive, but the patterns of reactivity obtained with the cytotoxic cells were not identical with the serologically recognized Bw35 and Bw53 or any other HLA antigen. The lymphocytes of donors who were negative for the Bw35 and/or Bw53 antigens were not lysed.

the HAM minor and major antigens so far only in relation to the effector phase of the homograft response. That is the only part for which some limited evidence is available.

MHC-restricted immunity against non-HLA and HLA determinants does not occur spontaneously; in other words, it must be induced *in vivo.* Almost no systematic information is available on the conditions under which MHC-restricted immunity can arise, but it is assumed that this stimulus must be strong; i.e., it will occur only after many blood transfusions or graft rejection, or both. In practice, this means that MHC-restricted immunity will arise only when the recipient is repeatedly challenged with MHC and non-MHC incompatibilities, in which the MHC incompatibilities provide "help" for the recognition of the non-MHC incompatibilities.

5. Discussion and Conclusions

We certainly have not been able to give an all-encompassing answer to the question why some poorly matched kidneys survive so well, but we have made a preliminary inventorying of the different factors other than *HLA-A* and *-B* matching that (might) influence graft survival.

In our opinion, blood transfusion is one of the prime variables. Even after a single pretransplant blood transfusion, the homograft reaction seems to be significantly weakened. The mechanism by which this occurs is unclear, but could be due to the induction of an (aspecific?) suppressor cell (Thomas *et al.*, 1977) or to the activation of cell clones that are capable of forming enhancing antibodies, or to both. On first sight, it might seem improbable that a single blood transfusion would be capable of inducing antibodies that would be able to enhance the survival of kidney grafts from almost any donor. Immunization against the determinants of a single locus, e.g., *HLA-DR,* is incompatible with the induction of such broad-reactive enhancing antibodies (van Rood *et al.,* 1979). However, if we take the MLC inhibition test as an *in vitro* analogue of *in vivo* enhancement, then a possible explanation offers itself (Albert, personal communication; Bach, personal communication). Jonker and van Rood (1978) and Albrechtsen *et al.* (1977) have shown that not only anti-DR but also anti-HLA-A and -B antibodies can inhibit the MLC reaction. The question then becomes what the chance is that a blood-transfusion donor will differ for one of the HLA-A, -B, -C, or -DR antigens with the recipient, while sharing it with the kidney donor. Assuming that cross-reacting antigens can be counted as one, then it can be calculated that in about 75% of the recipients of one blood transfusion, the blood-transfusion donor will share a cross-reacting HLA-A, -B, or -DR antigen with the kidney donor, while this antigen is absent in the recipient. This percentage of "enhanced" grafts can be added to the 20–30% of the grafts that do well even if no blood transfusion is given and would then result in the high percentage of well-functioning grafts we have indeed found. This hypothesis is open to experimental proof, because one would expect that such antibodies would be detectable. We have not been able to demonstrate their presence with the complement-dependent cytotoxicity test, but because more sensitive test systems have not yet been tried, their existence cannot be formally excluded.

If only one blood transfusion is given, we assume, but again have no hard data to evidence, that immunization against MHC-dependent or independent non-HLA antigens will not frequently occur. There are as yet insufficient data to assess the importance of (partial) matching for *HLA-DR* in the nontransfused patient or after only one blood transfusion.

If, on the other hand, many blood transfusions have been given before transplantation, immunity against HLA and non-HLA determinants will often ensue, and depending on the match of donor and recipient, this will influence graft survival. In our patient material, partial matching for *HLA-DR* improves graft survival significantly in this group of patients. CML nonreactivity can develop in a period of weeks posttransplantation independently of the *DR* match. This CML nonreactivity might be due to the induction of suppressor cells or clonal inactivation or both.

Many of the still-existing discrepancies might disappear if full characterization of the antibodies formed after blood transfusion were carried out routinely. This can be quite difficult and is certainly not possible if only a standard complement-dependent cytotoxicity test is used. It is depressing to come to the conclusion that more than 20 years after it was shown that non-complement-binding antibodies can cause enhancement instead of graft rejection, almost all centers study their patients' sera only with complement-dependent cytotoxicity assays. A complete analysis of the methods that should be used to detect antibodies in the sera of transplant recipients and to determine their specificity has yet to be made. Such an analysis will, apart from the technical problems, also be hindered by our incomplete knowledge of the immunogenetics of the *HLA* and especially the non-*HLA* systems. A beginning of the inventorying of the non-*HLA* systems that are relevant in kidney transplantation and the way they exert their influence has been made. It should be stressed that it is so far only a beginning.

ACKNOWLEDGMENTS. The authors would like to thank Professor John S. Thompson for his critical reading. This research was in part supported by the Dutch Organization for Health Research (TNO) and the Dutch Foundation for Medical Research (FUNGO), which is subsidized by the Dutch Foundation for the Advancement of Pure Research (ZWO); the J.A. Cohen Institute for Radiopathology and Radiation Protection (IRS); and the Dutch Kidney Foundation.

References

Albrechtsen, D., Solheim, B.G., and Thorsby, E., 1977, Antiserum inhibition of the mixed lymphocyte culture (MLC) interaction: Inhibitory effect of antibodies reactive with HLA-D associated determinants, Cell. Immunol. 25:258.

Albrechtsen, D., Flatmark, A., Jervell, J., Solheim, G., and Thorsby, E., 1978, HLA-DR antigen matching in cadaver renal transplantation, Lancet 1:825.

Belzer, F.O., Perkins, H.A., Fortmann, J.L., Kountz, S.L., Salvaterro, O., Cochrum, K.C., and Payne, R., 1974, Is HL-A typing of clinical significance in cadaver renal transplantation?, Lancet 1:774.

Bradley, B.A., and Festenstein, H., 1978, Cellular typing, Br. Med. Bull. 34:223.

Brynger, H., Frisk, B., Ahlmén, J., Blohmé, I., and Sandberg, L., 1977. Blood transfusion and primary graft survival in male recipients, Scand. J. Urol. Nephrol. Suppl. 42:76.

Claas, F.H.J., van Rood, J.J., Warren, R.P., Weiden, P.L., Su., P.J., and Storb, R., 1979, The detection of non-HLA antibodies and their possible role in bone marrow graft rejection, Transplant. Proc. 11:423.

Cochrum, K., Perkins, H.A., Payne, R.O., Kountz, S., and Belzer, F., 1973, The correlation of MLC with graft survival, Transplant. Proc. 5:391.

Dausset, J., Hors, J., Busson, M., Festenstein, H., Oliver, R.T.D., Paris, A.M.I., and Sachs, J.A., 1974, A joint analysis performed by France-Transplant and the London Transplant group, N. Engl. J. Med. 290:979.

Diepenhorst, P., Sprokholt, R., and Prins, H.K., 1972, Removal of leukocytes from whole blood and erythrocyte suspensions by filtration through cotton-wool. I. Filtration technique, Vox Sang. 23:308.

Festenstein, H., Sachs, J.A., and Paris, A.M.I., 1976, Influence of HLA matching and blood transfusion on outcome of 502 London Transplant group renal-graft recipients, Lancet 1:157.

Fotino, M., and Allen, F.H., 1972, A shared HL-A haplotype seems to make a cadaver donor satisfactory for kidney transplantation, Vox Sang. 22:309.

Goulmy, E., Bradley, B.A., Lansbergen, Q., and van Rood, J.J., 1978, The importance of H-Y incompatibility in human organ transplantation, Transplantation 25:315.

Hamburger, J., Crosnier, J., Descamps, B., and Rowinska, D., 1971, The value of present methods used for the selection of organ donors, Transplant. Proc. 3:260.

Histocompatibility Testing 1977 (W.F. Bodmer et al., eds.), 1978, Munksgaard, Copenhagen.

Hors, J., Busson, M., and Dausset, J., 1974, Rôle des incompatibilités HL-A et de la pre-immunisation en transplantation rénale, in: Proceedings of the 5th International Course on Transplantation, Lyon, 1973 (J.P. Revillard, ed.), pp. 19–30, Simep-Editions, Villeurbanne.

Hurme, M., Hetherington, C.M., Chandler, P.R., and Simpson, E., 1978, Cytotoxic T-cell responses to H-Y: Mapping of the Ir genes, J. Exp. Med. 147:758.

Iwaki, Y., Terasaki, P.I., Park, M.S., and Billing, R., 1978, Enhancement of human kidney allografts by cold B-lymphocyte cytotoxins, Lancet 1:1228.

Jeannet, M., 1970, Histocompatibility testing using leukocyte typing and mixed lymphocyte culture in kidney transplants, Helv. Med. Acta 35:168.

Jonker, M., and van Rood, J.J., 1978, Can anti-HLA-A and -B antigens inhibit the MLC test?, Tissue Antigens 11:251.

Martins-da-Silva, B., Vassalli, P., and Jeannet, M., 1978, Matching renal grafts, Lancet 1:1047 (letter to the editor).

Moraes, J.R., and Stastny, P., 1977, A new antigen system expressed in human endothelial cells, J. Clin. Invest. 60:449.

Morris, P.J., Bishop, M., Fellows, G., Ledingham, J.G., Ting, A., Oliver, D., Cullen, P., French, M., Smith, J.C., and Williams, K., 1978, Results from a new renal transplantation unit, *Lancet* **2**:1353.

Oliver, R.T.D., Sachs, J.A., Festenstein, H., Pegrum, G.D., and Moorhead, J.F., 1972, Influence of HL-A matching antigenic strength and immune responsiveness on the outcome of 349 cadaver renal grafts, *Lancet* **2**:381.

Opelz, G., and Terasaki, P.I., 1978, Improvement of kidney-graft survival with increased numbers of blood transfusions, *N. Engl. J. Med.* **299**:799.

Opelz, G., Sengar, D.P., Mickey, M.R., and Terasaki, P.I., 1973, Effect of blood transfusions on subsequent kidney transplants, *Transplant. Proc.* **5**:253.

Oriol, R., Cartron, J., Yvart, J., Bedrossian, J., Duboust, A., Bariety, J., Gluckman, J.C., and Gagnadoux, M.F., 1978, The Lewis system: New histocompatibility antigens in renal transplantation, *Lancet* **1**:574.

Paul, L.C., van Es, L.A., van Leeuwen, A., van Rood, J.J., de Graeff, J., and Brutel de la Rivière, G., 1979, Antibodies directed against antigens on the endothelium of peritubular capillaries in patients rejecting renal allografts, *Transplantation* **27**:175.

Persijn, G.G., van Hooff, J.P., Kalff, M.W., Lansbergen, Q., and van Rood, J.J., 1977, Effect of blood transfusion and HLA matching on renal transplantation in the Netherlands, *Transplant. Proc.* **9**:503.

Persijn, G.G., Gabb, B.W., van Leeuwen, A., Nagtegaal, A., Hoogeboom, J., and van Rood, J.J., 1978, Matching for HLA antigens of A, B and DR loci in renal transplantation by Eurotransplant, *Lancet* **1**:1278.

Persijn, G.G., Cohen, B., and van Rood, J.J., 1979, Eurotransplant: Improved graft survival through HLA-A, -B and -DR matching and prospective blood transfusion policy, *Dialysis Transplant.* **8**:493.

Shearer, G.M., 1974, Cell-mediated cytotoxicity to trinitrophenyl-modified syngeneic lymphocytes, *Eur. J. Immunol.* **4**:527.

Solheim, B., Flatmark, A., Jervell, J., and Arnesen, E., 1977, Influence of blood transfusions on kidney transplant and uremic patient survival, *Scand. J. Urol. Nephrol. Suppl.* **42**:65.

Starzl, T.E., Marchioro, T.L., Hermann, G., Brittain, R.S., and Waddell, W.R., 1964, Renal homografts in patients with major donor–recipient blood group incompatibilities, *Surgery* **55**:195.

Stenzel, K.H., Shitsell, J.C., Cheigh, J.S., Riggio, R.R., Stubenborg, W.T., Sullivan, J.F., Rubin, A.L., and Fotino, M., 1974, Effects of HL-A matching and immune responsiveness on cadaver kidney graft survival, *Transplant. Proc.* **6**:89.

Stiller, C.R., Sinclair, N.R., Sheppard, R.R., Lockwood, B.L., Ulan, R.A., Sharpe, J.A., and Hayman, P., 1978, Beneficial effect of operation-day blood transfusions on human renal-allograft survival, *Lancet* **1**:169.

Storb, R., Prentice, R.L., and Thomas, E.D., 1977, Treatment of aplastic anemia by marrow transplantation from HLA identical siblings: Prognostic factors associated with graft-versus-host disease and survival, *J. Clin. Invest.* **59**:625.

Termijtelen, A., Bradley, B.A., and van Rood, J.J., 1977, The influence of HLA-A and -B associated gene products on typing for HLA-D by the HTC and PLT methods, *Tissue Antigens* **10**:161.

Thomas, J., Thomas, F., and Lee, H.M., 1977, Why do HLA-nonidentical renal allografts survive 10 years or more?, *Transplant. Proc.* **9**:85.

Thompson, J.S., Jackson, D., Greazel, N.A., Parmely, M.J., and Severson, C.D., 1976, Antileukocyte antibody in postpartum and renal transplant subjects: A comparison of capillary agglutination and lymphocytotoxicity reactions, *Transplantation* **21**:85.

Thompson, J.S., Corry, R.J., Lawton, R.L., Bonney, W.W., and Kaloyanides, G.J., 1977a,

Effect of prospective HLA-haplotype matching on renal transplantation, *Transplant. Proc.* **9**:205.

Thompson, J.S., Severson, C.D., Greazel, N.A., and Ferrone, S., 1977b, Detection of HLA (Ia) and non-HLA specificities by "B-cell" antisera, *Transplant. Proc.* **9**:597.

Ting, A., and Morris, P.J., 1978, Matching for B-cell antigens of the HLA-DR series in cadaver renal transplantation, *Lancet* **1**:575.

Transplantation Proceedings, 1977, Vol. 9.

Troup, G.M., Jameson, J., Thomsen, M., Svejgaard, A., and Walford, R.L., 1978, Studies of HLA alloantigens of the Navajo Indians of North America. I. Variance of association between HLA-DRw (WIA) and HLA-DW specificities, *Tissue Antigens* **12**:44.

van Es, A.A., Marquet, R.L., van Rood, J.J., Kalff, M.W., and Balner, H., 1977, Blood transfusions induce prolonged kidney allograft survival in rhesus monkeys, *Lancet* **1**:506.

van Hooff, J.P., Hendriks, G.F.J., Schippers, H.M.A., and van Rood, J.J., 1974, The influence of possible HL-A haploidentity on renal graft survival in Eurotransplant, *Lancet* **1**:1130.

van Hooff, J.P., Kalff, M.W., van Poelgeest, A.E., Persijn, G.G., and van Rood, J.J., 1976, Blood transfusions and kidney transplantation, *Transplantation* **22**:306.

van Rood, J.J., 1967, A proposal for international cooperation in organ transplantation: Eurotransplant, in: *Histocompatibility Testing 1967* (E.S. Curtoni, P.L. Mattiuz, and R.M. Tosi, eds.), pp. 451–458, Munksgaard, Copenhagen.

van Rood, J.J., van Leeuwen, A., and Bruning, J.W., 1967, The relevance of leucocyte antigens for allogenic renal transplantation, *J. Clin. Pathol. Suppl.* **20**:504.

van Rood, J.J., van Leeuwen, A., Termijtelen, A., and Bradley, B.A., 1978, HLA-D rally won by serology, in: *Histocompatibility Testing 1977* (W.F. Bodmer, J.R. Batchelor, J.G. Bodmer, H. Festenstein, and P.J. Morris, eds.), p. 403, Munksgaard, Copenhagen.

van Rood, J.J., Persijn, G.G., van Leeuwen, A., Goulmy, E., and Gabb, B.W., 1979, A new strategy to improve kidney graft survival: The induction of CML non-responsiveness, *Transplant. Proc.* **11**:736.

von Boehmer, H., Fathman, C.G., and Haas, W., 1977, H-2 gene complementation in cytotoxic T cell responses of female against male cells, *Eur. J. Immunol.* **7**:443.

Wonigeit, K., and Pichlmayr, R., 1977, Specific defect in the capability to generate cytotoxic effector cells *in vitro* after organ transplantation in man, *Dialysis Transplant.* **6**:58.

Zinkernagel, R.M., and Doherty, P.C., 1974, Restriction of *in vitro* T cell-mediated cytotoxicity in lymphocytic choriomeningitis within a syngeneic or semiallogeneic system, *Nature (London)* **248**:701.

14

Histocompatibility Antigens and Susceptibility to Disease—Genetic Considerations

Lars P. Ryder, Per Platz, and Arne Svejgaard

1. Introduction

Since the discoveries in 1972 by Russell *et al.* (1972) and Falchuk and Strober (1972) that psoriasis and coeliac disease are strongly associated with certain HLA antigens, it has become clear that the HLA system is involved in the etiology or pathogenesis, or both, of a variety of diseases. These relationships between HLA and disease are of considerable clinical and theoretical importance because they provide new ways for the study of etiology, genetics, and nosology of HLA-related diseases, and in a few cases they may have diagnostic and prognostic implications. One of the most fascinating aspects of this research involves attempts to establish the mechanisms by which HLA confers susceptibility or resistance to disease. Such mechanisms have been dealt with in detail abundantly elsewhere (Dausset and Svejgaard, 1977; McDevitt and Bodmer, 1972; Svejgaard *et al.*, 1977). However, at this time, there have been very few definite explanations established for the HLA–disease associations. Accordingly, in this survey, we shall focus solely on a somewhat more neglected field: the contribution of HLA studies to our knowledge of the genetics of diseases. First, we shall give a general concept of genetic disorders and discuss how studies of genetic markers may help determine the mode of inheritance of disease susceptibility and resistance. Next,

Lars P. Ryder, Per Platz, and Arne Svejgaard • Tissue-Typing Laboratory of the Blood-Grouping Department, State University Hospital (Rigshospitalet), DK-2100 Copenhagen Ø, Denmark.

we shall summarize the present knowledge about HLA and disease associations and finally describe examples that illustrate how this knowledge may guide our interpretation of disease-inheritance patterns.

2. General Considerations

All diseases are genetic in the ultimate sense that gene products are involved in all disease processes in all organ systems, but when discussing the genetic background of a disease, we shall consider as genetic only those disorders in which the genetic variability within the human species plays a role in the variability in the manifestations of that disorder (Roberts, 1970).

Familial clustering has usually been the first observation suggesting a genetic element of a disease, but probably all diseases are influenced by environmental factors, although there are enormous variations, and relatives also share environmental factors. At one end of the spectrum, we have the completely genetic diseases, on which the environment has little effect; i.e., given the genotype, the phenotype will always be expressed. However, even in the case of such diseases, environment or other genes may influence the development of disease.

At the other end of the spectrum we have diseases by which virtually all individuals will be affected if exposed to the proper environmental factor; i.e., any genotype will express the diseased phenotype. Examples are some infectious diseases such as rabies and measles. Again, other environmental factors or the genotype may modify the phenotype, as does malnutrition in measles infections.

The majority of diseases fall between these two extremes, and with a few notorious exceptions, this is also true for the diseases that have been found to be associated with HLA. They usually show familial clustering but no clear mode of inheritance, suggesting that environmental factors are also involved. In general, it may be stated that these not completely genetic disorders are not inherited as such: it is the various degrees of susceptibility and resistance that are inherited.

Simple Mendelian inheritance operates with the classic all-or-none concepts of dominant and recessive expression of genes, which in turn gives rise to the Mendelian segregation ratios in families and the Hardy–Weinberg predictions at the population level (Cavalli-Sforza and Bodmer, 1971; Li, 1961). In our context, let us consider a disease with a simple Mendelian inheritance governed by a disease locus with two alleles d and D. A simple dominant inheritance (let D be the dominant allele) would thus mean that all individuals of the genotypes D/d or D/D, and only these individuals, get the disease, while in the recessive

Mendelian case, all individuals of the genotype d/d, and only these individuals get the disease.

The relative incidences of the disease in different groups of relatives to the propositi have often pointed toward a mode of inheritance: (1) the same relative incidence in parents, siblings, and children is found in the *dominantly* inherited diseases; and (2) a higher incidence in siblings than in both parents and children is suggestive of the *recessive* mode of inheritance.

Only a minority of the more common diseases with a genetic component show a simple Mendelian inheritance, and a wide variety of more and more complex genetic models have been put forward to explain the apparent non-Mendelian inheritance of the remaining diseases.

Some of the models are elaborations of the Mendelian theme, but involve the combined action of Mendelian genes at different loci. This kind of inheritance may be called complex Mendelian as opposed to simple Mendelian inheritance. Other models consider the manifestation of disease as a result of a continuous variable, a liability, exceeding a certain threshold, and the genetic models are formulated to predict the quantitative inheritance of this liability in terms of the combined effects of multiple factors (Cavalli-Sforza and Bodmer, 1971; Falconer, 1965). An obvious difficulty with these models is that the liability is usually not a measurable quantity, but a mathematical abstraction.

If genes at many loci are supposed each to give a small contribution to the determination of the liability, the inheritance is called "polygenic" or "multilocal," while the narrower term "oligogenic" or "pauci-local" is used when only a few loci each exert a major effect (Elston and Rao, 1978). The broader concept "multifactorial" covers involvement of both environmental and genetic factors.

Common to these threshold models is the property that even the knowledge of an individual's genotype at the relevant loci does not tell whether the individual will get the disease, but it may indicate the risk that he will get the disease (which is related to the penetrance of the genotype concerned).

This would also be the situation in the complex Mendelian case if the genotype was known for only a part of the relevant loci, and often the consequences of the two kinds of models are indistinguishable (Smith, 1971). Only studies of the concordance rate between monozygous twins would allow discriminating between the models, because complete concordance should exist only for the Mendelian diseases, whether simple or complex. Noncomplete concordance reflects the involvement of environmental factors.

Despite the generality of these models, they have apparently not contributed decisively to solving the genetics of many common diseases such as diabetes mellitus. This is due partly to insufficient data—a thorough analysis requires large bodies of very complete data on familial segregation and population occurrence of the disease—and partly to computational difficulties. The use of genetic markers, such as blood groups, can in some instances greatly help to reduce both the stringent requirements of the data and the amount of computation needed to obtain insight into the mode of inheritance (Edwards, 1955). The efficiency of the various marker systems varies greatly and increases in general with increasing numbers of alleles and increasing proportions of heterozygotes. This is why the HLA system is for the moment one of the most efficient marker systems, both at the level of the individual *HLA* loci and, for some applications, even more so when considering *HLA* haplotypes. Moreover, the role of the HLA system in many immune responses makes it even a good candidate as a causal factor in diseases with "aberrant" immunity.

In general, it is entirely unknown whether the HLA factors known to be associated with a disease are themselves responsible for the disease susceptibility or whether these known HLA factors show association only because they are controlled by genes in linkage dysequilibrium with other genes controlling as yet unknown factors directly involved in disease susceptibility.

As long as this uncertainty endures, we may view the influence from the HLA system as a risk factor of the disease for each *HLA* genotype. This risk factor must thus take into account both the situation of a disease-susceptibility locus in linkage dysequilibrium with the HLA factors and the conceivable direct disease-disposing action of the HLA factors.

Various approaches have been taken to utilize the efficiency of the HLA markers in studies of the inheritance of disease:

- Association of disease at the population level
- Distribution of HLA phenotypes within patient samples
- Proper formal linkage and segregation analysis on pedigrees
- Distribution of HLA identity among pairs of affected siblings

We shall discuss briefly the information given by each of these methods and their limitations.

2.1. HLA Association at the Population Level

This is generally investigated by HLA typing a random sample of patients with a given diagnosis and concurrently a sample of normal individuals from the same homogeneous background population, i.e., a case-control study. The numbers of individuals positive or negative for the various antigens are counted in the two groups. For each antigen, these figures are compared in a 2×2 contingency table yielding an estimate of the relative risk and a statistical significance. If several independent association studies have been performed, these 2×2 tables for each antigen can be subjected to a combined analysis giving the weighted overall relative risk and the statistical significance of its deviation from unity, and a test can be done on the heterogeneity among the individual 2×2 tables (Woolf, 1955; Haldane, 1956; Ryder and Svejgaard, 1977).

This is, of course, a rather crude way of analyzing such data, but it is often the only practicable way and often the data are given only in this form in publications. Another statistical approach has been proposed (Smouse and Williams, 1978) that in a stepwise procedure provides first a broad test of disease association with the *HLA* complex that, if significant, may be further analyzed to see whether this is due to a single allele. In this method, every individual is scored twice, corresponding to each of the two alleles. Strictly, this requires data on the genotypes of all investigated individuals, but phenotypes can be used if one can assume a negligible null-allele frequency. The method has another drawback in that it is not easily extended to a combined analysis on several case-control studies.

The mere observation of an *HLA* association indicates the existence of a disease-susceptibility *(DS)* locus (or loci) of major effect within the HLA system or in linkage dysequilibrium with the HLA markers, but it does not give information on the actual mode of inheritance: unilocal, pauci-local, or multifactorial; dominant or recessive.

2.2. Distribution of HLA Phenotypes within the Patient Sample

This can provide hints on the mode of inheritance because, as described below, for the one-*DS*-locus model with two alleles, only a completely recessive inheritance of the disease is compatible with a Hardy–Weinberg equilibrium among the patients, irrespective of the penetrance.

When sampling a group of normal individuals from a panmictic population, the distribution of phenotypes follows the Hardy–Weinberg equilibrium: the proportion of individuals with a given phenotype is determined by the probability of ascertaining from the general population individuals of genotypes corresponding to the phenotype (allowing for null-alleles and super-/subtypic relationships). In the general population, the frequency $p(a_i, a_j)$ of a genotype a_i, a_j can be found by little algebraic manipulation from the expression $[p(a_1) + p(a_2) + \ldots]^2$ by identifying the terms involving $p(a_i)$ and $p(a_j)$. This expression is the heart of the Hardy–Weinberg law; in fact, any expected pattern that can be expressed in this form can be said to have a Hardy–Weinberg structure.

When sampling a group of patients with a disease associated with some HLA markers, the expected distribution of *HLA* genotypes depends on the underlying genetic model of the disease susceptibility.

Let us assume the existence of one *DS* locus with two alleles *d* and *D* in linkage dysequilibrium with *HLA*, and let us for simplicity consider only a single *HLA* locus with three alleles a_1, a_2, a_3.

At the *DS* locus, three genotypes are possible: *d/d*, *d/D*, and *D/D*. Each of these occurs with a certain frequency in the population and each has a certain probability of disease (penetrance):

DS genotype	Frequency in population	Penetrance
d/d	$p^2(d)$	f_0
d/D	$2p(d)p(D)$	f_1
D/D	$p^2(D)$	f_2

The frequency, F_D, of disease in the population is thus given by $F_D = f_0 p^2(d) + f_1 2p(d)p(D) + f_2 p^2(D)$, and patients ascertained randomly through their disease are distributed correspondingly with respect to genotypes at the *DS* locus. Each of the three genotypic classes at the *DS* locus can be further partitioned with respect to the HLA-marker genotypes by inserting $p(d) = p(a_1, d) + p(a_2, d) + p(a_3, d)$ and $p(D) = p(a_1, D) + p(a_2, D) + p(a_3, D)$ into the expression for F_D, and the expected genotype proportions at the marker locus are found by isolating the respective terms.

When $f_0 = f_1 = 0$ and $0 < f_2 < 1$ (i.e., complete recessivity with complete or incomplete penetrance), it follows that $F_D = f_1 p^2(D) = f_2[p(a_1,D) + p(a_2,D) + p(a_3,D)]^2$, which implies that in the sample of patients, the Hardy–Weinberg structure will be expected at the marker locus, but the expected proportions will involve the *marker-DS* haplotype frequencies and thus differ from those in the general population due to the linkage dysequilibrium between the *marker* and *DS* alleles.

In the case of any other combination of values for f_0, f_1, f_2, the marker genotypic proportions cannot be expressed in quadratic form and the Hardy–Weinberg structure will not be expected among the patients except for the two trivial cases: (1) if $f_0 = f_1 = f_2$, i.e., no genetic influence by the *DS* locus; and (2) if there is no linkage dysequilibrium between the markers and the *DS* alleles.

The completely recessive hypothesis can be tested by computing the goodness of fit chi-square between the observations and the expected Hardy–Weinberg proportions by standard methods. This test has deficiencies: (1) it is not very efficient because quite large numbers of individuals may be required to obtain a valid test; and (2) deviations from the Hardy–Weinberg expectations may have several causes, e.g., serological pitfalls, population stratification. Thus, it would probably be wise to investigate both a sample of normal controls and the patients simultaneously by identical methods to exclude such systematical errors. Also, if more than one DS gene is involved in the susceptibility, it may become more difficult to distinguish the situation from recessivity.

2.3. Linkage Studies

Studies of linkage between *HLA* and simple Mendelian disorders are very efficient due to the pronounced polymorphism of *HLA*. For such disorders, even families with one affected member may provide information. However, the task of performing a sound analysis of linkage between *HLA* and the *DS* locus for a not completely genetic disease (as are most of the *HLA*-associated diseases) is far from straightforward. The reasons for this may be worth mentioning without going into the theory of linkage analysis, for which the reader is referred to the following references: Cavalli-Sforza and Bodmer (1971), Hill (1975), Lange *et al.* (1976), Ott (1974, 1978), and Smith (1975). An efficient linkage analysis of such diseases requires data on whole families with two or more affected members. This may in itself be a problem for the rare disorders and introduces the possibility of a classic ascertainment bias if the chance of a family's being included in the analysis depends on the number of affected members. The ascertainment bias may be compensated if it is known exactly how this chance is a function of the number of affected members. The validity of the analysis depends on the validity of this correction, but it seems difficult to devise a test of the validity of the correction. One way to overcome the ascertainment bias is to have a complete ascertainment of all affected individuals in a well-defined population.

Another problem arises because a characteristic of the not completely genetic diseases is a reduced (or incomplete) penetrance; i.e., an apparently healthy individual may have the "disease genotype," and this will of course seriously blur the familial pattern, and necessitates complicated mathematical treatment of the data. A related complication occurs for diseases with a variable age of onset: an individual scored as nonaffected at the time of investigation may develop the disease later.

These reservations are especially pertinent when attempts are made to estimate the genetic map distance between the marker *HLA* loci and the supposed *DS* locus.

2.4. Affected Sibpair Method

This method is a less pretentious way of merely demonstrating genetic linkage without estimation of the map distance (Day and Simons, 1976; Thomson and Bodmer, 1977; Suarez, 1978). Simple Mendelian inheritance of the HLA markers predicts (see Table 1) that a pair of sibs have the following probabilities: $p = 1/4$ of sharing no parental *HLA* haplotypes, $p = 1/2$ of sharing exactly one parental haplotype, and $p = 1/4$ of sharing both parental *HLA* haplotypes (i.e., they are *HLA*-identical by descent).

When a sibling sample is ascertained through both being affected by a given disease, deviations from these proportions may occur if a *DS* locus is closely linked to the *HLA*-marker loci. The statistical significance of the deviation can readily be evaluated by a chi-square test.

It might intuitively be seen that for a very low *DS*-allele frequency P_D, all sibpairs affected with a simple recessive disease are expected to be *HLA*-identical *by descent* (due to the extreme polymorphism of *HLA*, it is very rare to see the segregation of two different haplotypes carrying the same set of alleles within one family). Among sibpairs with a simple dominant disease, 50% are expected to be identical and 50% to share one *HLA* haplotype. With increasing P_D, it becomes more and more likely that several different *HLA* haplotypes within the same family carry the *DS* allele and thus give rise to *HLA*-nonidentical affected sibpairs.

Under the assumption of simple inheritance, further information can be gained from such data. It has been shown (James, 1971; Suarez, 1978) that the magnitudes of the proportions in general depend on (1) the gene frequency P_D of the disease allele in the general population and (2) the penetrances (f_0, f_1, f_2) of the three possible genotypes at the *DS* locus (0, 1, or 2 disease alleles present), i.e., the mode of inheritance.

It has been pointed out (James, 1971; Suarez, 1978) that because the *three* proportions depend on *four* factors, it should be possible to find infinitely many combinations of values for the four factors that can completely fit the data (not all solutions may be reasonable, because only parameter values between 0 and 1 are allowed). However, if, for example, a certain mode of inheritance is assumed (i.e., if f_0, f_1, and f_2 are fixed), the expected proportions depend only on P_D, and it will not always be possible to fit the observed values. On the other hand, it can then be tested whether any value of P_D gives an acceptable fit, and the P_D giving the best fit may be found by various methods (by maximum likelihood or almost equivalently by minimizing the chi-square).

Special attention has been focused on two modes of inheritance: completely recessive susceptibility with reduced penetrance and completely dominant susceptibility with reduced penetrance. In the completely recessive model, only individuals homozygous for the disease allele have any risk of disease ($f_0 = f_1 = 0, f_2 > 0$), while the completely dominant model states that individuals carrying one or two disease alleles have *equal* risk of disease and those carrying no disease allele have no risk of disease ($f_0 = 0, f_1 = f_2 > 0$). In both these special cases, the expected proportions are independent of the values of the nonzero penetrances because they cancel out in the expressions for the proportions, which thus depend only on P_D, the gene frequency of the disease allele (Table 1).

This sibpair method can with a little effort be expanded to include sibships of any size.

It should be noted that the above approach will give misleading results if recombinations occur between the HLA markers and the *DS* locus and if the penetrance differs between sexes.

Before leaving this section, we should mention the problem of

TABLE 1. Segregation of *HLA* Haplotypes in Pairs of Affected Sibs[a]

Model	Expected proportion of sibpairs sharing i *HLA* haplotypes[b]		
	$i = 0$	$i = 1$	$i = 2$
No relationship between disease and *HLA*	1	2	1
One *DS* locus with two alleles, closely linked to *HLA*	$1 - \delta_0$	$2 - \delta_1$	$1 + \delta_2$
Completely recessive case	$P_D{}^2$	$2P_D$	1
Completely dominant case	$P_D(4 - 4P_D + P_D{}^2)$	$2 + 2P_D(1 - P_D)$	$2 - P_D$

[a] The deviations δ_i are dependent on: P_D, the gene frequency of the susceptibility allele D; f_0, the risk of being affected for a genotype with no D's; f_1, the risk of being affected for a genotype with one D; f_2, the risk of being affected for a genotype with two D's.

Two simple special cases have been treated: (1) completely recessive susceptibility: $f_0 = f_1 = 0; \ 0 < f_2 \leq 1$; (2) completely dominant susceptibility: $f_0 = 0, \ 0 < f_1 = f_2 \leq 1$. In both these cases, the deviations δ_i from the segregation ratio 1 : 2 : 1 depend exclusively on P_D. For a very rare disease, $P_D \approx 0$, the ratios are the well-known 0 : 0 : 1 [(1) above] and 0 : 1 : 1 [(2) above], while for increasing P_D, the deviations δ_i decrease and become zero for $P_D = 1$.

[b] $\delta_i \geq 0, i = 0,1,2$.

disease heterogeneity, i.e., the phenomenon that apparently identical diseases or conditions may be caused by different genes (genocopies) or solely by environmental factors (phenocopies). If this is the case, the results of family studies should be interpreted with caution because familial cases may not be representative of all cases in the population. However, the *HLA* association may help solve this problem because it can be investigated whether the association is of the same order in familial and in sporadic cases. None of the associations between *HLA* and disease is absolute (for example, about 10% of patients with ankylosing spondylitis do not carry HLA-B27). In the enthusiasm over the associations, the absence of the disease marker in some patients is very often explained by the existence of as yet unknown *HLA* factors. However, one should not forget the possibility that an *HLA*-associated disease perhaps could develop in some patients irrespective of the *HLA* polymorphism.

3. Relationships between *HLA* and Specific Diseases

Table 2 summarizes most of the positive findings from *HLA* and disease studies in Caucasians. The data have been extracted from the third report of the HLA and Disease Registry (Ryder *et al.*, 1979). It appears that a variety of different diseases are associated with various *HLA* antigens. Most of the associations are very highly significant, but a few have *p* values higher than 10^{-5} and may be due to chance deviations. The strengths of the associations, as expressed by the relative risk, vary from zero (no risk) for diabetes in Dw2-positives through 1.2 (slightly increased risk) for Hodgkin's disease in B8-positives to 87.4 for ankylosing spondylitis in B27-positives. The B27 antigen is associated with various arthropathies, but not with rheumatoid arthritis, which shows an increase of HLA-D/DRw4. The HLA-D/DRw3 antigen(s) is associated with a number of diseases, most of which are characterized by some element of "aberrant" immunity, if not autoimmunity. At the time of writing, it is uncertain whether it is the HLA-D/DRw3 antigen itself that confers susceptibility or another still unknown HLA factor that is associated with D/DRw3 in the population. It is of interest to note that some of the D/DRw3-associated diseases are associated with other D factors in Japanese. This might indicate that it is still unknown HLA factors that are more directly involved. In contrast, the B27 associations have been seen in all ethnic groups studied.

In the following sections, we shall give some examples illustrating how relationships between *HLA* and disease may clarify the inheritance of disease. The first two conditions (C2 deficiency and congenital adrenal hyperplasia) were known in advance to be simple Mendelian recessive, but are included for the sake of completeness.

TABLE 2. HLA and Disease Associations in Caucasians[a]

Disease	Antigen	Frequency of antigen (%) Controls	Frequency of antigen (%) Patients	Relative risk	Significance (p)	Number of studies	Number of patients investigated
Arthropathies							
Ankylosing spondylitis	B27	9.4	90	87.4	$< 10^{-10}$	29	2022
Reiter's syndrome	B27	9.4	79	37.0	$< 10^{-10}$	9	341
Reactive arthritis	B27	Increased in *Yersinia*, *Salmonella*, and *Shigella* arthritis.					
Psoriatic arthritis	B27	9.4	29	4.0	$< 10^{-10}$	5	177
	B16	5.9	15	2.8	10^{-3}	3	138
Juvenile arthritis	B27	9.4	32	4.5	$< 10^{-10}$	10	596
Rheumatoid arthritis	Dw4	19.4	50	4.2	$< 10^{-9}$	3	152
	DRw4	28.4	70	5.8	$< 10^{-5}$	1	53
Eye diseases							
Acute anterior uveitis	B27	9.4	52	10.4	$< 10^{-10}$	5	341
Optic neuritis	Dw2	25.8	46	2.4	$< 10^{-3}$	2	103
Skin diseases							
Psoriasis vulgaris	B13	4.4	18	4.8	$< 10^{-10}$	11	836
	B17	8.0	29	4.8	$< 10^{-10}$	11	836
	B37	2.6	11	4.4	$< 10^{-6}$	5	323
	Cw6	33.1	87	13.3	$< 10^{-10}$	1	40
Dermatitis herpetiformis	Dw3	26.3	85	15.4	$< 10^{-10}$	2	61
	DRw3	25	97	56.4	$< 10^{-10}$	1	29
Behcet's disease	B5	10.1	41	6.3	$< 10^{-10}$	7	147
Intestinal diseases							
Coeliac disease	Dw3	26.3	79	10.8	$< 10^{-8}$	2	47

(continued)

TABLE 2. (cont.)

Disease	Antigen	Frequency of antigen (%)		Relative risk	Significance (p)	Number of studies	Number of patients investigated
		Controls	Patients				
Liver diseases							
Chronic autoimmune hepatitis	B8	24.6	75	9.0	$< 10^{-10}$	5	161
	DRw3	19	78	13.9	$< 10^{-6}$	1	18
"Systemic" diseases							
Bürger's disease	B12	24.4	3	0.1	$< 10^{-4}$	2	64
Myasthenia gravis	B8	24.6	57	4.1	$< 10^{-10}$	6	328
Sicca syndrome	Dw3	26.3	78	9.7	$< 10^{-9}$	2	54
Systemic lupus erythematosus	B8	24.6	41	2.1	$< 10^{-10}$	11	554
Hemochromatosis	A3	28.2	76	8.2	$< 10^{-10}$	7	191
	B14	3.8	16	4.7	$< 10^{-10}$	6	156
		Behaves as a recessive trait closely linked to HLA in family studies.					
Endocrine diseases							
Juvenile and/or insulin-dependent diabetes	Dw2	25.8	0	0.0	$< 10^{-6}$	2	115
	Dw3	26.3	44	2.2	$< 10^{-5}$	2	201
	Dw4	19.4	49	4.0	$< 10^{-10}$	2	232
Graves's disease	Dw3	26.3	57	3.7	$< 10^{-9}$	3	126
Idiopathic Addison's disease	Dw3	26.3	69	6.3	$< 10^{-5}$	1	30
Congenital adrenal hyperplasia	B5	10.1	29	3.6	$< 10^{-4}$	2	55
		Close linkage to HLA-B in family studies.					
Neurological diseases							
Multiple sclerosis	Dw2	25.8	59	4.1	$< 10^{-10}$	9	932
Cerebellar ataxia		Perhaps linked to HLA in family studies.					
Manic–depressive disorder	B16	5.9	13	2.3	$< 10^{-4}$	5	313

Disease	Antigen						
Allergy							
Ragweed hay fever	B7	25.8	56	3.6	$< 10^{-3}$	2	65
	Perhaps linked to *HLA* in family studies.						
Infections							
Leprosy	Type of leprosy (lepromatous, tuberculoid) apparently linked to *HLA* in family studies.						
Tuberculosis	B8	20	57	5.1	$< 10^{-6}$	1	46
Recurrent herpes labialis	A1	32.0	56	2.7	$< 10^{-10}$	2	292
Subacute thyroiditis	B35	14.6	70	13.7	$< 10^{-10}$	4	105
Malignant diseases							
Hodgkin's disease	A1	32.0	40	1.4	$< 10^{-10}$	25	2669
	B8	24.6	28	1.2	$< 10^{-4}$	25	2670
Acute lymphatic leukemia	A2	53.3	62	1.4	$< 10^{-6}$	15	1099

[a] The data are from the HLA and Disease Registry (Ryder et al., 1979). The frequencies in controls are mainly from a Danish population sample, but when only one study had been reported, the actual figures are given.

3.1. Complement Factor 2 Deficiency

This is a simple Mendelian recessive trait (for reviews, see Lachmann and Hobart, 1978; Jersild et al., 1977). It is not a disease as such, but merely a condition that may or may not lead to overt diseases such as glomerulonephritis, lupoidlike syndromes, or severe infections. The heterozygous carriers can usually be detected by special laboratory investigations showing decreased levels of complement factor 2 (C2) in their blood. The condition is most easily explained by the existence in the population of a "blank" or amorph $C2^0$ gene that has no detectable gene product. HLA family and population studies have established two important facts: (1) C2 deficiency is closely linked to HLA and (2) there is a strong association between the $C2^0$ gene on the one hand and the HLA-Dw2, B18, and A25 genes on the other, with the strength of association decreasing in the order of HLA genes mentioned. Indeed, it is striking to note that the association between C2 deficiency and Dw2 is one of the strongest associations observed between an HLA factor and a condition even though $C2^0$ and Dw2 are not identical. This illustrates the necessity of caution when attempts are made to extrapolate from the strength of an association to a causative role for a disease-associated factor. In the general population, there is striking linkage dysequilibrium among A25, B18, and Dw2, although this is not a frequent haplotype. It is tempting to speculate that the mutation giving rise to the $C2^0$ gene took place on an A25, B18, Dw2 haplotype and that it has slowly been removed from the A25 and B18 genes by crossing over. It has been calculated that this hypothetical mutation took place about 1700 years ago (Svejgaard and Ryder, 1979).

3.2. Congenital Adrenal Hyperplasia Due to 21-Hydroxylase Deficiency

This is another simple Mendelian recessive condition closely linked to HLA (Dupont et al., 1977). It may appear as in utero virilization in girls, while boys are often not diagnosed until a later age. After the discovery of the HLA linkage, it has become possible to identify heterozygous carriers of the 21-hydroxylase-deficiency gene among the relatives of the patients by means of HLA typing, and this has been confirmed by biochemical investigations. The HLA linkage opens the possibility of antenatal "diagnosis," but it should be stressed that HLA typing of amniotic cells is not an easy task.

Congenital adrenal hyperplasia provides a good example of genocopies because this condition may also be due to lack of other enzymes, e.g., 11-hydroxylase, the gene for which has been shown not to be closely linked to HLA.

3.3. Idiopathic Hemochromatosis

Although this condition is also a clearly metabolic disorder—characterized by excess absorption and deposits of iron—its inheritance is not a simple one: both autosomal recessive and dominant modes of inheritance with incomplete penetrance have been suggested. Genetic studies have been complicated by the varying, often late, onset of the disease. The first *HLA* studies of unrelated patients showed a striking association with HLA-A3 and a less pronounced association with B14. These two antigens are not associated in the general population. Patients show no pronounced increase of *A3* homozygosity, which would favor a recessive inheritance. Nevertheless, *HLA* typing of affected sibpairs revealed a striking excess of *HLA*-identical pairs, indicating recessivity (Simon *et al.*, 1977). Kravitz *et al.* (1979) studied in an elegant linkage analysis a large pedigree with many relatives suffering from idiopathic hemochromatosis and concluded that this condition is a recessive disorder closely linked to *HLA*. This is in accordance with a very close fit to the Hardy–Weinberg structure at *HLA-A* and *-B* loci in a series of 198 unrelated patients (R. Fauchet, personal communication).

3.4. Ankylosing Spondylitis

With this disorder, we move into the group of diseases that are characterized not only by unclear modes of inheritance but also by largely unknown etiologies. Emery and Lawrence (1977) performed family studies and found that the polygenic hypothesis would best explain their findings. Nevertheless, this disease is so strongly associated with HLA-B27 that one is tempted to assume that one *HLA* gene is of major effect in relation to this disorder. The mere observation that almost all B27-positive patients with ankylosing spondylitis are B27-heterozygous suggested that the *HLA*-linked susceptibility is inherited as a dominant trait. Further strong support for this assumption was obtained by Thomson and Bodmer (1977) and by Kidd *et al.* (1977). Thomson and Bodmer (1977) tested the proportion among B27-homozygous, B27-heterozygous, and B27-negative patients and could reject the possibility of a recessive mode of inheritance. Kidd *et al.* (1977) came to the same conclusion on the basis of a similar analysis of their own data. Moreover, Kidd *et al.* (1977) studied the frequency of ankylosing spondylitis in B27-positive individuals drawn from the general population and in B27-positive relatives of probands, which enabled them to provide an estimate for the frequency of the *HLA*-linked "disease-susceptibility" *(DS)* gene of about 0.022, and for the *B27,DS* haplotype of 0.020. As pointed out by these authors, the majority of individuals carrying the *DS* allele do not develop ankylosing spondylitis, and this incomplete penetrance may be due to environmental factors or to epistasis with an allele at an independent locus. Kidd *et al.* (1977) also mention the possibility of disease heterogeneity.

3.5. Insulin-Dependent Diabetes

The inheritance of diabetes mellitus has occupied geneticists for many years without a solution being reached. The first contribution of HLA studies to this problem came from population studies that showed that the juvenile- and maturity-onset forms are two distinct entities because only the former shows a strong association with HLA. Both HLA-B8 and -B15 are increased in juvenile—or rather insulin-dependent—diabetes, and by analyzing phenotype data, we found that *B8/15* heterozygotes have about twice the risk of developing this disease that individuals carrying only B8 or B15, whether heterozygous or homozygous, have. We took this as evidence that there are two different *HLA* genes that confer susceptibility to juvenile diabetes, each by its own mechanism, and that they interact to further increase the risk when present together. Later, it was found that the associations with B8 and B15 are secondary to increases of Dw3 and Dw4, respectively. Interestingly, the HLA-Dw2 antigen seems to be totally absent in insulin-dependent diabetes. It has also been shown that *Dw3/4* heterozygotes have a higher risk than individuals carrying either of the corresponding antigens.

Family studies revealed a strikingly high frequency of *HLA* identity among affected sibpairs, and this was taken as evidence that juvenile diabetes is a recessive *HLA*-linked condition with 50% penetrance (Rubinstein *et al.*, 1977). This degree of penetrance has been challenged because concordance data from twin studies generally give smaller estimates (about 35%). By analyzing all available *HLA* data on affected sibpairs, we found that a recessive model is indeed more compatible with the observations than a dominant one (Table 3 and Fig. 1). However, the lowest gene frequency fitting the data is so high (0.20) that the penetrance would have to be rather low (about 5%) to account for the data on population prevalence.

The problem of the inheritance of juvenile-onset diabetes has not yet been solved, but the *HLA* associations have brought us much closer to a solution now. The answer is most probably going to come from additional *HLA-D* and *-DR* studies of more cases without biased ascertainment. There is evidence that the *HLA* associations differ according to the mode of ascertainment and the age at onset, and between familial and nonfamilial cases, suggesting further heterogeneity within the insulin-dependent-diabetes group.

TABLE 3. Segregation of *HLA* Haplotypes in Pairs of Siblings with Juvenile Diabetes

	HLA haplotypes shared			
	0	1	2	
Observed number of sibpairs[a]	5 (4.2%)	44 (37.3%)	69 (58.5%)	
Expected proportions 1. No relationship between disease and *HLA*	29.5 (25%)	59.0 (50%)	29.5 (25%)	$\chi^2 = 77.1$ (2 df, $p < 10^{-15}$)
2. Completely recessive case (for the P_D giving best fit)	6.3 (5.3%)	41.9 (35.5%)	69.8 (59.2%)	$\chi^2 = 0.38$ for $P_D = 0.30$ (1 df, $p > 0.1$)
3. Completely dominant case (for the P_D giving best fit)	4.3 (3.6%)	58.5 (49.6%)	55.2 (46.8%)	$\chi^2 = 7.1$, for $P_D = 0.04$ (1 df, $p < 0.01$)

[a] For references, see Ryder *et al.* (1979).

Note added in proof. A substantial number of insulin-dependent diabetes patients were investigated in the Eighth International Histocompatibility Workshop, and the conclusions reached corroborate the above arguments (Svejgaard *et al.*, 1980).

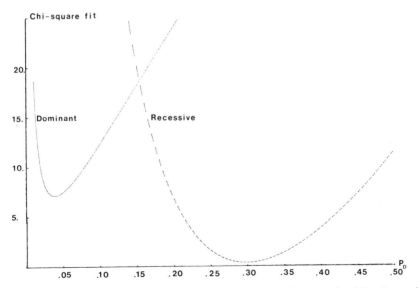

Figure 1. Sibpair analysis in juvenile diabetes. Graph of the chi-square fit of the observed data in Table 3 compared to the expected values (cf. Table 1) for varying gene frequencies (P_D) under the assumption of a dominant and a recessive model. It appears that the dominant model gives a significantly bad fit for all values of P_D, while the recessive model is acceptable for values of P_D between 0.2 and 0.4.

3.6. Multiple Sclerosis and Optic Neuritis

Shortly after the first reports on *HLA* and diseases, three groups (Bertrams *et al.*, 1972; Jersild *et al.*, 1972; Naito *et al.*, 1972) independently reported an association between HLA-A3 and -B7 and multiple sclerosis (MS), and these results have now been confirmed by many authors (see Ryder *et al.*, 1979). Later studies have established that the Dw2 antigen shows the strongest association (for a review, see Platz *et al.*, 1979). It has also been observed that the disease progresses significantly faster in Dw2-positive MS patients compared to Dw2-negatives.

These results have once again changed the view on the genetics of MS. Originally, familial occurrence of MS was considered exceptional, but studies in the 1950's showed that the familial prevalence of MS was approximately 20 times higher than that of the general population (Schapira *et al.*, 1963; Mackay and Myrianthopoulos, 1966). Classic genetic studies failed, however, to convincingly establish a genetic element in MS. In particular, twin studies showed no significant difference between the concordance rate in mono- vs. dizygotic twins.

The major contribution of the *HLA* studies in MS has thus been finally to confirm that genetic factors *do* play a role in the pathogenesis of MS. However, several important questions remain to be answered, including (1) what is the mode of inheritance and (2) by what mechanism do these genetic factors operate? To answer the first question, we have to look at family data. As previously stated, familial MS is rare and *HLA* data on familial MS are even more sparse.

There are available, however, some data on sibships with MS (Table 4) that provide evidence based on the sibpair method discussed in Section 2.4. It appears that the frequencies of sibpairs sharing two, one, or null haplotypes are 40.3, 42.6, and 17%, respectively, and these frequencies do not deviate significantly from the expected 25, 50, and 25% distribution. These data thus neither suggest strong linkage with *HLA* nor allow discrimination between modes of inheritance (Fig. 2) and seem to stand in contrast to the strong association with Dw2 found in most populations studied.

How can this apparent discrepancy be explained? Most of the previous hypotheses on the genetics of MS have assumed that we were dealing with a rare *DS* gene that under the influence of unknown environmental factors leads to overt MS. The 17% of *HLA*-nonidentical affected sibpairs speaks against this assumption, but as discussed in Section 2.4, the proportions of affected sibs sharing two, one, or null *HLA* haplotypes change with increasing gene frequency. Figure 2 shows that both a dominant and a recessive model can fit the observations; however, the recessive fits only for very high values of P_D. If we use as

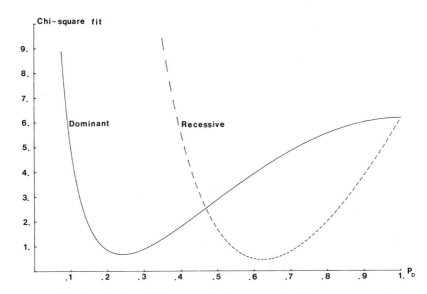

Figure 2. Sibpair analysis in MS (see the Fig. 1 caption). In this case, the analysis cannot discriminate between a dominant and a recessive model.

an example the gene frequency of HLA-Dw2, which in the Danish population is approximately 0.15, the expected proportions for the dominant model of the three different types of sibpairs are very close to those observed (Table 4, expectation 3), while the recessive model is not acceptable.

If further *HLA* family studies in MS confirm the tendency shown in Table 4, an alternative hypothesis could be that the *HLA*-linked MS *DS* gene(s) (HLA-Dw2 or genes linked to Dw2) has a high frequency in the normal population, and that only under certain environmental situations does it give rise to the rare disease MS.

If this hypothesis is true, further understanding may be reached by investigating different immunological functions in Dw2-positive and -negative individuals, both MS patients and normals, to find differences that under certain environmental conditions would allow the MS process to be triggered.

Next, it might be predicted that MS in Dw2-positive individuals differs from MS in Dw2-negative individuals, and the aforementioned differences in the progression of the disease may be a hint in this direction. Another related approach is to study acute monosymptomatic optic neuritis (ON), which often precedes MS by several years. It appears (see Table 2) that Dw2 is increased in ON patients and nearly to the same extent as in MS. Results concerning the prognostic value of Dw2

TABLE 4. Segregation of *HLA* Haplotypes in Pairs of Siblings with Multiple Sclerosis

	HLA haplotypes shared			
	0	1	2	
Observed number of	8	20	19	
sibpairs[a]	(17.0%)	(42.6%)	(40.3%)	
Expected proportions				
1. No relationship between	11.75	23.50	11.75	$\chi^2 = 6.2$
disease and HLA	(25%)	(50%)	(25%)	(2 df, $p = 0.04$)
2. Completely recessive case	7.0	22.3	17.7	$\chi^2 = 0.47$ for $P_D = 0.63$
(for the P_D giving best fit)	(14.9%)	(47.4%)	(37.7%)	(1 df, $p > 0.1$)
3. Completely dominant case	7.2	22.8	17.0	$\chi^2 = 0.67$ for $P_D = 0.24$
(for the P_D giving best fit)	(15.3%)	(48.6%)	(36.1%)	(1 df, $p > 0.1$)
4. Completely recessive case	0.8	10.67	35.53	$\chi^2 = 80.7$
(for $P_D = 0.15$)	(1.7%)	(22.7%)	(75.6%)	(2 df, $p < 10^{-15}$)
5. Completely dominant case	5.2	22.9	18.9	$\chi^2 = 1.9$
(for $P_D = 0.15$)	(11.1%)	(48.8%)	(40.1%)	(2 df, $p = 0.4$)

[a] For references, see Platz *et al.* (1979).

have, however, been conflicting. In one prospective study (Sandberg-Wollheim *et al.*, 1975), an equal number of Dw2-positive and Dw2-negative individuals developed MS in the observation period, whereas a significant correlation between Dw2 and later development of MS was observed in two retrospective studies (Stendahl-Brodin *et al.*, 1978; Compston *et al.*, 1978).

4. Concluding Remarks

The inheritance of diseases in man is a topic that has occupied geneticists for many years. Familial clustering of various disorders has been taken as evidence that genetic factors are involved in the disease processes, but such clustering may also occur because relatives share more environmental factors than do unrelated individuals. In some cases, however, family studies have revealed clear-cut simple Mendelian—recessive or dominant—modes of inheritance, but for most common diseases, this has not been the case, and the concept that these disorders have a genetic element was mainly based on different concordance rates in mono- vs. dizygotic twins. Twin studies are also very informative in estimating the degree of penetrance, but they do not reveal the detailed mode of inheritance. This has now become possible with the discovery that some genetic markers—particularly those of the HLA system—are strongly associated with a variety of diseases. In a few cases, simple

Mendelian disorders (e.g., C2 deficiency and congenital adrenal hyper-plasia) have been shown to be closely linked to *HLA*. Other diseases, not simply inherited diseases (e.g., hemochromatosis and ankylosing spondylitis), that were previously considered "polygenic" have now been found to be based on a genetic background largely dependent on *HLA* factors, although environmental factors must also play a role. In still other cases (e.g., insulin-dependent diabetes), *HLA* factors also appear to play an important role in the disease susceptibility, but the precise mode of inheritance still remains to be clarified. The associations between *HLA* and multiple sclerosis and between *HLA* and rheumatoid arthritis demonstrate for the first time the involvement of genetic factors in the susceptibility to these two disorders, but it seems likely that environmental factors play a larger role.

Thus, it appears that HLA markers provide a powerful tool in clarifying the genetic background of a number of diseases. *HLA* studies are also helpful in sorting out problems of disease heterogeneity, and it should be kept in mind that *HLA*-associated diseases might develop without polymorphic HLA factors being involved.

Finally, the associations are probably going to be very useful in the unraveling of the unknown pathogenetic pathways of the *HLA*-associated disorders, but a major breakthrough in this field has not yet been achieved.

In this context, one of the most promising recent developments has been the emerging picture of the role of the major histocompatibility complex (MHC) in antigen presentation initiated by the discovery of the "MHC restriction" at the level of both the T cell–monocyte cooperation and the cytotoxic-T-cell response. This may lead to fundamental new insight into the biological function of the MHCs in general and of *HLA* in particular and thus into the eventual role of *HLA* itself in the disease processes.

ACKNOWLEDGMENTS. Our thanks are due to Mrs. Christina Törner for excellent secretarial assistance. The HLA and Disease Registry is sup-ported by grants from EEC, the Danish Medical Research Council, and WHO.

References

Bertrams, J., Kuwert, E., and Liedtke, U., 1972, HL-A antigens and multiple sclerosis, *Tissue Antigens* **2**:405.

Cavalli-Sforza, L.L., and Bodmer, W.F., 1971, *The Genetics of Human Populations,* W.H. Freeman, San Francisco.

Compston, D.A.S., Batchelor, J.R., Earl, C.J., and McDonald, W.I., 1978, Factors influencing the risk of multiple sclerosis developing in patients with optic neuritis, *Brain* **101**:495.

Dausset, J., and Svejgaard, A., 1977, *HLA and Disease,* Munksgaard, Copenhagen.

Day, N.E., and Simons, M.J., 1976, Disease susceptibility genes—their identification by multiple case family studies, *Tissue Antigens* **8**:109.

Dupont, B., Oberfield, S.E., Smithwick, E.M., Lee, T.D., and Levine, L.S., 1977, Close genetic linkage between HLA and congenital adrenal hyperplasia (21-hydroxylase deficiency), *Lancet* **2**:1309.

Edwards, J.H., 1955, The meaning of the associations between blood groups and disease, *Ann. Hum. Genet.* **29**:77.

Elston, R.C., and Rao, D.C., 1978, Statistical modeling and analysis in human genetics, *Annu. Rev. Biophys. Bioeng.* **7**:253.

Emery, A.E.H., and Lawrence, J.S., 1977, Genetics of ankylosing spondylitis, *J. Med. Genet.* **4**:239.

Falchuk, Z.M., and Strober, W., 1972, HL-A antigens and adult coeliac disease, *Lancet* **2**:1310.

Falconer, D.S., 1965, The inheritance of liability to certain diseases, estimated from the incidence among relatives, *Ann. Hum. Genet.* **29**:51.

Haldane, J.B.S., 1956, The estimation and significance of the logarithm of a ratio of frequencies, *Ann. Hum. Genet.* **20**:309.

Hill, A.P., 1975, Quantitative linkage: A statistical procedure for its detection and estimation, *Ann. Hum. Genet.* **38**:439.

James, J.W., 1971, Frequency in relatives for an all-or-none trait, *Ann. Hum. Genet.* **35**:47.

Jersild, C., Svejgaard, A., and Fog, T., 1972, HL-A antigens and multiple sclerosis, *Lancet* **1**:1240.

Jersild, C., Rubinstein, P., and Day, N.K., 1977, Complement and the major histocompatibility systems, in: *Biological Amplification Systems in Immunology* (S.B. Day and R.A. Good, eds.), pp. 247–275, Plenum Press, New York and London.

Kidd, K.K., Bernoco, D., Carbonara, A.O., Daneo, V., Steiger, U., and Ceppellini, R., 1977, Genetic analysis of HLA-associated diseases: The "illness-susceptible" gene frequency and sex ratio in ankylosing spondylitis, in: *HLA and Disease* (J. Dausset and A. Svejgaard, eds.), pp. 72–80, Munksgaard, Copenhagen.

Kravitz, K., Skolnick, M., Cannings, C., Carmelli, D., Baty, B., Amos, B., Johnson, A., Mendell, N., Edwards, C., and Cartwright, G., 1979, Genetic linkage between hereditary hemochromatosis and HLA, *Am. J. Hum. Genet.* **31**:601.

Lachman, P.J., and Hobart, M.J., 1978, Complement genetics in relation to HLA, *Br. Med. Bull.* **34**:247.

Lange, K., Spence, M.A., and Frank, M.B., 1976, Application of the lod method to the detection of linkage between a quantitative trait and a qualitative marker: A simulation experiment, *Am. J. Hum. Genet.* **28**:167.

Li, C.C., 1961, *Human Genetics: Principles and Methods,* McGraw-Hill, New York, Toronto, London.

Mackay, R.P., and Myrianthopoulos, N.C., 1966, Multiple sclerosis in twins and their relatives, *Arch. Neurol.* **15**:449.

McDevitt, H.O., and Bodmer, W.F., 1972, Histocompatibility antigens, immune responsiveness and susceptibility to disease, *Am. J. Med.* **52**:1.

Naito, S., Namerow, N., Mickey, M.R., and Terasaki, P.I., 1972, MS-association with HL-A3, *Tissue Antigens* **2**:1.

Ott, J., 1974, Estimation of the recombination fraction in human pedigrees: Efficient computation of the likelihood for human linkage studies, *Am. J. Hum. Genet.* **26**:588.

Ott, J., 1978, A simple scheme for the analysis of HLA linkage in pedigrees, *Ann. Hum. Genet.* **42**:255.

Platz, P., Ryder, L.P., Thomsen, M., Svejgaard, A., and Fog, T., 1979, HLA and multiple sclerosis: Genetic considerations, in: *Humoral Immunity in Neurological Disease* (D. Karcher, A. Lowenthal, and A.D. Strosberg, eds.), pp. 131–145, Plenum Press, New York.

Roberts, J.A.F., 1970, *An Introduction to Medical Genetics,* Oxford University Press, London, New York, Toronto.

Rubinstein, P., Suciu-Foca, N., and Nicholson, J.F., 1977, Genetics of juvenile diabetes mellitus, *N. Engl. J. Med.* **297:**1036.

Russell, T.J., Schultes, L.M., and Kuban, D.J., 1972, Histocompatibility (HL-A) antigens associated with psoriasis, *N. Engl. J. Med.* **287:**738.

Ryder, L.P., and Svejgaard, A., 1977, Histocompatibility associated diseases, in: *B and T Cells in Immune Recognition* (F. Loor and G.E. Roelants, eds.), pp. 437–456, John Wiley, London, New York, Sydney, Toronto.

Ryder, L.P., Andersen, E., and Svejgaard, A. (eds), 1979, HLA and Disease Registry. Third Report, Munksgaard, Copenhagen.

Sandberg-Wollheim, M., Platz, P., Ryder, L.P., Nielsen, L.S., and Thomsen, M., 1975, HL-A histocompatibility antigens in optic neuritis, *Acta Neurol. Scand.* **52:**161.

Schapira, K., Poskanzer, D.C., and Miller, H., 1963, Familial and conjugal multiple sclerosis, *Brain* **86:**315.

Simon, M., Bourel, M., Genetet, B., and Fauchet, R., 1977, Idiopathic hemochromatosis: Demonstration of recessive transmission and early detection by family HLA typing, *N. Engl. J. Med.* **297:**1017.

Smith, C., 1971, Discriminating between different modes of inheritance in genetic disease, *Clin. Genet.* **2:**303.

Smith, C.A.B., 1975, A non-parametric test for linkage with a quantitative character, *Ann. Hum. Genet.* **38:**451.

Smouse, P.E., and Williams, R.C., 1978, An alternative assessment strategy for HLA–disease associations, *Ann. Hum. Genet.* (submitted).

Stendahl-Brodin, L., Link, H., Möller, E., and Norrby, E., 1978, Optic neuritis and distribution of genetic markers of the HLA system, *Acta Neurol. Scand.* **57:**418.

Suarez, B.K., 1978, The affected sib pair IBD distribution for HLA-linked disease susceptibility genes, *Tissue Antigens* **12:**87.

Svejgaard, A., and Ryder, L.P., 1979, HLA markers and diseases, in: *Genetic Analysis of Common Diseases: Applications to Predictive Factors in Coronary Heart Disease* (C. Sing and M. Skolnick, eds.), p. 523, Alan R. Liss, New York.

Svejgaard, A., Platz, P., and Ryder, L.P., 1977, Associations between HLA and some non-rheumatic diseases and possible explanations, *Clin. Rheum. Dis.* **3:**239.

Svejgaard, A., Platz, P., and Ryder, L.P., 1980, Insulin-dependent diabetes mellitus, in: *Histocompatibility Testing 1980* (P.J. Terasaki, ed.), p. 638, UCLA Tissue Typing Laboratory, Los Angeles.

Thomson, G., and Bodmer, W.F., 1977, The genetics of HLA and disease associations, in *Lecture Notes in Biomathematics: Measuring Selection in Natural Populations* (F.B. Christiansen and T.M. Fenchel, eds.), pp. 545–564, Springer-Verlag, Berlin, Heidelberg, New York.

Woolf, B., 1955, On estimating the relation between blood group and disease, *Ann. Hum. Genet.* **19:**251.

Index